T0319364

Migration and the Globalisation of Health Care

Migration and the Globalisation of Health Care

The Health Worker Exodus?

John Connell

Professor of Geography, University of Sydney, Australia

Edward Elgar

Cheltenham, UK • Northampton, MA, USA

Published by
Edward Elgar Publishing Limited
The Lypiatts
15 Lansdown Road
Cheltenham
Glos GL50 2JA
UK

Edward Elgar Publishing, Inc.
William Pratt House
9 Dewey Court
Northampton
Massachusetts 01060
USA

A catalogue record for this book
is available from the British Library

Library of Congress Control Number: 2009940636

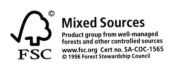

Mixed Sources
Product group from well-managed
forests and other controlled sources
www.fsc.org Cert no. SA-COC-1565
© 1996 Forest Stewardship Council

FSC

ISBN 978 1 84720 737 1

Printed and bound by MPG Books Group, UK

Contents

Figures

Abbreviations

ADB	Asian Development Bank
APEC	Asia-Pacific Economic Cooperation
CHW	community health worker
EU	European Union
GATS	General Agreement on Trade in Services
GDP	gross domestic product
HIV/AIDS	human immunodeficiency virus/acquired immune deficiency syndrome
ICU	intensive care unit
ILO	International Labour Organization
IMF	International Monetary Fund
IMGs	international medical graduates
IT	information technology
MDGs	Millennium Development Goals
MOH	Ministry of Health
MOU	Memorandum of Understanding
MSF	Médecins sans Frontières
NAFTA	North America Free Trade Agreement
NCDs	non-communicable diseases
NGO	non-governmental organisation
NPC	non-physician clinician
OECD	Organization for Economic Co-operation and Development
OHS	occupational health and safety
PEPFAR	President's Emergency Plan for AIDS Relief
PHC	primary health care
PNG	Papua New Guinea
POEA	Philippines Overseas Employment Administration
SARS	severe acute respiratory syndrome
SHW	skilled health worker
SSA	sub-Saharan Africa
TBA	traditional birth attendant
THC	Township Health Centre
UAE	United Arab Emirates
UK	United Kingdom

UNDP	United Nations Development Program
USA	United States of America
WHO	World Health Organization
WTO	World Trade Organisation

Preface

In recent years the migration of skilled health workers has grown dramatically. At the same time there has been growing demand for evidence-based health policy; hence this book seeks to document and analyse the evidence on one of the most important global trends in contemporary health care – the international migration of health workers – and trace what this might mean for policy, practice and, above all, health outcomes. Health workers have been caught up in an age of accelerated globalisation, and health cannot be seen simply in terms of national challenges. It has become a global public good.

In its 2006 annual report the World Health Organization estimated that there was a global shortage of over 4 million health workers. This is a massive figure, even compared with roughly 60 million employed health workers, and it has increased by about half a million since then. Some 57 countries, many in sub-Saharan Africa, experience a critical shortage of health workers, although migration is not the only reason for that. Substantial differences in health status have emphasised a North–South divide, but accentuated by migration.

Human resources – people – are central to health care systems and essential for the delivery of care and services to patients. The most familiar terminology of the profession, such as 'bedside manner', testifies to the critical role of people in diagnosis, cure and care. Health systems are being stretched and stressed by high costs of treatment and training, increased demands upon them, demographic shifts and by the mobility of health workers.

The emphasis of this book is on the provision of human resources in the global South, here generally referred to by the slightly outmoded, presumptuous and indefinable terms 'developed', 'developing' or 'less developed' countries. Like all concepts, these pose problems particularly in middle-income countries like South Africa, Israel or Turkey. I have also tried to refer to people, at least as much as to 'human resources' and 'human capital', although sometimes these are unavoidable. Unless otherwise stated, currencies are in US dollars. While the book aims at a global coverage, this is necessarily impossible; even allowing for linguistic incomprehension, very little has been written on Latin America while the tiny nations of the Pacific have generated a literature out of proportion to their size, but indicating the gravity of health care issues in small island states. Moreover, not only had I previously worked there, but in mid-2009 I again visited Fiji, Tonga and Samoa to examine certain health issues, this time clutching the final draft of the book; hence if it reflects outwards from the Pacific, this is no surprise. Similarly, although the book attempts to cover the international migration of a range of skilled health workers, including specialised workers such as pharmacists, radiologists and lab technicians, most research and most literature has focused on nurses and then doctors; hence this book inevitably follows suit. In the absence of many other global studies on related issues, a wide range of examples has been included to provide breadth of coverage, although at times this collage and mosaic of fragments may border on the indigestible, and not all data meet a gold standard. My hope is that it may still play one small part in the development of a more equitable system of health care provision that is also efficient and accountable.

I could not have accomplished this alone. Pascal Zurn and Barbara Stilwell introduced me to many of the ideas (and directions to much of the grey literature) that are here. Lorraine Kerse guided me through the practicalities of migration and health in the Pacific islands. David Evans, Stuart Rosewarne, Joel Negin, Pascal Zurn, Jim Buchan, Kurt Iveson and Richard Brown read parts of the text and Alex Collie produced the maps. Thantida's table and love were great supports. I am grateful to WHO for permission to reproduce two maps and to Jim Buchan for his assistance with data for a third map. I would like to thank Felicity Plester of Edward Elgar for her continued patience and enthusiastic support for the book. The idiosyncrasies, inaccuracies and gross generalisations (that make the vague 'some' and 'many' all too frequent adjectives) are as always my own.

John Connell
University of Sydney
July 2009

Epigraphs

When Petra Kalivodova, a 31-year old nurse, was considering whether to renew her contract at a private clinic [in Prague] special perks helped clinch the deal: free German lessons, five weeks of vacation, and a range of plastic surgery options, including silicone-enhanced breasts. 'I would rather have plastic surgery than a free car' said Ms. Kalivodova, who opted for cosmetic breast surgery that would normally cost about $3,500 as well as liposuction on her thighs and stomach. These were physical enhancements, she said, which she could not afford on her $1400 a month salary. 'We were always taught that if a nurse is nice, intelligent, loves her work and looks attractive, then patients will recover faster'. Critics lament the plastic surgery inducement, saying it is the most drastic sign of an acute nursing shortage that health officials say is undermining the Czech health care system. In the past year alone nearly 1200 nurses have migrated to countries like Germany or Britain in search of better wages. Health analysts estimate that this has contributed to a shortage of 5000 nurses in an already overstretched public sector. The nursing shortage is part of a worrying global trend that doctors and nurses say is hurting patient care and potentially risking lives. (Bilefsky 2009, p. 12)

Dr Piotr Robinski's second life begins every other Friday at 4am. He has got a very long day ahead. Having worked from Monday to Thursday in his Polish surgery, he is already tired. Six hours later, after a long drive to the airport, Dr Robinski is finally airborne. 'If there will be no cheap flights I could not afford to fly to Scotland . . . But for me it's just like taking a bus to work now,' he laughs. Dr Robinski flies to Scotland every other weekend to work for the NHS in Aberdeen. He says he is only doing the same as most of his contemporaries. 'Doctors in Poland work in more than one job so it is completely normal for me to take another job somewhere else. If I [didn't] go to Scotland, I would find [a] second job here in Poland.' Doctors in former Eastern Bloc countries, such as Poland, can expect to earn less than the average wage, which is around £300 a month. Dr Robinski can earn the same amount in one shift in the UK. He arrives in Aberdeen at 15.50, just long enough to grab half a hamburger and a shower. By 18.00 GMT Dr Robinski is back at work – this time on home visits. Each fortnight he works a five-hour shift on Friday and nine-hour shifts on Saturday and Sunday. By the end of his first shift, Dr Robinski will have been on the go for around 19 hours, but he says he's not too tired to work. Dr Robinski is doing what he can to provide for his family while he is young. 'I'm not sure that when I get older whether I shall have so much fun in travelling to another place all the time. Maybe I'll just stay here in Poland'. He is one of many doctors from Poland who are commuting to Britain to fill out-of-hours shifts. Ironically, British GPs say they opted out of providing out-of-hours care because they were too tired. (BBC News, 15 January 2009)

1. Introduction

Globalisation has become mundane, a cliché grown ever more banal through meaningless repetition. It is everything and nothing, somehow pervasive in everyday life: a marker for our times. Largely associated with the relatively recent spread of capitalism – commercialism, consumption, global corporations, industrialisation and trade, each with seemingly Western characteristics – abetted by political, technological and cultural shifts, it has produced, and is part of, great transnational flows and circulations of people, goods, services, information and capital, creating new global divisions of labour and ever-expanding deterritorialised communities – bound together by social ties and economic transactions across ever more complex networks. The contemporary world is a site of multiple interdependencies, whether of transnational corporations, international production chains, global financial markets or real and potential pandemics. Globalisation also involves growing and evolving patterns of international migration of skilled health workers with complex consequences for service provision, at home and abroad. This book seeks to draw together much still-emerging work on the international migration of health workers – just one part of a wider flow of skilled and unskilled (or low-skilled) migrants. In practice, although the book attempts to consider a range of skilled health workers (simply defined as those with more than a year's health training), it largely focuses on nurses and doctors, although in some contexts the migration of small numbers of specialised workers, including managers, is of particular importance. Which people move, what happens to them and the effects of their mobility are at the core of the book.

The international migration of skilled health workers (SHWs), the first significant 'brain drain', parallels a seemingly similar migration of other professions, notably IT workers (Xiang 2007; Millar and Salt 2007) but also financiers (Beaverstock and Smith 1996), teachers (Voigt-Graf 2003), sportsmen (Lanfranchi and Taylor 2001), engineers, geologists and various others. This steady growth in skilled migration reflects the expansion, internationalisation and accelerated globalisation of the service sector in the last two decades (e.g. Iredale 2001; Findlay and Stewart 2002), rising demand for skilled workers in developed countries (where sophisticated training is increasingly costly) and their supply in countries where once they were absent. New flows exist: small and distant island states such as Fiji provide military and security personnel for Iraq and Kuwait, while Thai restaurateurs open restaurants in Nigeria. Such professional services as health care are part of the new internationalisation of labour, and have increasingly been demand driven (or at the very least facilitated), resulting in the growing global integration of health care markets. Demographic, economic, political, social and, of course, health transformations have had significant impacts on global, regional and local migration flows. Migration has consumption and investment benefits, affecting population size, composition and health status, and the ability of countries, through their populations, to engage in global economy and society. Health workers directly improve the quality of life for others, who can then contribute more to wider society. Ultimately health workers are different from other skilled workers: they literally keep people alive and ensure the well-being of communities and nations.

A SHORT HISTORY?

From early colonial times health workers have migrated, often in support of colonial administrations, and long before most other groups of skilled workers. Half a century ago, in the 1960s, when the international migration of SHWs first became important, doctors – mostly men – were the main migrant group, but nurses – mostly women – have gradually become more numerous, and migration has taken on a gendered structure unlike other components of skilled migration. There are both new pressures and new opportunities for women to work, that challenge simplistic representations of migrant women as passive and unskilled (Kofman and Raghuram 2006). Nurses form the majority of all SHWs: they have become the quintessential skilled migrants, transforming domestic, emotional labour in the West, while sometimes producing a vacuum in sending countries (Brush and Vasupuram 2006). Health workers share important elements of this emotional labour.

Relative declines in public sector funding have enhanced the perception that working in that sector is less desirable. A greater range of jobs for women now exists, outside a sector that is seen by some as dirty and dangerous (and unrewarding), sometimes difficult and demanding, and even perhaps degrading, especially where HIV/AIDS has become significant. In many developed countries, as the children of the 'baby boom' generation have grown up, fewer national workers now enter the workforce. Partly in consequence, demand for nurses far exceeds that for doctors and other health workers, so that in some countries male doctors have retrained as nurses to secure migration opportunities.

Restructuring, usually externally imposed, has affected health systems of developing countries, notably in some sub-Saharan and small island states, contributing to static or declining budgetary support for health (see Chapter 2). Declining funding has inevitably raised concerns over wages, working conditions, training and other issues, all of which have stimulated migration, enhanced by more active recruitment. Accelerated demand and recruitment by developed countries, where populations are ageing, expectations of health care increasing, recruitment of health workers (especially nurses) is not easy and attrition considerable, has increased the volume of migration and the number of countries that are involved, raising complex ethical, financial and health questions. Technology cannot easily replace workers, while the rise of HIV/AIDS and more chronic diseases has put new demands on workforces.

Public health provision emerged historically as a key policy of most nation states, a crucial element of state responsibility for the welfare of its citizens and typified in variants of the post-war British welfare state. The role of the state in health care has significantly altered with the rise of migration. To a greater extent than for the international migration of other skilled workers, the state plays a crucial role in its organisation and regulation: through defining standards, the domestic production of skills, the formulation of migration criteria (skills and points), structured bilateral labour movements and, less directly, by the establishment of skill mixes, wage levels and working conditions. States bond scholarship holders and seek to direct SHWs to particular regions and specialities. Recruitment agencies, licensed by the states and partially regulated by national and international codes, play an increasing role in stimulating and directing migration flows. The economic logic of market forces is both blunted and restructured by the institutional barriers and channelling mechanisms of state policies, within which context individuals and their families make critical choices over occupations and destinations. Significantly, the health sector is also somewhat different from most other skilled sectors since the bulk of employment usually remains in the public sector, with the singular prominent exception of the USA, but where conditions have tended to worsen (relatively and sometimes absolutely) with restructuring and inadequate funding. Virtually ubiquitously there has been movement of workers and patients from the public to the private sector.

The first significant wave of international migration of SHWs in the 1960s was of doctors, from large Asian states like the Philippines and India, and also Iran, mainly to the USA. With training oriented to overseas needs, the Philippines had already contributed the largest number of overseas doctors in the USA. Doctors and nurses from the Philippines and South Asia had started to go to the Gulf and the UK (Mejia et al. 1979). Over time, what were then relatively simple migration flows, usually reflecting linguistic, colonial and post-colonial ties, became steadily more complex, more obviously perverse (being away from areas of greatest need, nationally and internationally), and stimulated by active recruitment. As health care has become more commercialised, so too has migration. Migration routes came to encompass most countries, some as both sources and destinations, with few parts of the world unaffected. China and East European countries have recently become important sources and Japan a destination. The countries most affected by emigration are mainly anglophone states in sub-Saharan Africa alongside some small island states in the Caribbean, Atlantic and Pacific (although numbers have been greatest from such Asian countries as India and the Philippines). In many source countries national economies are often performing poorly, and populations still growing steadily, thus putting increased pressures on health systems. The major recipient countries are the developed nations, including the USA, Canada, the UK, Australia and New Zealand, but also several in the Gulf, notably Saudi Arabia, Kuwait and the United Arab Emirates.

Increasingly, global migration is linked to skill status. Skilled professionals constitute a growing proportion of all migrants, as new technologies enable and promote a global labour market, and production of skilled workers is inadequate in most developed countries, which therefore seek to hire, regulate and recruit skilled migrants. Many of the relatively affluent Organization for Economic Co-operation and Development (OECD) countries have eased legislation on the entry of highly skilled workers (OECD 2005). Countries like Canada, Australia, New Zealand, and more recently the UK, have developed and expanded migration points systems that favour skills to regulate and facilitate entry, and the EU has moved towards a 'blue card', to expedite the movement of skilled workers. The migration of health workers is a key element of these global changes, as health skills are in international demand, linking countries through waves of increasingly diverse migration in a now global and hierarchical health care chain.

A WIDENING CONTEXT

Health workers may be skilled but their migration is not necessarily distinct from that of others. In south India, the Philippines and many small island states, migration of SHWs has occurred over more than one generation, and is embedded in a context where it has become pervasive, based on established historical precedent and widely accepted as an appropriate means of achieving economic and social well-being. It is thus nurtured and enhanced by the presence of overseas or otherwise distant kin, and the incomes and prestige attached to migration, to the extent that it has become normal and expected. In such circumstances a 'culture of migration' exists (Connell 2008b), which extends equally to skilled and unskilled workers. Policies that discourage migration may be scarcely feasible.

Migration of SHWs usually occurs in a wider cultural and mobility context, even involving the creation of extended household 'transnational corporations of kin' (Marcus 1981), with great significance for the creation of human capital and the flow of remittances to home countries and households. Migration is a response to rising expectations over what constitutes a satisfactory standard of living, a desirable occupation, a suitable mix of accessible services and amenities for workers and their children, and, perhaps, even a chance to live in a pleasant place. Since health workers do not necessarily make individual decisions to migrate, but are part of extended households, influences on migration coming from within the health sector may sometimes be trivial. While 'push' and 'pull' factors usefully explain particular migration decisions, such choices are better seen as part of a fluctuating household dynamics, where migration diversifies livelihoods within an evolving transnational network. Cultural and political complexities permeate what might otherwise be merely a 'new economics' of migration.

Health workers move primarily for economic reasons, in much the same way as many other migrants, and increasingly choose health careers because they offer migration prospects, and social and economic mobility. Because of relatively high incomes in the health sector, international salary differences are greater than for unskilled workers, hence the likelihood of becoming an 'economic migrant' may also be greater. Tertiary health training can provide a passport to distant prosperity. A substantial element of the migration of SHWs represents a strategic investment in education as part of a broader investment in migration within a globalising world. Otherwise health workers, in most respects, are little different from many other migrants – they take account of extended-family locations and aspirations in choosing destinations and migration strategies, and play a key role in sending remittances.

The globalisation of migration is simply a new form of what has long been referred to as step migration, often via intermediate 'transit stations' and 'stepping stones', as health workers engage in 'cascade migration', often culminating in the USA, or more dramatically along a 'global conveyor belt' or 'medical carousel', that transfers professionals from poorer to richer countries, and 'from the bottom to the top' (Schrecker and Labonté 2004; Kingma 2006). Seemingly inexorable, the ever-shifting carousel, that a century ago took missionaries to developing countries, now draws health workers from just those countries to richer countries. In recent years it has even begun to take health workers from the richest countries, such as France and Germany, to the UK and elsewhere, alongside commuter migration (see Epigraphs). The more ethical migration of the missionary era has evolved into a more materialistic contemporary migration.

POLICY AND PRACTICE

Health care ministries and national and regional governments throughout the world have had to respond to new migration flows, even where they instigated them, through policies that seek to train and retain skilled staff, or encourage them into new places or positions, while ensuring the effective delivery of care. The particular significance of health care has posed ethical issues and led to pressure for international codes of practice for recruitment. Globalisation (and also urbanisation, with half the world's population now being urban) has increased migration flows, of people (whether as refugees, migrant health workers or medical tourists) and diseases (notably HIV/AIDS, but also SARS, swine flu and avian flu), emphasised new forms of inequality and provided (and demanded) opportunities for a global commitment to improved health, evident in the Global Fund, PEPFAR, the Global Health Programme of the Bill and Melinda Gates Foundation and other similar initiatives. A greater concern for social justice and equity, evident in the Alma Ata declaration of 1978 and the initial WHO Health for All slogan and strategy, has entered most debates on globalisation and health, and been enshrined in the United Nations Millennium Development Goals (MDGs), where health issues have some prominence, and a renewed focus on primary health care.

Despite the growth and significance of migration, in numbers, impacts (medical, economic, social and political), few books examine the overall situation in any detail, despite past studies (Gish 1971; Mejia et al. 1979) and recent work on the migration of nurses (Kingma 2006). Similarly, most of the literature on health-worker migration from particular regions, such as SSA, has tended to focus on migration towards the USA, the UK and Canada (Hagopian et al. 2005; Mullan 2005; Ross et al. 2005). Little has been documented on the extent of migration to the Gulf, Australia or New Zealand, although the last has one of the highest proportions of overseas trained health workers in the world (Zurn and Dumont 2008). Good data on migration flows are largely absent, even for most countries where migration is significant. Despite the impact of health worker migration on the functioning of health systems, there is a remarkable paucity and incompleteness of data, much of which is collected in quite different ways in sources and destinations. It is therefore difficult to determine the real extent of migration from, and within, most source countries, and thus develop effective forecasting or remedial policies (Stilwell et al. 2003). For a decade the 'fact' that there are more Malawian doctors in Manchester than in the whole of Malawi has been widely circulated but without supporting data. Less visible health workers, such as pharmacists and radiologists, whose migration may be as critical as that of better-documented nurses and doctors, have largely been ignored. Without better data, reaching definitive conclusions on the structure and impact of migration is challenging, and evidence-based policy formation problematic.

A growing number of studies have examined the migration of skilled workers from the perspective of human resources but relatively few have examined migration from the migrants' perspectives. While the human resource context is central to migration (and its outcomes), rather more attention is given here to the migrants themselves and their aspirations. A distinctive feature of the migration of mainly women health workers is that high earnings, comfortable status and accelerated professional status, the outcomes for many skilled migrants (Favell et al. 2006: 18), are less frequent for skilled nurses. Moreover, social costs have followed, especially as women workers are separated from families. Yet migration meets individual, household and, increasingly, even national aspirations. New skills and experience are acquired and remittances support extended families at home. This book seeks therefore to provide new, interdisciplinary reflections on such core issues as the brain drain, gender roles, remittances and sustainable development at a time when there has never been greater public and political interest in the migration of health workers.

Migration has been at some economic cost, has left gaps and depleted workforces, diminished the effectiveness of health care delivery and reduced the morale of the remaining workforce. In many source countries, but in SSA especially, failure to invest adequately in health systems and professional health education, the rising death toll from AIDS, and consequent migration of SHWs, are all major factors contributing to the ongoing health workforce crisis, and explain contemporary emphasis on 'scaling up': the substantial global expansion of education and training (Global Health Workforce Alliance 2008). Overall shortages tend to be aggravated by uneven distribution within countries, the movement of health workers from rural to urban areas, and from the public to the private sector, alongside attrition and retirement. As demand in rich countries increases, such shortages are likely to persist, and unless there is greater recruitment into the health workforce, less attrition, or significant policy changes, migration too is likely to continue. Changing expectations will place further demands on health systems.

Countries have sought to implement national policies on wage rates, incentives and working conditions to gain and retain workers, sometimes with desperate strategies (see Epigraphs), but most recipient countries have been reluctant to establish effective ethical codes of recruitment (itself made easier by instantaneous access to websites through the Internet), or modes of compensation. In a context of existing shortages, migration has further weakened fragile health systems, and been perceived as a financial subsidy from the poor to the rich. Yet migration may increase further, diminishing the possibility of achieving the MDGs, challenging workforces to manage HIV/AIDS and exacerbating existing inequalities in access to adequate health care.

Where needs are greatest, and where recruitment has been significant throughout this century (Connell and Stilwell 2006; Rogerson and Crush 2008), words such as 'poaching', 'looting', 'stealing', and even the 'new slave trade', a 'tug of war' (Hamilton and Yau 2004) and the 'great brain robbery' (Patel 2003) have entered the literature. Richards has argued that migration is not so much a drain but 'a positive suction on the part of many developed countries' (2002: 112). No less than Nelson Mandela spoke out in 1997 about Britain's poaching of nurses from South Africa, while also accusing the migrant health workers of being 'cowardly and unpatriotic citizens', perpetuating a 'fundamental betrayal of the nation'. More sober concepts of brain and skill drain have become common alongside more polemical newspaper articles. In May 2005 the English newspaper *The Independent* splashed across its front page, above the photo of an obviously sick child, the banner headline 'An African Child Four Weeks Old Disabled by Britain' which was attributed to Britain's 'voracious demand for Third World doctors nurses and midwives' so that too few remained in Ghana (27 May 2005). Three months earlier *The Times* had a headline 'NHS Strips Africa of its Doctors' (22 February 2005). More sober academic accounts have referred to 'fatal flows' (Chen and Boufford 2005) and 'care drains' (Kittay et al. 2005); Kingma (2006) has queried whether a 'global treasure hunt' will be a 'disaster in the making' and Mullan et al. have argued that the approximately 5000 international medical graduates (IMGs) who join the permanent physician workforce in the USA alone each year 'represent the equivalent of the entire graduating classes of some 50 medical schools around the world' (1995: 1521). A group of academics later asked 'Should active recruitment of health workers from sub-Saharan Africa be viewed as a crime?' and argued that it should (Mills et al. 2008). In the same year the Ugandan Minister of Health argued that

'Rich nations are snatching our doctors' (quoted in Wasswa 2008: 579). Such phrases and negative perspectives can be repeated seemingly indefinitely. It is widely argued that the excessive migration of health workers is unethical and challenges goals of redistributive justice and universal access to adequate health care, since the erosion of human capital that migration usually entails has a direct impact on the provision of welfare, measured through static or falling health indicators in primarily source countries. Yet amidst all such emotion and argumentation migrant health workers are themselves choosing to move, even if from challenging socioeconomic contexts in circumstances only partly of their own choosing. This book makes some effort to examine these assertions, rectify past omissions, distinguish anecdote from data, balance polemic with argument and provide a more comprehensive perspective.

Chapter 2 examines the need for health workers and the broad relationship between disease burdens and the actual distribution of health workers, with SSA emerging as a region of unresolved need, where migration is none the less significant. Chapter 3 discusses the lengthy history of migration and the transition from a more evidently colonial migration towards needy places, to a more perverse, complex and global migration away from them. Chapter 4 assesses the extent to which developed countries have stimulated demand for SHWs, as demographic shift produces ageing societies and ageing health workers, and attrition takes its toll on the workforce. The following three chapters shift attention to developing countries, initially examining why people become health workers, and what role opportunities for migration play in this (Chapter 5), the broad rationale for migration, from discontent with salaries and working conditions to the blandishments of recruitment agencies (Chapter 6), and the effect that migration has on health care provision and on health workers in sending societies (Chapter 7). These impacts lead into an assessment of the brain drain, which seeks to balance the economic costs of migration, largely from training, with the rewards from remittances and return migration (Chapter 8). Since many, but not all, countries recognise costs to migration, a range of policies has been developed to discourage migration, increase the gains from migration, regulate it more effectively or even stimulate it, although few policies have had enormous success (Chapter 9). Finally the Conclusion points to the distinctiveness of the skilled migration of health workers and reflects on the remarkable and recent globalisation of health care that has produced new forms of uneven development.

2. The geography of need

It would be reasonable to assume that the demand for health workers has some relation to need; hence this chapter examines the changing global and regional distribution of disease and ill-health burdens, the task of reducing these burdens and the role of SHWs. Although definition and measurement of needs and shortages are complex (Vujicic and Zurn 2006), and the competence and effectiveness of workers equally hard to assess, the need for health care is greatest in least developed countries and regions; most of these are tropical, with the greatest disease burdens. Disease burdens are also usually greater in rural areas. However, in a global example of the 'inverse health care law', national and regional needs are less well served than in developed countries. Why that should be so is considered here.

The provision of health workers is only one of many factors influencing health status, and there are significant variations in the health status of countries with similar ratios of health workers to population. The relationship between poverty, material deprivation and poor health is now well established, alongside a range of social determinants including gender, ethnicity, education, functional literacy, social capital (trust), drug use, malnutrition and social inequality, some of which, and notably the last, have been enhanced through contemporary processes of economic globalisation (Nguyen and Peschard 2003; Loewenson 2004). While inequalities tend to be more significant, critical and visible in developing countries, increasing geographical inequalities in health have also characterised many Western countries since the 1980s (e.g. Pearce et al. 2006). The basic relationships between social and economic determinants and health status are none the less universal. The relatively poor tend to be located in rural areas in most countries, especially in developing countries, and inadequate health status is correlated with some incidence of poverty (which in turn may reflect inadequate housing status, access to clean water, ability to pay for services etc.). A clear, and multidirectional, relationship exists between poverty, malnutrition and poor health (Jorgensen 2008; van de Poel et al. 2008), and poverty and malnutrition are effective proxies for health outcomes. Poverty, ill-health and the distribution of health workers are closely connected.

Quite simply, 'the great majority of health interventions depend for successful and sustained intervention on an infrastructure of basic health services, consisting of community based services, health centres and local hospitals. These can address most of the burden of ill-health' (Mills and Shillcutt 2004: 64). Implicitly they must be staffed and accessible – geographically, economically and culturally – but geography, poverty, culture and institutional constraints limit access to both health care and medicines. In many countries, especially in Africa, patients must either buy medicine from the private sector, where treatments are more expensive and frequently unaffordable, or must go without (Cameron et al. 2009). The presence of health workers is crucial to positive health outcomes, and the association between 'health workforce density' and health outcomes has been clearly demonstrated: lack of health workers contributes to poor health status, and provision of such basic functions as adequate coverage of immunisation or attendance at births, with negative outcomes on maternal, infant and under-five mortality rates (Anand and Barnighausen 2004, 2007; Sudhir and Barnighausen 2004; Zurn et al. 2004a; Mitchell et al. 2008; Léonard et al. 2009). As the density of health workers increases, infant and maternal mortality fall, irrespective of other factors. What health workers do and what skill mix exists is also significant, and relationships are not always clear-cut, because of the variable role of health workers who are neither doctors nor nurses (Kruk et al. 2009). Moreover it is not only the availability of SHWs, but also the presence of family, and various physical resources, that is crucial to the effectiveness of health care.

GLOBAL DISEASE BURDENS

The incidence and intensity of disease – the disease burden – is especially great in SSA, and is particularly hard on children. In Africa as a whole 46 per cent of all deaths are of children aged under 15 years; the comparable percentage in South-east Asia is 24 per cent, whereas in high-income (mainly OECD) countries only 1 per cent of deaths are of children (WHO 2008a: 7). North and South America contain only 10 per cent of the global burden of disease, yet almost 37 per cent of the world's health workers live in this region, whereas SSA, with 11 per cent of the world's population, has 24 per cent of the global burden of disease but less than 3 per cent of the health workforce and less than 1 per cent of global financial resources (WHO 2006a: 8; Scheffler et al. 2008). A substantial and basic inequality in the disease burden correlates with the resource deficits.

Geography affects disease prevalence. Many infectious diseases are endemic to tropical and subtropical zones, including malaria (carried by mosquitoes) and helminthic infections. Although epidemics of 'tropical' diseases have occurred sporadically elsewhere, it is more difficult to control diseases where transmission takes place year round and affects a large part of the population. Contemporary mobility has substantially changed what were once more localised diseases, evident in the global (and regional) diffusion of HIV/AIDS along major transport corridors, the rapid diffusion of SARS from Hong Kong and south China to countries that were trading partners or sources of tourism, and the global incidence of the swine flu pandemic. Previously localised tropical diseases can quickly now become global, and their management correspondingly more complex.

In low-income countries the dominant causes of death are still infectious and parasitic diseases (including respiratory infections, diarrhoea, HIV/AIDS, tuberculosis and malaria), whereas in middle- and high-income countries the leading causes of death are non-communicable diseases (NCDs). Among children in low-income countries the main causes of death are respiratory infections, diarrhoea, prematurity and low birthweight, and neo-natal infections. Cardiovascular diseases and injuries are common causes of death among adults in most of the world, but AIDS is the main cause of adult mortality in SSA. While not necessarily contributing to mortality, a significant disease burden, including that from malnutrition, typhoid, malaria etc., reduces the capacity to function effectively and so achieve other of the MDGs, such as education. Such disability rates are higher in low-income countries and highest in Africa, with the years of healthy life lost by virtue of being in a poor state of health being at least twice as high in SSA as in any other region. South-east Asia and Africa together thus bear about 54 per cent of the global disease burden although they account for about 40 per cent of the world's population (WHO 2008a: 40). Children bear more than half the disease burden in low-income countries.

Countries are at various stages of the epidemiological (or health) transition, from a situation where the causes of morbidity and mortality are dominated by infection, acute respiratory disease and undernutrition, to one where NCDs, or 'lifestyle diseases', especially cardiovascular disease, diabetes and cancer, and external causes (such as accidents), are the principal causes of ill-health. Such changes in most developing countries are a function of greater urbanisation and sedentarism, new patterns of expenditure and nutrition (oriented to imported, processed foods) resulting in inadequate diets, alcohol consumption and smoking. Chronic substance abuse has emerged as a global problem. In many regions NCDs have become extremely important as a cause of mortality and morbidity; they account for up to 70 per cent of all deaths in the Pacific region, and the world's most obese nations are all there: Nauru, Federated States of Micronesia, Cook Islands, Tonga and Niue (Connell 2009). The final stage of the health transition, the age of delayed degenerative diseases (Olshansky and Ault 1986), most evident in developed countries, is accompanied by the considerable ageing of populations and further pressure on health care. The whole epidemiological transition, alongside increasing life expectancies, ageing and growing populations (Chapter 4), has placed increased demands on health workforces.

Recent re-emergence of infectious diseases, notably tuberculosis, malaria and dengue, in developing countries has resulted in a 'double burden' of NCDs and infectious diseases. Despite the epidemiological transition being more evident in developed countries, in Pacific states, such as Nauru and Tonga, the incidence of NCDs surpasses that in developed countries. The rise of HIV/AIDS has shifted perceptions of the disease burden and intensified the demand for SHWs in developing countries, especially in SSA. HIV/AIDS and the health workforce crisis are closely connected, as an inextricable part of a vicious circle of weak health care systems, an ailing health workforce with a high attrition rate, and an inadequate response to the HIV epidemic (Bhargava and Docquier 2008; WHO 2006b: 3).

The outcome of diverse patterns of disease distribution (and the ability to access health care) is that life expectancies and infant mortality rates vary enormously between (and within) countries.

> Life expectancy in Swaziland is half that in Japan. A child unfortunate enough to be born in Angola has seventy-three times as great a chance of dying before age five as a child born in Norway. A mother giving birth in southern sub-Saharan Africa has 100 times as great a chance of dying in labor as one birthing in an industrialised country. (Daniels 2008: 333)

Of all the MDGs maternal mortality is the goal that has fallen furthest from its target:

> The highest rates are amongst the poorest women in remote rural areas of developing countries, and they are not the kind to demand their rights. No, they die in a dark mud hut with a terrified relative or on the back of a bicycle or a pick-up truck being rushed over bumpy roads to a hospital where there are neither the doctors nor drugs to treat them. (Bunting 2008: 19)

Exactly how such inequalities have come about, the means of reducing them, and what the role of SHWs might be in prevention and cure, varies from place to place.

Information on the distribution of disease burdens and mortality rates within countries is poor; hence it is impossible to determine where regional needs for medical care are greatest. Although 'modern' NCDs, such as HIV/AIDS, tend to be concentrated in urban areas, and some epidemics are more common there because of poor environmental health (Connell 1989), higher infant and maternal mortality rates occur in many outlying areas, emphasising the presence of the 'inverse care law' at local and regional scales.

THE DISTRIBUTION OF SKILLED HEALTH WORKERS: NATIONAL CONTEXTS

Based on the global assumption that countries need 2.3 SHWs for every thousand people, the WHO has estimated that some 57 countries have critical shortages, equal to a global deficit of 4 million health workers, including 2.4 million doctors, nurses and midwives (WHO 2006a), let alone pharmacists, dentists and others. Africa alone was short of a million nurses. Remarkably, despite having much the largest number of doctors and losing few, the USA is expected to have a projected shortage of 200,000 doctors by 2020 (Cooper and Aiken 2006), and some 340,000 new nurses will also be needed by 2020 (Auerbach et al. 2007). Other recent projections suggest American shortfalls as high as a million by 2010 (Caribbean Commission on Health and Development 2006). The Gulf states may have similar substantial needs, with Saudi Arabia seeking, from Pakistan alone, 'as many physicians as it can spare' (quoted in Talati and Pappas 2006: S57). Such projections imply both the need for local training and the potential for migration. Yet all projections and estimates of future needs vary enormously, depending on definitional issues, concepts of need, skill mixes and population changes.

Sub-Saharan Africa faces by far the greatest challenges, matched only by some island states, such as Haiti, and impoverished land-locked Asian states, such as Nepal. The rise of HIV/AIDS has intensified these challenges. Some 36 of 47 SSA countries fall short of the minimum WHO standard of 20 doctors and 500 nurses per 100,000 people (Figure 2.1). Several have fewer than five doctors and 50 nurses per 100,000 people. Uganda and Niger have six or seven nurses for 100,000 people, while the USA has 773, yet migratory flows are primarily from the former to the latter. The shortage of doctors, especially in SSA, is unlikely to be satisfied by 2015, the target year for the achievement of the MDGs (Scheffler et al. 2008). Anecdotal data support such statistical generalisations. Thus in 2005 it was estimated that there were somewhere around 1500 to 2000 paediatric cardiologists in the USA and just four in India (Anon 2005), a

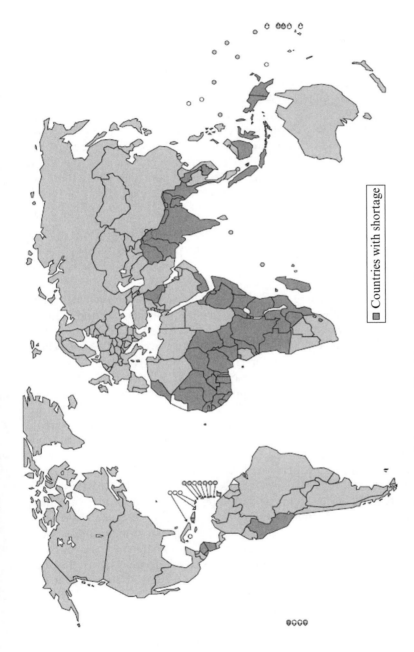

Figure 2.1   Countries with a critical shortage of health service providers

Source: WHO 2006a, p. 12.

country with five times the population and a higher birth rate. For other specialist positions, such as psychiatrists, a similar global distribution exists.

Numerical deficits are greatest in those Asian countries with large populations. Specialists are in shortest supply in least developed countries, where they are also more unevenly distributed, as is evident in the global distribution of psychiatrists (WHO 2007: 26–7). Even allowing for anecdotal exaggeration and miscalculation, the discrepancies and inequities are considerable. Moreover, health workers are far from equal in ability or effectiveness. The level of training in low- and middle-income countries is usually lower than in high-income countries. None the less, the world may be seen in terms of broad health clusters (Figure 2.2), where there are clear relationships between mortality rates and the availability of health workers.

REGIONAL CONTEXTS, URBAN BIAS AND THE INVERSE CARE LAW

The inverse care law, first formally proposed in 1971, argued that 'The availability of good medical care tends to vary inversely with the need for it in the population served. The inverse care law operates more completely where medical care is most exposed to market forces, and less so where such exposure is reduced' (Tudor Hart 1971: 405). The 'law' was developed from post-war circumstances in south Wales, where in areas with the greatest incidence of sickness and death, general practitioners had more work, longer patient lists, less hospital support, and inherited more clinically ineffective traditions of consultation than in healthier areas, while hospital doctors had heavier case loads with fewer staff and less equipment, and more obsolete buildings. Other studies have emphasised the broad continuity of the inverse care law in the UK (Pell et al. 1997; Stirling et al. 2001; McLean et al. 2006), Australia (Humphreys 1985, 1988), Greece (Tountas et al. 2005) and elsewhere. A national Australian study revealed that, despite higher rates of chronic disease and lower rates of preventive care uptake, patients in low socioeconomic-status areas received fewer and shorter consultations than patients in more advantaged areas (Furler et al. 2002). The intuitive logic of the inverse care law has meant that relatively few studies have otherwise referred directly to it and its general relevance is widely accepted.

Everywhere SHWs have long been concentrated in urban areas, especially in the often primate capital city, while rural and regional areas are relatively neglected (see below). By the 1960s, after the first global phase of

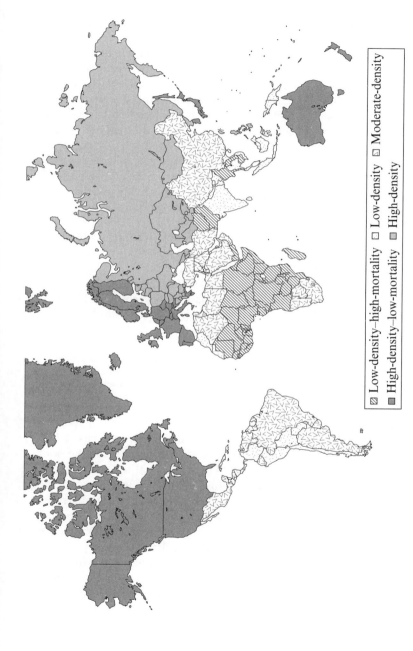

Figure 2.2   Health clusters worldwide, showing mortality rates and availability of health workers

□ Low-density–high-mortality □ Low-density ⊠ Moderate-density
■ High-density–low-mortality ■ High-density

Source: Joint Learning Initiative 2004, p. 30.

decolonisation, this uneven distribution of health care in developing countries was readily apparent, with doctors migrating to urban areas, despite their having 10 or 12 times the rural sector's level of medical provision. Disparities were greatest in poorer, larger and less densely populated countries (Lipton 1977: 265, 448–9; Horn 1977). While the uneven distribution of doctors was extreme, the distribution of other health workers, including nurses, and of facilities, such as beds, was not greatly different (King 1967; Sharpston 1972). In Ghana, where hospitals and doctors were in the main urban areas, a third to a half of the population had no effective access to curative services (Sharpston 1972: 27). In many developing countries government provision of facilities was even more concentrated in urban areas, and rural areas were often dependent on mission facilities and workers. Over time, uneven distribution has increased, with over 75 per cent of all doctors and over 60 per cent of nurses living in urban areas (especially capital cities) while just over half the global population (but fewer in developing countries) live in urban areas.

Economies of scale ensure that skilled human resources are invariably heavily concentrated in urban areas, especially with hospital-based systems of medical care (Zurn et al. 2004a), while skilled workers usually prefer urban life (see Chapter 6). Such conclusions have been reported from a range of contexts, including Somalia and Nigeria (Ojo 1990) and Mongolia (World Bank 2007b). Indeed, most countries have situations much like Sierra Leone, where there has long been

> a greater concentration of health care facilities in the towns, particularly in the capital, than in the countryside. Contributory to this is the unwillingness or inability of many wealthier and better educated people to settle away from the facilities of the city – hospitals, schools, social, recreational and economic opportunities. This includes doctors and their families. (Stevenson 1987: 404)

The distribution of SHWs in Ghana has remained much as it was in 1970. A single gynaecologist, and two surgeons, serve one-third of the country's land area and one-sixth of its population, in the three most deprived regions, while 35 per cent of all health staff are in just two teaching hospitals (Dovlo 2005: 6). In Sudan, nearly 70 per cent of health personnel work in urban settings, serving about 30 per cent of the national population, while two-thirds of all doctors are in the capital city, Khartoum. There are 12 specialists per 100,000 people in Khartoum but just 0.8 in West Darfur State (Badr 2007: 19). Every gynaecologist in Surinam is in the capital city. Managua, the capital of Nicaragua, contains one-fifth of the country's population but half of the country's health workers. In Tanzania, urban districts have twice the number of health workers as rural districts, and those with a small share have an even smaller share of the most skilled workers (Munga and Maestad 2009). In Zimbabwe, although less than 30 per cent of national health positions were filled in 2003, the Harare Central Hospital had an excess of doctors over positions, while provincial hospitals were better staffed than district hospitals. The average national nurse:patient ratio was 1:700, but in the health centres, the lowest level in the hierarchy, the ratios were over 1:3000 and workloads were substantially greater, with the inference that the heavy workload was one of the main reasons that nurses sought to move to larger places (Chikanda 2004). Even China experiences significant urban bias, both quantitative, with 70 per cent of doctors and nurses being in urban areas, and qualitative, since college-educated doctors are most likely to be in urban areas (Anand et al. 2008). As reported in Kenya there is a more substantial urban bias for doctors than for nurses (Mwaniki and Dulo 2008). Similar statistics can both be repeated seemingly indefinitely, and broadly replicate long-established patterns (Mejia 1987). In many countries this universal functional hierarchy is a legacy of centralised colonial times. Urban bias is particularly significant for the most skilled and within the poorest countries.

Centralisation has sometimes been extreme, with many hospitals having a very restricted radius of influence, or 'patient gradient', where transport unavailability and cost, and attitudes to hospitals discourage attendance (Lipton 1977: 266; see below). This is also a function of the focus of health care systems. Public, preventive health care has tended to be undervalued, and childbirth complications, nutritional deficiencies, dysentery and other chronic but low-key diseases, all more significant in regional areas, are relatively ignored. In the 1970s Rio de Janeiro had become the 'plastic surgery capital of the world', with hundreds of specialist surgeons, while rural areas had minimal health care (Horn 1977: 438). Such broadly institutional issues, as in Zambia, were and are often emphasised by the lack of recurrent expenditure, so that

> in many rural areas, health centres have been desperately short of or totally without such things [supplies, transport and staff]. Villages have not been visited by health staff for long periods because of lack of money to buy petrol. The shortage of spare parts for vehicles and the government's inability to buy them due to lack of foreign exchange are a major cause of transport problems. This in turn leads to a lack of field visits and supervision. (Akhtar and Izhar 1994: 231)

Somewhat similarly, in rural Ethiopia,

> Health-service staff complain of being demoralised, overworked, and underpaid, especially in remote locations. There is poor supervision and support, and

a lack of the most essential drugs and basic equipment. The health centre in Delanta reported a shortage of everything, and no funds or medication for at least three months each year. (von Massow 2001: 25)

Expediency has been more significant than any formal planning based on movement towards equity and the achievement of the MDGs. In turn this leads to the demeaning of rural health activities. Urban bias partly follows a shortage in supply. In Nigeria wages and salaries took up most of the health budget so that 'there was very little money left for the maintenance and running costs of facilities. Purchases of drugs and dressings also attracted an insignificant proportion and, to worsen the situation, wastage and irrational prescribing practices were common' (Iyun 1994: 252). Rural violence in countries like Sudan, Nepal, Pakistan, Bolivia and Sri Lanka has accentuated maldistribution at a time of growing rural needs. Doctors are unwilling to move to rural Pakistan because of 'thwarted growth of self and children, insecurity from threats, robberies and kidnappings and interference from community leaders' (Talati and Pappas 2006: S60). In the Southern Highlands of Papua New Guinea (PNG), where violence is rife, and 32 per cent of all patients are emergency surgery cases, no outside doctor has been willing to be posted there for 15 years (Pantenburg 2009). Female SHWs in particular cannot easily be posted to such areas, a growing concern as SHWs become more dominantly female (Chapter 4). Health workers are reluctant to work in areas with few amenities, especially where 'traditional' perspectives on health care are prevalent and cultures are different: a Ghanaian pharmacy student observed, 'the tribal issue is there; if you go to a place you are not from the treatment is not good' (quoted in Owusu-Daaku et al. 2008: 581). Low pay, lack of motivation, and inadequate training, mentoring and supervision have also resulted in high staff turnover. In developed countries like Canada, too, turnover rates are highest in rural areas. In British Columbia the lowest retention rates for health workers were in the smallest communities, with rates in communities of fewer than 4000 people being almost half those of places with 20,000–30,000 people (Thommasen 2000). Variants on these kinds of situation recur widely, as a function of a lack of resources (see below), minimal interest in remote concerns, or administrative failures, and universally explain part of the problem of retaining staff in rural areas and the rationale for internal migration (see Chapter 6). The outcome is the relatively poor status of rural health care.

Organisation of health administration is necessarily hierarchical, but emphasised by sometimes authoritarian and centralised administrative structures, inherited from colonial times, producing what has been described, at least in the Pacific, as a 'militaristic and inflexible bureaucracy' (Taylor 1990: 105) that may appear, and sometimes is, autocratic to those in subordinate positions. In such hierarchical systems centralised authorities tend to monopolise planning, budgeting and human resource recruitment and allocation functions, and may be reluctant to assist in devolution of specific functions, capacity-building and the appropriate development of outlying areas. Urban bias is not merely a geographical or technical phenomenon, but is part of the political economy of resource allocation.

At a broader scale, similar inequalities exist between regions. In China, India and Nigeria, the distributions of hospitals, hospital beds and doctors, relative to population, are all uneven, with the same states benefiting or losing out from uneven distribution. In Nigeria this multiple deprivation operated in favour of southern states and against the Muslim states of the north, in India it marginalised some 'tribal' and remote areas, and in China it was biased against low-income provinces (Anand et al. 2008), which also included most areas of minority ethnicity. In each country, within the states and provinces, additional urban bias existed (Okafor 1987; Akhtar and Izhar 1994). In small and fragmented states such uneven development is usually greater because the institutional structure is more centralised and decentralisation unusually difficult.

While it has been argued that officially the production of doctors in South Asia (Bangladesh, India, Nepal, Pakistan, Sri Lanka) is in excess of official requirements, their urban concentration means that there is a gross inequality in health provision, with underprovision in regional areas, exacerbated by socioeconomic status and gender biases (Adkoli 2006; Bhutta et al. 2004; WHO 2006a). In India, for example, urban bias in the distribution of health workers has existed from colonial times. In 1969, in a *Times of India* newspaper article, 'Brain Drain in Medicine', one of the first references to the brain drain in developing countries, an overseas trained and returned doctor wrote:

> While there may be one doctor for a thousand persons in the towns, there is often less than one doctor to a hundred thousand villagers in the remote parts of the country . . . but can one seriously expect a highly-trained specialist or surgeon to go and settle down in a rural hospital? He [sic] has been trained at great expense to himself and the country, to perform a specialised task and his talents and skills would be completely wasted in a rural dispensary. (Pandya 1969: 6)

In this era medical education remained firmly based on colonial traditions, which emphasised modern science and techniques rather more than healing, so that career orientations, as in Argentina, were oriented to modern urban institutions or migration to the USA, creating a rural deficit and an urban oversupply, to the extent that 'the more advanced and scientifically oriented the curriculum of medical schools in Argentina, the more obsolete it has become for the nature and location of actual health needs' (Portes 1978: 23), circumstances that existed in many other countries. In Iran, feelings were much the same as in India:

> While altruism might sustain the returning physician for a short while, it is, to say the least, unreasonable to expect him to ignore his years of training and to practise bush medicine with inadequate drugs or supplies: or to do without professional support and opportunity for continuing education and research. The near impossibility of supporting a family, and providing for their future on the meagre government salary – the only sources of income in rural practice – is of course a basic issue. (Joorabchi 1973: 45)

While there was some truth in this, and similar statements can still be made, what might have been seen as a plea for more intermediate skills in rural areas effectively went unheard. In Mexico the regional distribution of doctors was similarly inequitable, with a shortage of doctors in remote and marginal areas and underemployment and unemployment in urban areas; doctors were relatively absent from remote states that had no medical schools, and because of their preference for hospital posts, the inability of rural areas to satisfy their personal needs, the lack of economic incentives (accentuated by urban bias in government health policies) and inferior social services (Harrison 1998). Urban bias is particularly evident in middle-income developing countries where private sector health care has tended to prevail, rather than where government employment is the norm.

Irrespective of geographical and funding deficiencies, some health care systems are inequitable because of cultural and gender inequities, where minority cultural groups or women lack some forms of access, because of systemic problems (e.g. an unwillingness to open, operate or service clinics in 'different' areas) or cultural restrictions on access to 'modern' services. In rural areas of eastern Burma, for example, tribal groups such as the Karen experience some of the worst health conditions in the world, because of persecution and lack of access to modern health care, with unusually high child mortality rates from relatively easily curable diseases such as malaria, respiratory ailments and diarrhoea (Aglionby 2006). While persecution is not usually the lot of marginal, culturally distinctive groups, access to health care is rarely comparable to that of the dominant cultural group but, as among the Akha of upland Laos, modernity, in health as in other spheres, has sometimes produced new structures of exclusion, hierarchy and inequality (Lyttleton 2005). In rich countries, too, the peoples of peripheries, especially when they are culturally distinct, as in Canada or Finland, are similarly disadvantaged. In Australia, where the life expectancy of Aboriginal Australians, many of whom live in remote areas, is 17 years less than that of all Australians (63 years versus 80 years), extending adequate services, especially provision of SHWs, has proved exceptionally difficult.

Similar issues characterise migrant groups, whether within countries or internationally. Cultural disparities in access to health care are well documented for groups such as South-east Asian refugees in the USA, because of language differences, beliefs about the nature of suffering or the cause of medical conditions, stoicism, apprehension over techniques (especially invasive techniques) and treatment regimes, or the social, physical and economic distance of hospitals (Uba 1992). Such differences have led to attempts to develop better and more wide-ranging forms of cultural competence among practitioners (Betancourt et al. 2003; MacLachlan 2006). Cultural distinctions in resort to health care are more common and more substantial in developing countries, such as Bolivia (Forsyth 2008) or PNG (Hamnett and Connell 1981), less adequately understood, even less frequently remedied and sometimes beyond medical comprehension and the practice of health care. Cultural and geographical distance from urban 'modernity' mediates other facets of inequity, as environment, economics, politics, experience and culture are combined.

PATIENTS

While the inverse care law refers to the provision of health care and services, those who need health care services the most may use the services relatively infrequently, and least effectively (e.g. in terms of following treatment regimes). This is partly a function of distance and economics; the very earliest nineteenth-century studies in medical geography revealed the inverse relationship between admission to hospital and distance from it. In developing countries, distance (and transport facilities), lower incomes (and work commitments), the availability of alternative therapies and sometimes cultural differences discourage attendance at urban facilities. While there is a clear and predictable relationship between distance, mediated by travel cost, and attendance at health care facilities (e.g. Stevenson 1987; Stock 1987; Kissah-Korsah 2008), distance is only one criterion. Thus in Bangladesh access to maternal health services varied according to household income levels, distance to hospital and the educational status of women and their husbands, with the poorest households being least likely to access private sector facilities (Anwar et al. 2008). In Sierra Leone access to care varied by distance, but also by ethnicity, maternal educational status, occupation, religion, age and assumed disease aetiology (Gesler and Gage 1987). Because rural centres are least well staffed, provision of health care is less adequate and the frustrations for patients (and practitioners) much greater (Awases et al. 2004; Chikanda 2008). As in the Marshall Islands and PNG, health assistants in rural aid posts and dispensaries may often be absent, obtaining supplies, going for training, on leave or for social reasons (Connell 1997; World Bank 2007a: 58), reliable service is unpredictable. In Vanuatu the number of village health workers declined by two-thirds between 1991 and 1992 with the collapse of financial support for their activities (World Bank 1994: 279). Rural and regional areas thus tend to be the victims of financial shortages, disarray and cost squeezes. Patients are reluctant to use such overcrowded and inadequate facilities, and the staff have a propensity towards migration.

Transport in circumstances where infrastructure is particularly poor can be detrimental to health, especially with belated resort to distant facilities. Challenges to the mobility of patients are considerable. Sick and injured people are less able to move, travel can be costly and opportunity costs deter mobility (e.g. World Bank 2007a: 64; ADB 1996: 119–20). Invariably transport infrastructure is worst in remote areas. The concept of 'outer island', formally (but relatively recently) recognised in some Pacific island states such as the Marshall Islands and the Federated States of Micronesia, emphasises acute distinctions in service provision and, significantly, many such 'outer islands' are less than 100 km from the centre. Consequently urban hospitals tend to serve primarily urban patients. In Vanuatu, for example, some 98 per cent of all hospital inpatients come from the towns where the hospitals are located, because residents of distant islands incur high costs of travelling into towns, and consequently may also see hospitals as a place of last resort. Similarly, in Ethiopia rural people often reach hospitals when it is 'too late' (von Massow 2001: 25) and thus, as in parts of PNG, see them as a place of death. The poorest people tend to be rural. Unequal access emphasises urban bias and inequity in service provision.

In many less developed countries it is possible to trace a steady post-independence centralisation of health facilities despite primarily rural populations, official policies of decentralisation and commitments to primary health care. Rural facilities have often been underfunded, erratically staffed and poorly managed, and health workers prefer to work elsewhere. In several states, notably Kiribati, Fiji and Samoa, patients bypass rural and regional facilities where they can, at some real and opportunity cost to themselves, for what they perceive as better urban health care, thus resulting in a further run-down of rural facilities (World Bank 2007a; Connell 2009; see Chapter 7). Facilities have tended to move away from areas of need, partly inadvertently, through mismanagement, and partly through deliberate practices that conflict with national health policies. Ministries of health and finance are not always in agreement. Centralisation, urban bias, financial crises and the unwillingness of health workers to live in regional areas have created imbalanced and, perhaps, increasingly inappropriate health care systems.

INTERNAL MIGRATION

Most migration of SHWs is actually within countries, and almost every country experiences some internal migration, on balance from rural to urban areas and from poor regions to richer regions – analogous to the structure of international migration. The outcome is also often similar: a concentration of the professional workforce in the larger urban areas and scarcity in remote areas, reflecting economies of scale, the practical and financial difficulties of meeting the diverse needs of remote places and their peoples, the aspirations of professionals and their families and the task of organising an adequate structure of health care delivery in the face of financial constraints, staff shortages, restructuring and the intermittent absenteeism, attrition and mobility of personnel.

Internal migration tends to be greatest in countries that are particularly fragmented and where the existence of services of various kinds, including health services, is particularly poor in the periphery. This is particularly true of island states where remote islands have limited and irregular service provision, evident in Indonesia and the Pacific (Chomitz et al. 1998; Connell 2009). Skilled workers seek adequate services that are more accessible in urban areas. The task of retaining workers in rural areas, or encouraging them to move there, is exacerbated where relatively few were there in the first place. Long before contemporary international migration, SHWs were moving from rural to urban areas or simply choosing not to go there. In Ghana in the 1960s doctors 'prefer[red] to work in rich areas', which normally meant the capital city, because they could establish an additional private practice (although this was against the regulations) and their wives (since most doctors were male) were more likely to be able to find employment, while they had become 'modern':

> At the social and cultural level there are also good reasons for doctors pre-
> ferring to work in the major towns. A doctor may have come from the rural
> areas originally: but at the same time as he [sic] became a doctor he usually

also adopted the outlook of an urban professional man. Most of his professional colleagues and friends will live in the cities, and Ghanaians attach great
importance to social life. Further, as an urban man he will expect to be able to
enjoy the sophistications which only urban living can provide . . . as regards
the 'bright lights'. For the up-and-coming the rural areas are places to escape
from . . . In addition, as a professional a doctor will like to concentrate on the
'interesting' cases, rather than keep to a steady diet of malaria and infant malnutrition; and the facilities for studying the 'interesting' cases will be in big city
hospitals. Indeed not only does a Ghanaian doctor have urban professional
attitudes: he has usually adopted attitudes very close to those of a doctor in
Europe, and in Britain in particular. (Sharpston 1972: 214)

Bonding of Ghanaian doctors to work in rural areas was never rigorously
enforced and doctors who resented rural postings could easily leave for the
private sector (ibid.: 216). In Zambia in the early 1980s doctors were similarly reluctant to work in rural areas and many such areas were dependent
on mission and other voluntary personnel to provide medical services; in
the Western Province some rural health centres had to be closed because
there were inadequate numbers of doctors or nurses (Freund 1987). At the
same time in Nigeria 'a physician who moves to the rural area sentences
his [sic] family to cultural exile and poverty' (Ojo 1990: 634). While this
dates from an era when many doctors in newly independent developing
countries were trained in Europe and inculcated with different values
and 'professional attitudes', more than vestiges of such attitudes remain
firmly in place, and are factors in contemporary rural–urban migration.
Two decades later, Cameroon doctors resented rural work 'because they
believe that working in the villages is like punishment and does not allow
them the opportunity for private practice where they can earn more
money' (Fongwa 2002: 327). Indeed, in contemporary Tonga a doctor
with an urban practice can double the income obtainable from public
service employment, and thus double what is possible in the regions,
where private practice is not feasible. Fewer hours of work in the private
sector are needed to acquire the same income. Nurses, with fewer private
options, and less income-earning opportunity, are consequently more
mobile within the country and beyond it. For many decades, servicing
rural and remote areas has ubiquitously proved difficult.

   In a group of African countries, migration from rural to urban areas was
mainly a response to the lack of infrastructure in rural areas, few opportunities for professional advancement, limited opportunities for private
practice, and lack of basic equipment and drugs in rural health institutions (Awases et al. 2004). As an Ethiopian health worker said: 'There is
an obvious difference between rural and urban postings. Working in rural
areas involves helping the poor . . . in urban areas one can learn, have
more income, have good schools for one's children' (quoted in Serneels et

al. 2005: 1). In regional centres, which may be small towns no more than a couple of hundred km from capital cities, but seemingly a world away, it is more difficult to attract skilled staff, unless they originally came from the region. Few workers stay long in remote postings, and seek to return to the centre or go overseas, as in India, where the public health sector is particularly poorly funded, to the extent that there is a 'paradox of saturation' where Indian cities have too many doctors and the countryside almost none (Mullan 2004: 29). Chinese nurses are uninterested in moving to rural areas where needs are unsatisfied even though they cannot get jobs in what are regarded as 'oversupplied' urban centres (Xu 2003), and Cameroon nurses move to urban areas 'where their spouses reside and work' (Fongwa 2002: 327). Significantly, health managers are even more likely to migrate from regional areas than clinical staff. In South Africa and Togo they either left to work in the private sector (with NGOs or profit-making clinics) or were quickly promoted (Egger and Ollier 2007: 5). Internal migration is selective. In Mexico, women are less likely to migrate than men since they are more likely to train in their home state and be less specialised (Harrison 1998). The more highly skilled workers are the most likely to leave rural and regional areas (see Chapter 7).

Absenteeism of public service doctors and nurses is common in parts of rural India, but is difficult to prevent where village councils have no control or authority over the health staff whose salaries, transfers and promotions are controlled at the district and state levels. Urban-trained health workers are not anxious to work in what they perceive as small, remote and backward villages, and are not disciplined if they do not turn up. Those few who stayed in the villages usually sent their children to school in the city, or sent their entire families there. Many commuted from the city. As one such doctor said:

> When government doctors are posted here they want out as quickly as possible. Everyone wants to live in the city. I'd like a transfer to Udaipur. If not, I'll have to move my children there. I'm an educated person. What opportunity is there for my children here? If you allow them to mix with local children they begin to use the local bad words. (Dugger 2004: 12)

One consequence of the lack of village doctors and nurses, when they were too far away, or simply failed to turn up, was local recourse to alternative sources of health care that were both expensive and dangerous (Dugger 2004; Chapter 7). While rural–urban migration, and the reluctance to work in rural areas, are greatest in less developed countries – where poverty and infrastructure deficits are considerable – both are universal phenomena.

More developed countries such as Australia, New Zealand and Norway have long been short of doctors in rural areas (e.g. Barnett 1991; Isaacs

2007; Kristiansen and Forde 1992), and in most developed countries there has also been a rural–urban migration of SHWs. In Australia rural doctors have felt that, compared with their metropolitan counterparts, 'they had significant additional stress, including lack of junior resident medical officers and specialist back-up, lack of access to educational opportunities and locum support, isolation from professional colleagues, the lack of spouse employment opportunities and lack of adequate educational facilities for children' (McEwin and Cameron 2007: 13). Constraints to the employment of SHWs in regional areas of developed and less developed countries are structurally similar, and extend far beyond any limitations of the health sector. Consequently most developed countries, including Australia and Canada, have become increasingly dependent on immigrant doctors to meet health needs in remote areas, and seek to direct them there, although many move to large urban centres as soon as they can, in national versions of the 'medical carousel' (Durey 2005; Grant 2006; Gilles et al. 2008). Even the iconic Royal Flying Doctor Service in outback Australia is predominantly staffed by migrant doctors. In South Africa, too, foreign migrants, mainly from elsewhere in SSA, make up 78 per cent of rural doctors; without them there would be major problems so that, after an outcry from other SSA countries, South Africa shifted to Cuba as a source (Kingma 2006: 126). Elsewhere, too, migrant doctors and nurses are more likely to work in rural and remote areas than their local counterparts, as in the USA (Miller et al. 1998; Phillips et al. 2007; Thompson et al. 2009) and Canada, where not only are over a quarter of all doctors in rural areas overseas-educated but the smaller, more rural areas have the greatest dependence (Labonté et al. 2006: 3–4). Thus in the USA (like Australia and New Zealand), migrant doctors are in counties that 'are distinguished by a younger, poorer, more non-white population' than the counties where US graduates or other migrant doctors locate (Miller et al. 1998: 263–4). In New Zealand the impact of migration of international graduates 'seems to have been largely redistributive, with foreign trained doctors increasingly entering primary care and locating in areas avoided by indigenous medical graduates' (Barnett 1988: 1050). Similarly, half of all New Zealand's psychiatrists in 1994 were overseas graduates (Miller et al. 1998). Yet migrant SHWs are also reluctant to move to regional areas, and are consequently concentrated in certain favoured regions, as in the USA: Canadians in California, New York and Texas, and Australians and New Zealanders in California, Massachusetts and New York (McKendry et al. 1996; Miller et al. 1998). For all migrant doctors in the USA, New York, California and Florida were the key destinations, while relatively few were in inland states (Miller et al. 1998; Mick et al. 2000).

Rural and regional areas, whether in developing or developed countries, have invariably been least well served by health institutions and by SHWs, often accentuated by contraction after the early post-colonial period, with increasing scarcity of resources, especially in SSA, and an erosion in public trust (Streefland 2005). National and regional governments have intermittently sought a battery of distinct policies, within and beyond the health sector, to attract and retain SHWs (Chapter 9). Many such policies have limitations, and the resort to migrant workers has been common, although cultural and language differences, the lack of other migrants from the same area and therefore the absence of familiar goods and activities make such postings usually more difficult for migrants than for local people, and especially for 'trailing spouses' (Omeri and Atkins 2002; Durey 2005). Migration from regional areas has remained substantial and been both precursor of and accompaniment to international migration.

THE RISE OF THE PRIVATE SECTOR

The private sector has grown rapidly in recent years but in very different forms, related to national incomes and the extent and form of public funding of health services. Where there is a significant private health sector, urban bias tends to be greater, since there is dependence on user-pays financing and the more affluent users are urban. Developing even a small-scale private sector in rural areas, as in Tanzania, has proved difficult, because of high costs and limited ability to pay for services, hence, as elsewhere, the private sector is concentrated in large urban areas (Rolfe et al. 2008; Kida and Mackintosh 2005). Smaller urban populations, lack of means to pay, limited privatisation of health insurance and competition from the public sector (where most services have been virtually free) meant that few private practitioners could be supported in most developing countries until recently. Urbanisation and growing modernity, alongside rural–urban and international migration, have resulted in a parallel movement of SHWs from the public sector into the private sector (and in each context very little return migration). Wages and salaries – and charges – are invariably higher in the formal private sector. Where there are considerable income and other differentials (notably superior technology and working conditions), substantial movement from the public sector may diminish its ability to provide services. In Zambia, for example, private doctors' salaries were more than double those in the public sector; midwives' salaries were almost one-third higher and laboratory technicians' salaries were more than three times higher. As in many other contexts, especially in SSA, NGO salaries were also up to 50 per cent more than those in the government. Incentive payments further boosted such differentials (McCoy et al. 2008: 678). Coverage by the private sector is usually quite limited. In South Africa it consumes 60 per cent of health expenditure but is responsible for just 18 per cent of the population (Pillay 2009). In some middle-income states, such as Malaysia, private sector health care expenditure is greater than in such developed countries as the UK and Germany (Rasiah et al. 2009).

In developing countries, migration of SHWs into the private sector has been greatest in Asian states, such as India, Thailand and Malaysia, as an affluent middle class emerged, but it occurs in even the poorest African states, because of superior salaries and working conditions, including better supplies of drugs and equipment, shorter hours and fewer patients, constrained only by reduced job security (Awases et al. 2004; von Massow 2001; Stringhini et al. 2009). In the Bahamas, a relatively affluent Caribbean state, and Fiji, the regional centre of the Pacific, there has also been considerable migration to private clinics and hospitals (van Eyck 2005; Connell 2009). The Apollo Group in India has developed state-of-the-art hospitals, that have hired US, Bangladeshi and other doctors, to meet 'the huge unmet demand for medical services among the middle and upper class in large urban centres' (Rahman and Khan 2007: 144). By contrast, in much of SSA, private health care providers are government employees who run part-time clinics, many out of their own homes. Some SSA states are increasingly dominated by the private sector, with Nigeria having only 12 per cent of registered doctors working in the public sector (Healy and Oikelome 2007). In Zimbabwe, in 1997, just one-third (551) of the nation's 1634 doctors were employed in the public sector, and a high proportion of nurses had also moved into that sector, although, unlike doctors, they could not set up private practices on their own. Indeed, so many nurses were working in the private sector that it was widely believed that 'nurses in the public sector are engaging in a lot of part-time work in private clinics. By the time they come for their normal duties they will be too tired to work. That is why we get poor service when we visit the clinic', since 'the public sector is largely left with individuals who are less dedicated and poorly motivated to perform their work' (quoted in Chikanda 2004: 10). Continued migration of SHWs into the private sector is also evident in developed countries, with some 65 per cent of all Greek doctors being in the private sector (Tountas et al. 2005). Universally the private sector expands at the expense of the public sector, and in urban areas at the expense of the rural.

Migration of SHWs to the private sector has been particularly substantial where health tourism has developed, notably in Thailand, India and Singapore, contributing to a dual health care system where rich migrant patients (medical tourists) can secure better care than local people, and disproportionately more SHWs respond to their needs (Connell 2006). A number of Indian doctors have returned from overseas because of opportunities for earning high salaries in the elite private sector hospitals that cater to medical tourists. There, and in Thailand, many doctors have moved away from rural areas to provide more lucrative services for medical tourists, resulting in an 'internal brain drain'. The parallel shift to the private sector, alongside a shortage of doctors, also produced a situation where it was stated that doctors at private hospitals in Thailand spent half an hour with foreign patients but public doctors had just five minutes for local patients (Sarnsamak 2009). Private sector hospitals may also provide few facilities for diseases such as malaria and typhoid that tend to involve the poor (Rasiah et al. 2009). Privatisation has accentuated existing rural–urban migration and contributed to new inequalities in access to health care.

The private sector also extends beyond what seem the formal confines of health care since several large organisations, such as mining corporations and large hotel resorts, as in Fiji and the Seychelles, have attracted nurses with higher wage levels, their own clinics, less work and no night shifts. Although the private sector remains relatively small, it is growing even in the poorest states, where the contrasts between 'private affluence and public squalor' can be greatest, but supports a small proportion of the local population, sometimes dominated by expatriates, and provides a model where health care is accessible to the relatively affluent, and preventive care is less significant.

FINANCE

The central theme of this book is the relationship between health provision and migration, with the implication that migration may have an overall negative impact on health, as SHWs move perversely. Although migration has placed stress on many health systems, it is certainly not the only factor to do so, nor is it the most important factor. Moreover, in some countries, such as Malawi, the main cause of a health worker shortage is neither migration, nor necessarily even inadequate finance, but deaths of workers, mainly from AIDS (Hamilton and Yau 2004; Chapter 6). Shortages of health workers have multiple causes; in many countries, again like Malawi, 'the root cause is poverty' (Palmer 2006: 30). National and regional variations in the supply and distribution of SHWs are primarily a function of health care expenditure in relative and absolute terms. Ironically, where the ratio of SHWs to population is most problematic (Figure 2.1), even the proportion – let alone the actual amount – of the national budget spent on health is often tiny. For one reason or another – an absolute lack of resources, a failure to give priority to health spending, economic crisis etc. – finance has often been limited. Although aid donors have usually given priority to health, this has not necessarily enabled adequate financial support for the health sector, and therefore adequate numbers of effective health workers, especially in the least developed countries.

Even countries largely unaffected by migration have experienced problems of insufficient finance. In Vanuatu, for example, the number of health workers is inadequate to provide effective health care, and the ratio of health workers to people has deteriorated: 'The health system suffers from a lack of qualified staff, especially midwives, doctors and specialists. Basic service delivery is either stagnating or in some cases deteriorating' (ADB 2002: 2). A temporary volunteer surgeon has described the situation in similar terms:

> I am the only surgeon for the whole country. It is amazing how deficient the hospital appears when contrasted with the comparably obscene excesses we enjoy in Australian hospitals. Here there is no radiotherapy or chemotherapy. Patients who present with Hodgkins disease are simply sent home. There is no chemical reagent for AIDS/HIV testing and you cannot even get a thyroid function test. Some health centres on distant islands are without supplies for long periods. The surgical department performs about one leg amputation per week, mainly for diabetic gangrene, however there are no facilities for prostheses. (Freedman 2008: 22)

Similar situations exist in other least developed countries, such as Kiribati (Kienene 1993: 254), and flaws usually also exist elsewhere in the public service. In some Micronesian states, such as Nauru, the Marshall Islands and the Federated States of Micronesia, inadequate funding of high-school education (and cultural attitudes towards education and employment) have resulted in few school leavers able and willing to train or be employed as health workers (Connell 2009). The outcomes of restricted financial support are highly variable.

Recruitment, training and retention of adequate numbers of health workers are critical. Several countries devote inadequate resources to training enough health workers, either by choice or misfortune, hence the contemporary focus on 'scaling up' numbers and skills. Considerable variation exists in the amounts and proportions of national budgets that are devoted to health care (WHO 2006a). A longstanding assumption is that countries should spend 5 per cent of their budgets on health and, in the Asia-Pacific region, for example, relatively rich Japan and Australia both devote 9 per cent of their national budgets to health, whereas Singapore,

Vanuatu and PNG devote 4 per cent. However, although Cambodia spends 10 per cent of its budget on health, which represents about $4 per capita, PNG spends $24, and Japan and Australia over $2000. Outcomes are therefore quite different. Countries tend to devote a greater share of their national budgets to health care as the national income increases (and thus also a greater absolute expenditure). Low-income countries spend less than wealthier countries, and proportionately less on public health, resulting in fewer hospitals, clinics and beds, fewer health workers, and populations that are consequently more vulnerable to disease, disability and mortality.

Lack of financial support has meant that, for example, in the 12 SSA countries for which adequate data are available, 'workforce shortages are even more alarming than suggested by the existing literature . . . In at least 6 of the 12 countries pre-service training is insufficient to maintain absolute numbers even at their current level' and none would reach WHO targets by 2015 (Kinfu et al. 2009: 227). Remedying such disadvantages there and elsewhere requires policies such as task-shifting and 'aggressive retention policies' since the domestic financial basis for adequate national training programmes is unlikely soon to be forthcoming.

In many countries, including most of those in SSA, India and elsewhere, funding for the public health sector has declined in real and relative terms. In a labour-intensive area, wage costs are necessarily a substantial proportion of budgets. With low budgetary allocations, public service institutions also experience shortages of protective clothing, basic equipment and drugs; moreover, they are unable to offer their staff competitive salaries, especially where governments have been put under pressure by multilateral lending institutions to reduce public expenditure and especially the wage bill (Awases et al. 2004: 1). Recruitment of SHWs is then also particularly difficult since employment, where it exists, especially for nurses, is less obviously attractive (despite the possibility of migration). With inadequate funding, too few SHWs are produced, while low wages result in poor morale and productivity. This may be a prelude to international migration if national skills are recognised elsewhere. By the mid-1990s the World Bank had concluded that two distinctive features could be identified as the 'South Pacific health paradigm': 'damaging spending reductions' and 'its vulnerability to worker and/or skill shortages' (World Bank 1994: 19). The two were generally related: reduced spending meant fewer training courses and scholarships, fewer positions and interested competent entrants, less infrastructure and a decline in the morale of those who remained. Reduced spending was usually most evident in rural and regional areas, which became increasingly out of sight and out of mind. Workloads tended to increase, but they also increased irrespective of funding or migration, for example where the rise of HIV/AIDS has placed new demands on already busy staff. Systemic problems of low budgets, limited recurrent funding (for salaries, equipment and supplies), weak education and management systems, deliver health services that are not always adequate. Migration simply emphasises and draws attention to this.

Basic issues of inadequate funding, especially in regional areas, have been well described for Tonga:

> The lack of funds for hospital maintenance can be seen in the urgent need for dental equipment and furniture at Vaiola [central] hospital and in the fact that many of the beds, mattresses and bed linen at [regional] Vava'u Hospital are unfit for use. But the real impact of declining percentages spent on maintenance and drugs is to exacerbate the low proportionate spending on primary health care . . . The attraction for patients of Clinics and Centres lies not in the surgical or advanced diagnostic skills of the staff but in the advantage of a local clinic being able to prescribe basic drugs, use simple diagnostic equipment, undertake home and follow-up visits and travel the local district undertaking preventive and health education programs. These are precisely the activities restricted by declining budgets for drugs, equipment, maintenance, and other vital non-salary items. The result in Tonga has been a classic case of inadequate funding for the non-hospital part of the system, low utilization of health centres and clinics because of perceived low quality of treatment, pressure and overcrowding in hospital outpatient facilities, and a failure of the primary health care system to become better oriented towards the newer lifestyle diseases. (ADB 1996: 121)

Similar financial shortages and consequent urban biases towards hospitals occur elsewhere to the detriment of residents of remote areas, causing overcrowding in central hospitals and the gradual assumption that inequity is the norm.

In a number of developing countries, economic restructuring in the 1980s and 1990s, often externally imposed by international agencies, such as the International Monetary Fund (IMF), the World Bank and the Asian Development Bank, led to reductions in the public sector workforce and restrictions on hiring new workers. It also stimulated the third and largest phase of international migration (Chapter 3), as developed nations' policy prescriptions for public sector reduction in developing countries both cut local services and provided a pool of labour for their own health systems. In Trinidad and Tobago in the 1980s, falling oil prices led to IMF-imposed structural adjustment, resulting in declining salaries and massive emigration of nurses (Phillips 1996). Similarly in Haiti, the lack of resources in the Ministry prevented nursing posts from being established, and many either emigrated or went into the private sector (Malvarez and Castrillon Agudelo 2005). In 1985, Mali, one of the poorest countries, even in SSA, could employ only some 15 per cent of 53 new medical graduates, and in

1984, Zambia, with 57 new graduates and 747 vacant posts, recruited just 15 graduates (Mejia 1987: 40). Restructuring sometimes meant the deterioration of working conditions, rather than the greater efficiency it was intended to encourage, the inability to train enough SHWs, since training is usually the first activity to be cut, as in Namibia (McCourt and Awases 2007), or the impossibility of finding jobs for new graduates.

In this century the financial situation has changed somewhat, as more countries have achieved stable macroeconomic positions. However, while aid for health programmes expanded, the IMF continued to encourage prudence, with governments and individual departments having expenditure ceilings, especially in the 'heavily indebted poor countries', most of which were in SSA. IMF embargoes effectively prevented some African countries from employing all their nurses, and thus using money given by other international agencies to put in place new programmes to reduce the incidence of diseases such as HIV/AIDS. Ironically, although half of all nursing positions in Kenya are unfilled, one-third of all Kenyan nurses are unemployed, as IMF pressure encouraged national wage restraint and a public sector hiring freeze (Baird 2005; Volqvartz 2005) to the extent that a special aid-funded private sector emergency hiring plan had to be adopted to counteract HIV/AIDS (Adano 2008). Around the same time, South Africa was estimated to have 35,000 registered nurses, who for whatever reason were either unemployed or inactive, despite 2000 vacancies in the public sector (Hamilton and Yau 2004). Where structural adjustment has resulted in reduced services, the abolition of price controls, cost recovery or more emphasis on fees for services, rural areas and the relatively poor are the most vulnerable. Changes in the health sector take place in a wider context, where negative balances of payment and high levels of debt servicing place huge resource constraints on many developing countries. In several countries, lack of resources, or alternative priorities, has resulted in low wages and poor conditions, with simultaneous vacancies, unemployment and migration. Rather like several SSA countries, such as Kenya and South Africa, China has a statistical shortage of health workers – with a particularly low ratio of nurses to population – but has an effective 'surplus', because of the lack of job opportunities that has resulted from the limited budgets of public health facilities (Fang 2007). In each of these countries there is effectively a 'pseudo-shortage' of health workers – a function of various economic and social issues that discourage employment in the prevailing conditions, rather than an actual numerical shortage. Providing adequate resources is critical at both national and regional levels, may be accentuated by migration (and contribute to it), and aggravates uneven distribution of health services.

GEOGRAPHY, ECONOMICS, POLITICS, CULTURE AND EQUITY

The issues that affect health systems and contribute to a maldistribution of health workers are a function of other related problems: shortages of financial resources, inadequate government commitment to health in several states (despite the linkage between poor health and slower economic growth), and weak management capacity. Ultimately, political decisions are critical in allocating financial, physical and human resources. As one disgruntled migrant doctor has written of Australia:

> The shortage of doctors is a combined achievement. It should be credited to the Australian Medical Council, the Australian Medical Association, state registration boards and professional colleges. This credit should be shared by the medical bureaucracy and the nation's politicians, living in a symbiotic relationship with the leadership of the medical fraternity. As long as this symbiosis exists, the country will continue to suffer from a lack of doctors. A powerful, unrelenting medical lobby, acquiescent politicians and self-serving bureaucrats combine to protect the market for local graduates. (Galak 2009: 30)

While this particular interpretation is controversial, it points to the complex and politicised structures and contexts of training and allocation. Uneven burdens of disease, accentuated in large, fragmented, poor and weak states, and by the rise of HIV/AIDS (especially in SSA), are paralleled by the uneven response to health care, increasingly characterised by urban bias and the inverse care law, that have often worsened in postcolonial times. In some places this is also linked to an emphasis on central hospitals and advanced technology, privatisation and dependence on overseas facilities (such as education and training facilities and specialist hospitals), resulting in costly referrals (making the task of financing local health systems and organising more labour-intensive preventive health care more difficult), and rising expectations for the delivery of services and standards of living. Political and ethnic violence has worsened some contexts, while weaknesses in governance and political will (involving organisation at all levels), and, more generally, the lack of a 'stakeholder society', are common. The conjuncture of such problems has challenged policies directed towards developing regional and rural health care systems, with more emphasis on primary and preventive health care and with adequate workforces.

In many contexts, but particularly in developing countries, health needs are greatest in rural and remote areas and are least well served there, in terms of both health workers and supporting facilities (hospitals, technology, medicines etc.). The inverse care law is universal, and raises questions about distributive justice. Inadequate financial support for health care systems poses similar questions about equity, especially in the poorest countries, where small proportions of small budgets are spent on health care. SHWs are often reluctant to work in remote areas, and may have to be bonded to do so. Most prefer urban life, and regard themselves as ignored – even punished – in the periphery. Given the opportunity, they tend to migrate to urban areas. Migration, whether rural–urban or international, in turn tends to emphasise distributional issues in contributing to a perverse flow, rather than being restorative or recuperative. While more comprehensive philosophical examinations of equity and fairness within health sectors emphasise the difficulty of being precise about exactly what constitutes inequality of access to health services (Daniels 2008: 248–52), it is readily evident that in most contexts, the disease burden is greatest in developing countries and least well served by workers and facilities. Migration from disadvantaged regions and countries is far from new, but has significantly grown in recent decades, as a key element of globalisation. The extent of this migration can now be examined.

3. Phases of globalisation

The migration of health workers is scarcely new, even if the current phase is more comprehensively global and of greater social and economic significance than those that have preceded it. Migration has changed direction, acquired greater complexity and taken on different gender dimensions over the past century, with flows from developing countries becoming more important, quantitatively and qualitatively, than either migration to them or more established migration flows between developed countries. The rise of international migration has been neither steady nor inexorable, as a short-lived hiatus in the 1980s demonstrated, when many countries appeared to have an oversupply and human resource policies briefly went into reverse. In the present century, few countries are isolated from significant migration flows, and oversupply is highly unusual. This chapter distinguishes at least three broad phases of migration and examines their implications and consequences.

FIRST PHASE: EARLY DAYS, COLONIAL YEARS

The international migration of SHWs was largely ignored until the 1960s. But the colonial era constituted a first phase: the movement of health workers from Western nations, often in association with missionary activities as part of the colonial endeavour. In most parts of the world the provision of health by government authorities was at least as late as the mid-nineteenth century. Until well into the twentieth century, in the developing world, colonial authorities introduced 'modern' medicine, in the administrative centres (often serving little more than the needs of Europeans and their employees), emphasising clinical and curative medicine, until large-scale preventive campaigns got under way. With exceptions such as the Indian Medical Service, this often took little note of local conditions, let alone local practices, and partly served as a form of social control (Olumwallah 2002; Bala 1991). Colonial medicine depended on the efforts of practitioners, mostly men, trained in the metropoles. Yet in Britain alone between 1896 and 1966 the Colonial Nursing Association recruited 8400 nurses, single white British women, to work across the British Empire (Solano and Rafferty 2007). Missionary medical activities more than supplemented colonial efforts, especially in rural areas, where, even more than in urban centres, doctors were necessarily 'renaissance men' (Bell 1999) but women were no less valuable and equally multi-skilled. A handful were heroic figures, from Father Damien to Albert Schweitzer, and, somewhat differently, Mary Seacole and Florence Nightingale (Gourlay 2003). The first phase in the migration of health workers was therefore from metropolitan countries to their colonial peripheries.

In the colonies, health was poor and mortality rates high, especially in the tropics; infectious diseases were common, although health care was officially a priority in many colonies. Limited resources were often thinly spread and mission activities invaluable. As in large parts of Africa and the Pacific, missions made the more concerted efforts to provide health care in rural areas, where they were often the only source of care; most hospitals had been built by them and missionaries usually received some medical training. In large parts of the Pacific, for example, the relationship between the missions and health services was extremely close at least until independence in the 1970s and 1980s, when government services became dominant. In PNG, refugee doctors from Hungary, Poland, Ukraine and elsewhere (whose qualifications were not recognised in Australia) were also a substantial cohort of the post-war intake of doctors (Denoon 1989: 74). In its colonial phase the movement of these pioneer health workers was entirely from places with relatively good health to those where health care was greatly needed.

Only belatedly were indigenous populations trained as health workers, and initially as health assistants and nurses rather than as doctors. There were exceptions; in the late nineteenth century Filipino doctors were graduating from local and international Spanish universities (Choy 2003: 18). More frequently, European doctors were reluctant to train even medical assistants, considering local people racially and morally inferior, while simultaneously safeguarding their own professional prestige (Shapiro 1987; Bell 1999). Although small numbers of local people, as in Ceylon (Sri Lanka), were trained early in the 'scientific' techniques of the West, it was without real responsibility, authority or formal recognition: subordinate in every way. In the Philippines, too, the first nursing school was opened by the US colonial government in 1907 but, as much as anything, it 'provided white American women with a sense of purpose in the colony . . . an international avenue for heroism' (Choy 2003: 23), and nurtured and validated empire rather than created an effective autonomous workforce. None the less, a decade later elite Filipinos were working and training in the USA, as a prelude to a 'prestigious path to professional mobility on their return to the Philippines' (ibid.: 61). While doctors in

Ceylon gained recognition as early as 1905, nurses went formally unrecognised until 1949, a year after Sri Lankan independence (Jones 2004). Most developing countries had relatively few indigenous health workers, even as they became independent, while the lack of recognition of qualifications necessarily limited any transfer of skills abroad. Migration from developed countries thus continued, centred on the steady flow of doctors from Britain to developing countries (Gish 1971: 16) and parallel flows from other colonial powers such as France and Portugal. Despite the existence of such organisations as Médecins sans Frontières (which in 2007 was supplying over 26,000 mostly local, but many international, doctors, nurses and other medical professionals, water and sanitation engineers and administrators to over 60 countries), such flows have now largely ended, and the direction of flow has reversed. Even so, a number of countries, particularly those that have experienced difficult times, remain dependent on overseas volunteers; Liberia, for example, has 46 NGO doctors and just 30 Liberian doctors, while NGOs operate more than 70 per cent of the nation's health facilities (*New African*, February 2009: 43). Up to 5000 volunteer SHWs, most in MSF, were working in SSA in 2005 (Laleman et al. 2007). Cuba has become a substantial donor of SHWs. By 2005 these had reached sixty-eight countries, mainly in Africa, Latin America and the Caribbean, but also in the Pacific, and especially Timor Leste (East Timor), where there were 300 Cuban health workers in 2008, though language differences posed some problems (Ospina 2006, Anderson 2008, Connell 2009). For a period in the 1980s, Vietnam sent 'surplus' doctors to African countries such as Mozambique, Angola and Libya, but not all such movements were 'voluntary'.

Some more localised movements occurred elsewhere. British hospitals relied heavily on Irish workers for much of the first half of the twentieth century, until the 1950s when Caribbean nurses began to replace them. Even so, through the 1940s and 1950s, more nurses emigrated from Britain than arrived from overseas (Solano and Rafferty 2007). In the USA, the late 1960s marked a similarly profound racial and economic transformation, when the increasing migration of Filipino nurses ended decades of numerical domination of migration by nurses from Europe and Canada (Choy 2003: 1). With the first nascent flows of migrants from poorer countries to richer ones, the direction of flow began irrevocably to change.

SECOND PHASE: THE FIRST BRAIN DRAIN?

As the trickle of migrant workers to the UK and the USA from the Caribbean, Ireland and elsewhere became a flow by the 1960s, the first phase gradually gave way to a second phase marked by migration from emerging developing countries. The legacy of colonial training systems played a continuing role:

> The Indian doctors who collaborated with colonial rule were the ones who stepped into positions of power after 1947: by then their socialization into the model of western medicine was almost complete. The emigration of doctors, the failure to produce a coherent medical policy, and the absence of public medical and health facilities in rural areas followed almost inexorably. The Indian peasant . . . has been the main sufferer from these patterns. (Jeffrey 1979: 325)

The scale of changes in India, and the orientation of training towards a Western model, ensured that Indians were prominent in the early flows of migrant doctors, but similar trends in training and migration gradually became more widespread, ironically as superior training facilities were established in developing countries in the years before independence.

The direction of migration thus shifted radically, as the first movements began from a few developing countries to a handful of developed countries, typified by the recruitment of nurses from the Philippines for the Gulf (Mejia et al. 1979). Larger independent developing countries, such as India, Pakistan and Iran, were the sources of thousands of SHWs, mainly doctors, for Western countries such as the UK, Australia, Canada and particularly the USA. The first studies of this migration appeared in the 1960s, mainly concerned with movements between developed countries. Early interest and concern stemmed from the situation where as many as one-third of British medical graduates were leaving for the USA and Australia, with these emigrants being replaced mainly by doctors from larger Commonwealth countries. This new phase of migration was the start of what quickly became widely recognised as a brain drain, a term first applied in the 1960s to the movement of scientists, doctors and other highly qualified people, then largely between relatively developed countries (Gish 1969a, 1969b). However, as early as 1966, the Philippines Department of Labor produced a *Report on the Problem of the Brain Drain in the Philippines*, that partly focused on nurses. The apparent validity of the concept was quickly recognised in health contexts elsewhere, from Latin America to India (Gish 1971; Bartsch 1974; Gish and Godfrey 1979; Horn 1977; Joyce and Hunt 1982; Engels and Connell 1983).

More developed countries experienced bidirectional flows. The UK, Australia and Canada were already witnessing both the arrival of migrant doctors, mainly from the Philippines, India, Pakistan, Iran and Colombia, and emigration, mainly to the USA, out of frustration over the lack of desirable promotion opportunities (rather than in response to significant income differentials). During the five years to 1961, one-third of British medical school graduates had emigrated, mainly to North America and Australasia (Parkhouse 1979: 100–102). Relatively poor countries – many former colonies – experienced even greater emigration. By the 1970s the Philippines had already contributed the largest number of foreign doctors in the USA, with training increasingly oriented to overseas needs. By 1974 as many as 10,410 Filipino doctors were working in the USA (Goldfarb et al. 1984). Moreover, by 1970 more Filipino nurses were registered in the USA and Canada than in the Philippines itself (Mejia et al. 1979), and by the late 1980s the Philippines was the second-largest source of migrants to the USA after Mexico. By the 1970s Jamaica was said to be the world's largest exporter of nurses (Phillips 1996). In Britain immigration policies were relaxed (for the first but certainly not the last time for skilled workers) to allow a steady supply of trainee nurses from overseas, especially in the 1960s, mainly from Commonwealth countries, notably the Caribbean and Malaysia, where there were common nursing curricula (Smith and Mackintosh 2007). By the 1970s, too, doctors and nurses from South Asia, and also elsewhere in the Middle East, were beginning to go to the affluent Gulf states, primarily Saudi Arabia, and the United Arab Emirates, but also Qatar, Oman and Kuwait. Migration to the Gulf was typified by flows of nurses from the Philippines and later South Asia, and by doctors from other Middle Eastern countries. But part of that migration was of skilled workers from Western countries, attracted by much higher salaries and a temporary but quite different lifestyle. Increased demand in the Gulf partly reflected local unwillingness to work in the health sector, the absence of policies to encourage this, and gendered and social contexts that discouraged it. International flows were becoming more differentiated.

In the USA 'exchange nurses' became significant in the 1950s, as 'an inexpensive labor supply to alleviate growing nursing shortages in the post-World War Two period'. In 1962 the American Nursing Association distributed a brochure to 'professional nursing associations worldwide' entitled 'Your Cap is a Passport' (Choy 2003: 78, 90), and between 1956 and 1969 over 11,000 Filipino nurses participated in the programme. By the late 1960s exchange nurses were almost exclusively Filipinos (Choy 2003; Ishi 1987). Prestige, income generation and the experience itself were important, so that by the 1960s going abroad had already become a reason for becoming a nurse for as many as 80 per cent of prospective Filipino nursing students; between 1952 and 1965 rather more than half of all graduates from the University of the Philippines College of Nursing went abroad. Despite discrimination and exploitation, many stayed on indefinitely beyond the official two-year period (Choy 2003: 73–4). The Vietnam War and publicly subsidised Medicare in the USA through the 1960s significantly increased parallel US demand for doctors. The 1965 Immigration Act, which focused on occupational preferences rather than historic national (mainly European) origins, dramatically shifted the focus of all migration into the USA to developing countries.

Until the 1970s, however, the single most important international flow of doctors was probably still that from Ireland; some 71 per cent of all graduates from Ireland's medical schools between 1950 and 1966 had emigrated and as many Irish doctors were practising in Britain as in Ireland (Gish 1971: 20). Despite this Irish migration, a new ethnic distinctiveness of skilled migration into the UK was already evident, and a geographical pattern had emerged that scarcely changed in later years. Two-thirds of overseas-born doctors had come from less developed countries, with those from India, Pakistan and Sri Lanka making up 70 per cent of these and the remainder coming mainly from the Caribbean and the Middle East (ibid.: 32–3). By the late 1970s, of the estimated 15,000 nurses moving globally each year, over 90 per cent went to eight countries, but mainly to the USA, the UK and Canada, and the vast majority came from the Philippines (Mejia et al. 1979). What was still a relatively simple migration flow steadily became more complex.

Flows of SHWs largely reflected linguistic, colonial and post-colonial ties evident in the UK's links with Ireland, South Asia and the Caribbean. Filipinos, Koreans, Thais and Taiwanese moved to the USA, small numbers of Africans and others went to France, and some Indonesians went to the Netherlands. The orientation and curricula of training institutions, and administrative structures, alongside other patterns of migration, shaped the migration of health workers. Ironically, in the contemporary political context, many Iranians moved to the USA, whereas Indonesians, who might have been expected to migrate since structural conditions seemed to favour migration, largely stayed because of 'a lack of positive identification with any large foreign system [and] a strong sense of national feeling' (Gish 1971: 99). While politics and colonial heritage influenced migration, Filipinos at least were travelling more widely, and taking up employment in Germany, the Netherlands, Brunei, Laos, Turkey and Iran (Choy 2003: 90) as new migration flows emerged.

Early flows were characterised by the employment of migrants in the lower echelons of the health service; as Gish observed, 'it is no secret that professional chauvinism is likely to exclude outsiders trying to break into the "club"' and 'the less "fashionable" or modern the specialty', such as geriatrics, the fewer British graduates will be attracted (1971: 25, 49). As early as 1961, in a British House of Lords debate on migrant health workers, it was simply pointed out that 'They are here to provide pairs of hands in the rottenest, worst hospitals in the country, because there is nobody else to do it . . . we are not playing fair by them.' There was widespread agreement that, without migrant doctors, hospitals 'would be absolutely unable to function' (quoted in ibid.: 52). By then a quarter of doctors and up to 35 per cent of nurses in state hospitals were from overseas (Gish 1971). A decade later, most overseas doctors were 'in the more unpopular specialties and in the less agreeable parts of the country' (Parkhouse 1979: 95). And, with 20 per cent of all nurses coming from overseas, they 'were over-represented in hospitals dealing with mental illness, mental subnormality, mental handicap and geriatrics, and very few are to be found in the "prestige teaching hospitals". Overseas nurses are therefore used to compensate for the shortage of British recruits into notoriously underpaid and often unpleasant work . . . as a "reserve army"' (Doyal 1979: 206). And at the start of this first phase of global migration, active recruitment was already evident:

> The Caribbean has become a hunting ground for medical recruiters, particularly those from North America. Not only is advertising for health personnel common but the recruiters themselves come to the islands looking for candidates. The United Kingdom has long been taking large numbers of girls from the region for nursing training. (Gish 1971: 112)

A group of health workers was also emerging, mainly from West Africa and the Caribbean, who were training and working illegally by evading immigration restrictions (ibid.: 142). Dentists, pharmacists and opticians tended not to migrate, partly because of non-recognition of qualifications in various destinations. Surprisingly little has subsequently changed.

The ready acceptance of the term 'brain drain' was a measure of the recognition that, even by the 1960s, less developed countries were experiencing the greatest costs from emigration, because of the disparity in the number of medical workers per capita (one doctor for over 30,000 people in Nigeria compared with one for 860 people in the UK), the particular problem of a more rural population distribution, which made servicing more difficult (and costly), and a heavier burden of disease, alongside the obvious unavailability of financial resources (Gish 1971: 63–4). In volume alone, some of the flows were alarming. More than 90 per cent of graduates from one Iranian medical school were routinely going to the USA and the majority remained there (Ronaghy et al. 1975). By the 1970s one-third of all graduates from the Ibadan Medical School in Nigeria were abroad, as were 62 per cent of medical graduates from the National Taiwan University (Osunkoya 1974; Kuan 1970). Some 140,000 doctors (6 per cent of the global total) were then overseas, though fewer nurses were overseas. Both doctors and nurses were concentrated in the USA, Canada, the UK and Germany. The international migration of SHWs was seen to be of critical importance at a more global level in the early 1970s when the WHO sponsored a path-breaking study of some 40 countries (with 13 analysed in more detail) that responded to widespread concerns of uneven flows, 'and had its roots in the international disquiet over the "brain drain" of professional manpower [sic]' (Mejia et al. 1979: 4). Poorer countries experienced greater losses, income differentials were important for nurses (who also remitted more), migrants occupied junior employment positions, training regimes and curricula influenced migration, and return migration was limited and hard to influence (Mejia et al. 1979). Return migration was also problematic since most returnees remained in urban areas, acquired a distinct distaste for rural service, sought to practise high-level skills that had little bearing on national needs, and often quite quickly migrated again (Gish 1971: 71, 84, 98). Several longstanding critical issues were already evident.

Although the Philippines and India dominated out-migration flows, some smaller countries were becoming significantly involved. Thailand lost as many as 1500 doctors, 20 per cent of its stock, between 1960 and 1975, almost all to the USA, where salaries were then 15 times those in Thailand, and very few returned (Wibulpolprasert et al. 2004). Although Mejia et al. (1979) had rejected the primacy of economic explanations for migration, the evidence from less developed countries such as the Philippines and Thailand stressed that uneven development was a factor. By the 1980s the Philippines had embarked on an active labour marketing policy; the Philippines Overseas Employment Administration produced a series of booklets subtitled 'Able hands to foreign lands', one of which offered 'Filipino Medical Personnel', whose 'calibre and professional competence had earned the trust and respect of leading institutions throughout the globe'. It emphasised the diversity and international recognition of skills and concluded, 'Through a systematic recruitment program, foreign entities can now avail themselves of Filipino services at the most expeditious time. If you have a job that needs doing in the medical or health-related fields, we have the manpower to do it' (POEA n.d.). A broad economic rationale became more evident as incipient globalisation ensued. While the numbers from many developing countries were small, much smaller than those from Thailand, India or the Philippines, even the migration of quite small numbers was having a real impact on several states. Health workers were the forerunners in the gradual globalisation of skilled migration and, then as now, their migration was of greater concern than other skilled international migration flows, just as the idea of a brain drain was largely centred on the mobility of health workers.

THIRD PHASE: GLOBALISATION

From the 1960s the oil boom in the Gulf brought extensive development, the construction of new hospitals and other medical services, and an enormous inflow of international workers, initially mainly outside the health sector, even reducing the indigenous population to a minority in such states as Kuwait and the United Arab Emirates (UAE). Elsewhere, however, the end of the Vietnam War, and a global financial downturn from the late 1970s, most evident in Latin America, marked something of a downturn in the extent of skilled migration, and some return flows in the 1980s. Outside the Gulf an interregnum in international migration was evident, doctors were unemployed in several countries such as Pakistan and Egypt, and fears of overproduction existed elsewhere, but alongside optimism that losses of SHWs would not now be significant.

The pause was short-lived. By the 1990s a new phase of expanded migration had begun, as the global economy again expanded more rapidly, oil prices rose, the European Union (EU) granted cross-boundary recognition of qualifications and higher education became an 'export business' to attract overseas recruits, ushering in a new 'internationalization of nursing' (Iredale 2001). Demand in developed countries accelerated as populations aged, domestic training programmes proved inadequate, and jobs in the health sector were more often seen to be too demanding, poorly paid and lowly regarded (Chapter 4). By then several countries, notably in the Gulf, but including several large Western nations, had become exceptionally dependent on overseas workers. In Singapore, in 1998, the Minister of Health concluded that, without foreign nurses, 'some of our services would be decimated' (quoted in Choy 2003: 187). Singapore was far from unique.

Contemporary migration of health workers has continued the trends of the 1970s, but increasingly involving governments and recruiting agencies, and gradually becoming more global, more complex, and more dominated by women. New movements of nurses emerged between relatively developed countries, for example from New Zealand, South Africa and Finland to the UK. Ireland, once an exporter of SHWs, became an active recruiter (Buchan and Seccombe 2005; Yeates 2008). Important changes included the entry of China into the market as a supplier of nurses, and Japan as a somewhat reluctant recipient. Within four years China had become one of the most significant suppliers to the USA (Xu 2003; Brush 2008), Singapore and Saudi Arabia (Fang 2007). Its greater involvement could profoundly influence the future global care chain. India has grown dramatically as a global supplier in the present century, now especially for nurses, and it is likely that other parts of South Asia, especially Sri Lanka,

Bangladesh and Pakistan, will follow. Pakistan currently exports almost half of its annual production of 5000 medical graduates, two-thirds of newly graduated Bangladeshi doctors seek to move overseas and a quarter of newly graduated Sri Lankan doctors move overseas (Adkoli 2006; Talati and Pappas 2006). As in the Philippines, some Pakistani doctors have chosen to become nurses to facilitate migration.

Hitherto Japan, virtually alone of countries that have experienced substantial post-war economic growth, largely managed its health services without resorting to overseas workers, but has slowly become an importer. Japan has always been unwilling to accept immigration, but its various policies to reduce the demand for labour have limited applicability in the health sector. The Japanese health care system has consequently come under considerable pressure, especially as the population ages and demand increases, without access to migrant health workers. Although Japan, more than any other country, has taken particular advantage of the notion of medical tourism, encouraging citizens to use overseas health care, since the mid-2000s it has negotiated the immigration of health workers from the Philippines, and in 2008 signed an accord with Indonesia to accept 1000 nurses and nurse specialists over the following two years. Both Filipinos and Indonesians were officially 'trainees', working in either rural areas or nursing homes.

Both globally and regionally migration became more complex. For example, in Africa by the late 1980s, because of the devaluation of the local currency and poor working conditions, doctors were leaving Zambia for neighbouring African countries, including Zimbabwe and Botswana. Even then expatriate doctors from India, Pakistan and Bangladesh made up the major proportion of doctors in the country. In the 1990s as few as one-third of Zambian doctors were local people, some 20 per cent were Cuban and a small proportion were from Egypt and China (Akhtar and Izhar 1994). Most African states were experiencing some negative outcomes of migration. In Zambia the number of doctors was half what was considered necessary, and some provinces were especially disadvantaged, while issues of language and culture were surfacing as immigrant doctors replaced local workers (ibid.: 228, 230; see Chapter 7). In subsequent years such complexities intensified with significant intra-regional migration within SSA.

A substantial number of all migrant SHWs are in the Gulf, although in the present century most Gulf states have sought some degree of localisation of health workers, as more conservative regimes have become more liberal, through wider access to education (especially among women), a preference for health care within a particular cultural context, and growing numbers of dependants within local households. Thus in 2005 some 30 per cent of the Saudi Arabian health workforce were nationals, although only 12 per cent of doctors and nurses were nationals; the country had as many as 85,000 migrant nurses and doctors. The UAE has even fewer local workers – with just 10 per cent of nurses and of doctors being nationals. Most doctors were from Egypt, Iraq and India, and nurses were from India, Egypt and the Philippines, although Sudan was also a significant source for both categories (El-Jardali et al. 2009). In Kuwait, local nurses constitute only 6 per cent of the workforce, and this proportion is still declining since nurses are regarded as passive, unintelligent and mere maids and assistants (Al-Jarallah et al. 2009). By contrast, both Oman and Bahrain had a majority of local workers. The Gulf states overall employ over 20,000 doctors, mostly from South Asia, but also from neighbouring and poorer Middle Eastern states such as Egypt, Palestine and Yemen (which in turn gains doctors from Russia). In the midst of the Middle East, Israel is also a recipient of health workers from Russia and elsewhere.

Outside the Philippines, India and South Asia, Asia has experienced relatively limited international migration given its population size, although almost all areas of rapid economic growth, notably Singapore, Brunei and Macao (e.g. Chan et al. 2008), experience shortages of SHWs. This is partly a function of post-colonial ties and language, specifically the relative lack of English-language competence, the absence of significant migrant populations overseas and non-recognition of qualifications. By contrast, the much smaller Caribbean and Pacific island states, where English is usually the key medium of education, have experienced considerable losses of health workers, largely inseparable from other migration flows, and where some national populations themselves are falling (Connell 2007a). Rather like parts of Asia, Latin America has been somewhat aloof from more general global migration flows, despite the massive significance of mainly unskilled Hispanic migration to the USA. Indeed, in direct contrast to the movement of unskilled Mexican workers to the USA, the migration rate of doctors was exceptionally low (Hussey 2007), although Mexico is the largest supplier of nurse aides to the USA, with Haiti and the Dominican Republic in fourth and fifth places (Arends-Kuenning 2006). Some Latin American nurses have moved north to the USA or Europe, especially to Spain and to a lesser extent Portugal, for language reasons. Significant numbers of Peruvians and Ecuadorians have gone to Italy, and the smaller countries of El Salvador and Panama have lost half their stocks of nurses (Malvarez and Castrillon Agudelo 2005).

Alongside much greater complexity, the numbers of migrant health workers have significantly increased. Between 1970 and 2005 the number of foreign-trained doctors increased rapidly in most OECD countries (with the exception of Canada); hence the proportion of foreign-trained staff in the medical workforce increased dramatically (Dumont and Zurn 2007). The expansion of the EU in 2004, with the accession of ten new member states, brought increased migration to the West from Eastern states, although numbers were fewer than anticipated (Dumont and Zurn 2007; OECD 2008), partly, again, because of language constraints. In the USA, the number of foreign-trained doctors rose from 70,646 in 1973 (Mejia et al. 1979) to 209,000 in 2003 (Mullan 2005). By 2006, some 24 per cent of US doctors and 12 per cent of nurses were foreign born. About 30 per cent of this migrant health workforce came from other developed nations, which then recruited internationally to fill the gaps; some 70 per cent were from developing countries, mainly in Africa, the Caribbean, South Asia and the Philippines. In 2001, some 52 per cent of 8613 nurse migrants were from the Philippines, with 12 per cent and 6 per cent from Canada and Korea; and in 2004, some 50 per cent of the 100,791 nurse migrants were from the Philippines, with 20 per cent from Canada and 8 per cent from the UK. Most of these were concentrated in the urban areas of just five states: California (25 per cent), Florida (10 per cent), New York, Texas and New Jersey (Brush and Vasupuram 2006; Brush 2008). Very similar trends have occurred in other major recipient countries, such as Canada, Australia and the UK. In the UK, the total number of foreign-trained doctors increased from 20,923 in 1970 to 69,813 in 2003 (Mejia et al. 1979; Connell et al. 2007). In the seven years to March 2005, over 71,000 nurses educated outside the EU registered with the UK Nursing and Midwifery Council, representing fully 37 per cent of all new registrants. Most were from India and the Philippines, but numbers from SSA also rose sharply, with more than half from outside South Africa (Smith and Mackintosh 2007: 2217), notably from the larger, primarily anglophone states of Nigeria, Zimbabwe, Ghana and Zambia. The same complexities that were emerging within the source regions were developing in the recipient countries, although India and the Philippines continued to dominate global flows.

The proportion of foreign-trained SHWs in the workforces of developed countries has usually also risen: for example, in the USA and the UK foreign doctors now represent approximately 24 per cent and 33 per cent respectively of their medical workforces. Similar percentages occur in Australia and New Zealand, while comparable estimates are around 7 per cent in Germany and France (Connell et al. 2007). An estimated 10,000 African doctors are registered to practise in the UK, mainly from South Africa and Nigeria, representing approximately 15 per cent of all foreign-trained doctors. In comparison, the number of African-trained doctors in the USA is fewer, amounting to approximately 5500, some 3 per cent of foreign-trained doctors (Connell et al. 2007; Hagopian et al. 2004).

Following gradual geographical diversification of migration from Africa, Canada has acquired a substantial share of African-trained doctors, including some from francophone countries. Numbers are estimated at around 2000, but mainly from South Africa, representing approximately 15 per cent of all foreign doctors. Other OECD countries are less important destinations for African doctors.

Not at all paradoxically, as the numbers of SHWs being produced in developing countries increased, so migration also increased. During the 1980s and 1990s, two-thirds of all Ghanaian medical graduates had emigrated within ten years (Dovlo and Nyonator 1999). Thus in 1966 there were 215 Nigerian doctors in the UK, representing 1.5 per cent of all foreign doctors, while that figure had grown to 1922 in 2003, representing 3 per cent of foreign doctors (Connell et al. 2007). Roughly 40 per cent of all graduates from one medical school in Nigeria had migrated overseas (mainly to the USA, the UK and Ireland) within ten years of graduation (Ihekweazu et al. 2005). Substantial losses of nurses and midwives have only occurred since the mid-1990s in Malawi, but by the early 2000s more than 100 nurses a year were leaving (primarily to the UK) and, for about five years, this was outstripping the training rate of around 50 nurses per year (Record and Mohiddin 2006). While that is not atypical, as Botswana, Mauritius, Kenya, Zambia and Swaziland have each exhibited parallel trends and equivalent declines over a similar time period (Robinson 2007; Connell et al. 2007), there are many variations of regional and global trends.

Regional variations are evident from the situation in 2000, when about 65,000 African-born doctors and 70,000 nurses, representing 20 per cent and 10 per cent respectively of the stock of African doctors and nurses, were working overseas in a developed country. The percentages of both doctors and nurses working overseas range from near zero to over 70 per cent (Figures 3.1 and 3.2) but these may be underestimates since Gulf destinations were excluded and migrant SHWs not actually working overseas could not be counted. Countries that have experienced political and economic instability have experienced the greatest emigration. Language barriers and non-recognition of qualifications deter migration from francophone but not lusophone SSA (Clemens and Petterson 2008). Smaller countries are particularly prone to emigration, especially of nurses. While absolute numbers point to the particular significance of South Africa and Nigeria as sources of migrants, both countries are relatively large, each with over 50 million people. Comparing the number of African doctors in some significant receiving countries with the total number of doctors in those countries and in their countries of origin emphasises how migration from countries such as Mozambique, Zimbabwe and Kenya is important

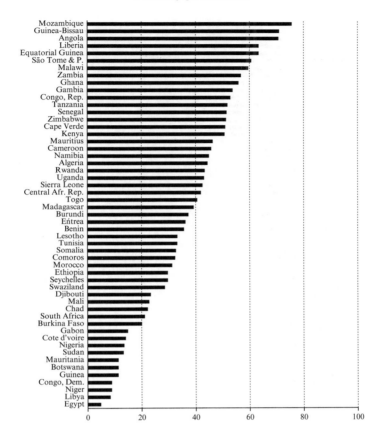

Figure 3.1 Percentage of African-born doctors residing and working abroad, 2000

Source: Clemens and Pettersson 2008, p. 5.

as the number leaving represents more than 50 per cent of doctors in those countries (Connell et al. 2007). As in most smaller countries, the actual number of migrants may be small, but their loss has a disproportionate influence on the national stock of skills.

Patterns of health worker migration from SSA have changed over the last 30 years. In the 1970s migrant health workers were from a relatively small number of African countries (the larger states of South Africa, Nigeria and Ghana) and predominantly went to a few developed countries outside Africa (Mejia et al. 1979). In the 1980s, structural adjustment programmes and high inflation reduced real wages, while non-wage benefits

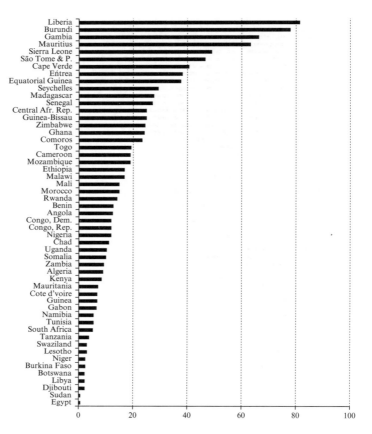

*Figure 3.2   Percentage of African-born nurses residing and working
          abroad, 2000*

Source: Clemens and Pettersson 2008, p. 6.

also fell in many SSA countries (McCoy et al. 2008), and salary compression, where the incomes of the most senior public servants became closer to those of the most junior, resulted in the migration of the more able. These changes set the scene for more rapid migration from SSA and movement towards a regional health workforce crisis. Migration has become much more complex, involving almost all SSA countries, including intra-regional and step migration (e.g. from the Democratic Republic of Congo to Kenya, and from Kenya to South Africa, Namibia and Botswana), and this has increasingly resulted from targeted recruitment, by both agencies and governments, as much as individual volition (Dumont and

Meyer 2004). Parallel trends in other world regions have not been well documented.

Training has also become more complex. For example, China sends nurses to undertake nursing degrees in Singapore, run by Australian nursing schools. The nurses who are trained in Singapore pay lower fees than they would in Australia but can then be recruited by Australia. Singapore meanwhile provides the clinical facilities and gets the services of the trainees (who speak the same language as most patients) at little cost, invaluable for a country where there is a nursing deficit (Gordon 2005: 382). Singapore also offers scholarships to nurses from China, with the obligation that they work in Singapore for six years after graduation. An increasing number of countries, from the Philippines to St Vincent, train nurses on the assumption that most will migrate.

Over the past 30 years the key receiving countries have remained remarkably similar, dominated by the UK and the USA. While demand in the Gulf has stabilised, other European and developed-country destinations (including Ireland, Canada, New Zealand and Australia) have grown in importance (OECD 2008). Migration to New Zealand was so rapid that between 2001 and 2004, at least, the number of registered immigrant nurses grew more rapidly than that of local graduates (North 2007: 224). Meanwhile Ireland, a long-established source of migrant workers, quickly reached immigration levels comparable to those of long-established recipient countries (Humphries et al. 2008). Over the same period, migration flows from developing countries significantly increased. In contrast to the 1970s, the number of countries experiencing emigration is substantially greater, as is the rate of migration. Thus Ethiopia, Angola and Uganda, which had very little emigration of doctors in the 1970s, now experience significant losses of doctors, nurses and pharmacists. Using different data from those of Clemens and Pettersson (2008), the 20 countries with the greatest emigration factors (the ratio of emigrant to resident doctors) include six in Africa (Ghana, South Africa, Ethiopia, Uganda, Nigeria and Sudan), three in the Caribbean (Jamaica, Haiti and the Dominican Republic), and the Philippines, India and Pakistan. Some of this cluster of countries are perhaps best characterised by crisis (Sri Lanka, Myanmar, Lebanon, Iraq and Syria), but others include New Zealand, Ireland, Malta and Canada (Mullan 2005). Several small Atlantic, Pacific and Caribbean states can also be included. By contrast, developing countries with higher 'physician migration densities' (the ratio of national doctors overseas to the population) are those with higher GNPs, greater female literacy and a high Human Development Index; they are not therefore the least developed countries, which lack medical schools and whose doctors lack complex skills and the knowledge and opportunities to migrate. These countries may be 'caught in an unfortunate dilemma: they have to tolerate poverty to retain their best and brightest, but they need to break out of poverty to increase their investments in their health workforce' (Arah et al. 2008: 152). Despite half a century and at least three phases of migration, the Philippines is still the world's largest exporter of nurses (with about 150,000 presently abroad) and India the largest exporter of doctors, and in both countries this export has reached critical proportions (Chapter 7).

Much of this migration, like other flows, remains dominated by post-colonial ties, especially where these link languages, training institutions, educational regimes, and where the migration of SHWs accompanies other migration flows. The presence of kin and new structures of recruitment encourage such consistencies, while geographical proximity helps. Language of training, kinship networks and geographical proximity are all correlated with the migration of doctors to the USA (Hussey 2007). Puerto Rican doctors are particularly useful in the continental USA since the substantial growth of the Hispanic population has increased the demand for Spanish-speaking doctors (Nieves and Stack 2008). Nicaraguan nurses move to Belize (Malvarez and Castrillon Agudela 2005), and nurses from Lesotho and Swaziland invariably go to South Africa. In the major global source country for nurses, the Philippines, migration is inextricably linked to its colonial heritage: 'the origins of Filipino nurse migration to the US lie in the early twentieth century US colonialism in the Philippines' and are bound up with language, religion, professional training, work culture, popular culture and even gendered notions of nursing as women's work (Choy 2003: 6–7). The UK's ties to the Commonwealth are evident in many migration flows. For France, migration from formerly francophone North Africa is significantly more important than from SSA, accounting for around 40 per cent of all overseas trained doctors (Connell et al. 2007). Senegalese (francophone) nurses in Canada are all in Quebec (Labonté et al. 2006: 5). Romanian nurses make up over half of all overseas SHWs in Italy (Chaloff 2008; Palese et al. 2008). In Portugal many of the foreign doctors are from Portuguese-speaking African countries, that were former Portuguese colonies, notably Angola and Guinea-Bissau. Francophone Africa is thus linked to France (and also Belgium and Canada), lusophone Africa to Portugal, anglophone Africa to the UK and North America, and Latin America to Spain. Mauritius has lost a particularly large number of nurses relative to its size because Mauritian nurses speak both French and English and therefore have a great range of potential destinations. Italy has relatively few foreign-born doctors, and most of these either trained in Italy or are German speakers working in the German-language province of South Tyrol, since Italian is rarely spoken elsewhere (Chaloff 2008). Similarly, Finland has few migrants since few outsiders speak Finnish, and

Finland has sought to be self-reliant (OECD 2008). In those parts of the world where European colonial languages never became significant, as in parts of Asia and the Middle East, skilled migration has been more limited or more localised. Unsurprisingly, regional preferences and cultural similarities have meant that two-thirds of all Lebanese migrant nurses are in Gulf states, while the remainder are in North America, and many Pakistani doctors are in Saudi Arabia or other Gulf states (El-Jardali et al. 2008a; Talati and Pappas 2006). Language proficiency is more crucial in the health sector than in perhaps any other arena of migration, skilled or unskilled, further emphasising colonial and post-colonial flows.

CAROUSELS WITHIN THE DEVELOPED WORLD

Long before migration from developing countries expanded the work-forces of developed countries, many individual migrants moved within the rich world, reflecting the great migration journeys of the nineteenth century and before, as countries such as Canada, the USA, South Africa and Australia were populated by migrants from the Old World, especially Ireland and the UK. Some of these were health workers whose skills were much welcomed in the New World. Their legacy remains.

Much international migration of SHWs is still between rich-world countries, as much for short-term experience as for longer-term income or lifestyle reasons. Doctors are more likely to move between rich-world countries because of superior training and professional opportunities. More than a quarter of overseas doctors in Belgium are from the Netherlands, and Norwegians make up half of all overseas doctors in Denmark (Wiskow 2006: 16). New Zealanders move to Australia and both they and Australians move to the UK. South Africans move to the UK, Belgians to France, and French to Switzerland and Luxembourg. Neighbouring countries such as the USA for Canadian nurses, Portugal for Spanish nurses, Switzerland for French and German nurses and Australia for New Zealanders are all key destinations. Language, culture and geography are again combined, but often within a wider 'carousel of migration' that necessitates replacement from poorer countries. Through such carousels, steps and 'conveyor belts', new immigrants replace emigrants, both internally and internationally.

The gradual expansion of the EU, especially across the once 'Iron Curtain', brought significant new westwards migration in Europe, particularly from Poland, Estonia, Latvia and Lithuania (Jinks et al. 2000; Czupryniak and Loba 2005; Wiskow 2006; Dumont and Zurn 2007). Although widespread intentions to migrate did not necessarily become reality, aspirations to migrate substantially increased (Smigelskas et al. 2007; Krajewski-Siuda et al. 2008). Czech doctors had started intensive West European language courses even before accession (Mareckova 2004), and countries like Estonia and Lithuania had to rapidly adopt new policies to retain their health workers (Buchan and Perfilieva 2006). Slovakia, where inefficient resource allocation had meant a lack of capital investment, obsolete equipment and facilities, low salaries, but an oversupply of doctors, balanced against wages in France and the UK that were ten times local wages, became a new source of SHWs in the West (Williams and Balaz 2008: 1926–7). After EU membership in 2004, more than twice as many certificates were issued to Slovakian doctors registering to work abroad as graduated annually. Destinations were again influenced by proximity, existing social networks and language competence; in Slovakia this resulted in migration to Germany, Austria, Switzerland and the Netherlands, but some English competence enabled more limited migration to the UK, the USA, France and Oman. Migrants from further east, Ukraine, Romania and Bulgaria, filled emerging gaps; in just six months in 2003 more than 1000 SHWs left Moldova (Wiskow 2006). Destinations thus shifted from the state socialism years, which largely involved either migration exclusively within the Eastern bloc, or no mobility at all.

In middle-income European countries like Greece, as many as half of all 'sole-agent' nurses (a function similar to that of nurses aides or carers in other places) are from overseas. In very recent years more affluent countries, such as Germany, which had 'a glut of doctors' until well into the twentieth century (and thus a phase of commuter migration of doctors to the UK), began to experience a shortage. Countries such as the UK and the Scandinavian countries, where training is insufficient to meet local needs, use 'aggressive government-sponsored recruitment campaigns' to attempt to lure doctors from elsewhere (Kopetsch 2009), alongside commuter migration from further east (see Epigraphs). As German doctors have moved away, so new private recruitment agencies emerged to recruit from Poland, the Czech Republic, Slovakia and Ukraine, mainly for Eastern Germany, where in some hospitals three-quarters of the medical staff are foreign nationals (Kopetsch 2009). In turn, Eastern European countries have looked even further eastwards. The new complexity of international migration is evident in Poland, as much a sending country as a recipient, where the main source countries are Eastern European countries (Ukraine, Belarus, Russia, Lithuania) and the Middle East (Syria, Yemen, Iraq) while in Denmark, key source countries are Germany, Iraq and Eastern European countries (Russia, Lithuania, Poland, Romania, Bosnia-Herzegovina) and in Finland, Eastern European countries (Estonia, Russia, Poland), but alongside Sweden and Germany.

In North America, migration took Canadians to the USA. Canadian doctors who had moved were more likely to be specialists than those who remained in Canada, and influenced by a range of factors, including postgraduate training and the climate. Australian and New Zealand migrants in the USA were also more likely to be specialists than those who remained at home (Miller et al. 1998). Family reasons were highly influential for remaining in Canada: 'the preferences of those living in Canada emphasize patriotism and family attachment, whereas the preferences of those in the US create a profile of independent, career-minded individualists' (McKendry et al. 1996: 180). This migration led to shortages in some Canadian surgical and medical specialisms (McKendry et al. 1996; Phillips et al. 2007) and, as in Europe, created a demand that rippled far beyond the continent.

Broadly similar reasons influence the migration of doctors within developed countries as in relatively poor countries (Chapter 6). Polish doctors, with salaries one-tenth of those in Western Europe, quickly moved when they could (Czupryniak and Loba 2005). German doctors began to move away more rapidly in this century, particularly to the USA, the UK, Switzerland and Austria because of concerns over salary levels and the lack of time available for leisure or families. They sought the better working conditions (including more regular working hours, flatter hierarchies and more curative work) and the reduced bureaucracy and administrative burden offered abroad (Kopetsch 2009). French doctors moved to the UK for similar reasons, including poor pay, limited career prospects and inadequate recognition and support within hospitals (Duverne et al. 2008). 'The dramatic collapse of Iceland's economy after the global financial crisis brought the loss of many skills. By the middle of 2009 many doctors had gone to the UK, the USA and Canada, lured by incomes, previously comparable with those in the USA; but by then just a quarter of them' (Jackson 2009). Here is the newest carousel, as, from some of even the richest countries, new flows of SHWs have become evident, and as they move others have replaced them.

CHAINS, STEPS AND NETWORKS

The greater complexity of migration is evident in the interlocking chains and hierarchies of recruitment and supply, although some were in place 30 years ago (Mejia et al. 1979). Thus Canada recruits from South Africa (which recruits from Cuba) as it supplies the USA; Australia and New Zealand recruit from the Pacific island states (which recruit from the Philippines, Burma and China) as they in turn supply the UK. Slovak doctors and nurses go to the Czech Republic, Czechs go to Germany and Germans go to the UK. All are variants of cascade migration. At the same time step migration takes SHWs to several places. Fiji loses nurses to the Marshall Islands and Palau; many move on to the USA, the UK, the UAE, the Bahamas and Bermuda. Kenyan nurses first went to Southern African countries such as Botswana, Zimbabwe and South Africa, and then moved on as step migration to Britain. In the Caribbean, Guyanan nurses move to several countries, including St Lucia and Jamaica, while Guyana has recruited from India (Anderson and Isaacs 2007), and Jamaican nurses similarly travel to several places, such as the Virgin Islands, but also to the USA and Canada. Most Jamaican nurses now live overseas, and Cubans have partly replaced them. In 2004, Bermuda was concerned about the loss of nurses to the USA; six months later Jamaica fretted over recruitment of nurses by Bermuda. Dependent territories, such as Anguilla in the Caribbean and Guam and American Samoa in the Pacific, gain workers from nearby independent states. The international migration of health workers has extended and expanded most national diasporas.

Many countries are both sending and receiving countries, particularly such large states as the UK, Canada, Australia and New Zealand, but also smaller states such as Barbados, the Netherlands Antilles and Fiji, and intermediate states such as Chile and Poland (van Eyck 2004). Pakistan is a major exporter but also imports doctors from China, the Philippines, the Caribbean and former Russian republics (Talati and Pappas 2006). Even tiny Niue, most of whose SHWs are overseas, has had to recruit doctors from Samoa, New Zealand, Ukraine and elsewhere (Connell 2007b). New transport technology and reduced costs have produced variants of 'commuter migration', with Jamaican nurses flying to Florida for five- to ten-day shifts and returning home, Samoan nurses flying to American Samoa for the working week, Botswanan nurses spending periods of 'sick leave' in South Africa, and German and later Polish doctors working long weekends in the UK.

An emerging hierarchy characterises global migration chains, for example from relatively poor Asian states and the small and poor island states of the Atlantic, Caribbean and Pacific, to the developed world, culminating in the USA. Parallel hierarchies link Eastern European countries to Western Europe, and SSA to the North. Norway and Austria have both become importers of SHWs, as recently as this century. Ireland went from being a major exporter to an importer, as membership of the EU enabled a booming economy, but a contemporary slump has ended recruitment. As demand in developed countries has increased, the structure of recruitment has grown and extended. A decade ago US hospitals recruited in the Philippines, Ireland and Canada to find English-speaking nurses but more recently they have turned to India. A growing number of countries, notably the Philippines, deliberately produce excess numbers of nurses to supply overseas markets. Migration and hierarchies are thus constantly in flux depending on market demands, domestic pressures and national production, new forms of global legislation and codes of practice, recruitment activities, economic crises and even perceptions of amenable and profitable destinations.

While 'English has become the universal language of migration' as migratory health workers largely maintained post-colonial ties, non-English-speaking migrants were virtually forced to learn English, and recruitment agencies 'fine tuned the accents and pronunciation of new recruits' so that nurses would 'communicate in English and be accent-free' (Brush and Vasupuram 2006: 183). In the late 1990s, when UK recruiters were encouraged to go beyond the Commonwealth, they targeted the Philippines (as also did Singapore) since, as one recruiter said: 'The Philippines seems a natural place to start – there is a culture of young people going abroad to work and the standard of English among potential recruits is excellent' (quoted in Choy 2003: 187). Greater complexity has produced new migration streams – for example from the Philippines to Japan – that have less to do with English (or another mutually intelligible language), while Korean nurses, hitherto noted as having considerable English-language difficulties (and problems of cultural transition) in the USA, have none the less increasingly been recruited there in substantial numbers (Brush 2008) and also for other destinations such as Australia. English remains dominant but new structures of migration have extended far beyond the anglophone world.

While SHWs may migrate without family members, almost all go to destinations where kin or members of their own cultural or national group are present (hence, no doubt, the frequent references to Malawians in Manchester), and often travel as groups. They thus follow established migration routes and consolidate existing beachheads, with kin acting like 'magnets' (Ryan 2008). Even where SHWs were effectively recruited by particular countries, or hospitals, and thus 'had little control of their labour', they none the less exercised 'connective autonomy' determining where, when and how they migrated within the context of familial ties and networks formed through nursing (George 2005; Ryan 2008). Unsurprisingly, migrants choose familiar routes in classic patterns of chain migration. Yet chain migration may be just as evident in alternative migration pathways. Thus the migration of Filipino nurses to the Netherlands from the 1960s centred on social ties. Conversely the movement of nurses from Kerala to Vienna largely cut across language and religious ties, but was facilitated by the presence of a particular Catholic religious order in Austria that supported the early migrants who then provided a beachhead for others to follow (Hintermann and Reeger 2005). In multiple flexible and innovative ways, large numbers of health workers gradually moved beyond what were assumed to be traditional migration routes.

The initial overseas destination of SHWs may not always be the intended final destination, especially for health workers in the Gulf. SHWs may first take advantage of familiarity, proximity, social ties, political connections and demand to move more easily to certain countries, notably in the Gulf, before moving on to superior destinations. Filipinos seek to move on to the USA (Ball 1996) as do Lebanese nurses, working in the Gulf for the relatively high wages and experience that would enable them to move to superior positions there (El-Jardali et al. 2008a). Indian nurses from Kerala use their stay in the Gulf to save money and take advanced courses 'to reach the much prized west', with the Gulf merely the first step in 'the "true" emigration': 'a necessary passage to get the experience and resources for further migration to the west' (Percot and Rajan 2007: 321, 323; Percot 2006: 155; George 2005; Thomas 2008). One Kerala student nurse described such a strategy:

> After graduation, I'll work here [in India] for two years. That is the minimum experience required for the Gulf and it will give me the time to save up for the fare. Once I am there I will work for two years and then I'll get married [having saved enough for the dowry]. My husband will come to work with me in the Gulf. After two years it will be possible to have children. During that time we will have the time to save money and I'll have the time to pass the TOEFL and maybe the CGNFS [the language and nursing qualifications necessary for work in the USA]. So it will be possible for us to go to England or to Connecticut where I have some family. (Quoted in Percot 2006: 163; see Chapter 5)

Many other SHWs had worked in such African countries as Zambia and Nigeria and various European countries before moving on to the USA (George 2005: 51). For Filipino nurses, 'nursing is seen as a way to move the whole family from the Philippines to the United States' (Ong and Azores 1994: 173), just as it is for Indian doctors. Filipino and Indian health workers in the UK and Ireland also seek to move on to the USA (Buchan 2008; Yeates 2008), as do Fijians in the Marshall Islands and the Gulf (Rokoduru 2008; Connell 2009), and Korean and Hong Kong nurses in Australia (Chung 2007; Ho 2008). 'Filipino nurses in Ireland usually seek to move onwards to Canada or the USA, less because of employment conditions, but in order to achieve stability with their families, rather than be insecure in terms of the possibility of family migration, reunion and citizenship in Ireland)' (Humphries et al. 2009b). As in so many other contexts, the USA is the alluring, ultimate destination of this step migration, as it is for cascade migration. Even other developed countries are rarely the ultimate goal.

Step migration is partly a function of ease of migration. Nurses moving to many African and Gulf countries from India or the Philippines were typically recruited in their country of origin, and had all their travel expenses paid; they did not require sponsorship or exhaustive tests, and often received holiday travel expenses, while in some Gulf countries living expenses were also covered. Although the high wages and lack of taxes were attractive, the sense of insecurity stemming from fixed-term contracts and the lack of citizenship and permanent residence options 'ultimately led them to emigrate to the United States' (George 2005: 53, 228). While step migration may lead, seemingly inexorably, to the USA, it is only one element of the complexity that also includes the uncertainties of return migration.

THE GLOBAL SHIFT

No phases of migration are discrete. They overlap, and exhibit regional variations. Even the first phase retains a localised presence. Many developing countries, such as those in the Pacific, continue to benefit substantially from the assistance of doctors and others from developed countries, on a short- or long-term basis (Connell 2009: 35–8). Several NGOs support the short-term return migration of SHWs. Some doctors come from Cuba, which had some 3000 health workers overseas in 2004, and also from Taiwan; both countries have pursued a policy of providing medical care to developing countries, with both humanitarian and political objectives (de Vos et al. 2007), adding new complexities to the globalisation of health care.

While the second phase accompanied the recognition of a widespread brain drain, the third phase drew in areas that were remote from metropolitan regions of demand and hitherto had relatively few SHWs, including much of SSA and the Pacific islands, and marked the full florescence of globalisation. The outcome has been the wide-ranging and expanding role of migration in shaping health workforces, as is true in all 31 OECD countries since the 1970s (OECD 2008: 34), alongside an astounding complexity and diversity of migration streams, symbolised by the global origins of nurses in London. As the means of recruitment of SHWs have diversified to include a 'combination of active international recruitment, employment of nurses who apply on their own initiative and tapping into local labour markets for IRNs [internationally recruited nurses] already in this country', the diversity of sources has multiplied to include 68 countries,

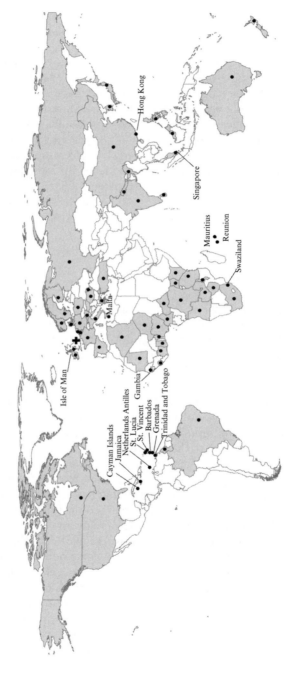

Figure 3.3   National sources of nurses in a London hospital trust, 2001

Source: Buchan 2002.

including most of Europe and SSA, in the case of a single London hospital trust (Buchan 2002; Figure 3.3). Similarly, a single Saudi Arabian hospital had nurses from 40 different countries in 1997 (Luna 1998). The number of countries from which nurses sought official US accreditation grew from 90 in 1983 to 139 in 2005. Between 2001 and 2005, nurses who passed the licensing examination came from at least 63 countries (Pittman et al. 2007; Figure 3.4). Recruitment and migration, even in anglophone countries, extended beyond more familiar anglophone colonial linkages, although the English language remained dominant.

In the third phase of migration the balance shifted firmly towards nurses, and thus the feminisation of migrant SHW flows, accentuated by the feminisation of the health workforce. (Between 1990 and 2005, the proportion of female doctors in OECD countries grew by more than a quarter, from 29 to 38 per cent.) As the gender basis of migration changed, so the economic rationale for migration simultaneously became even more evident. Yet social ties are critical for supporting the ambitions of migrants, and choices of destination are usually linked to existing social networks and structures of chain migration (Chapter 5). Simultaneously the increased volumes of SHW migration paralleled a global transition from unskilled to skilled workers, and a wider active recruitment of them. Countries like the UK, the USA and Australia, consistent destinations for migrants, both became more aggressive and global recruiters and developed structured immigration programmes designed to enable easy integration into the workforce, for example through language acquisition programmes (Kopetsch 2009). Once a safety valve for high population densities, migration gradually became a safety valve for stagnant economies, political crises and social change. Skilled workers are relatively easily able to migrate, and crises quickly provoked their migration, as in Fiji, Zimbabwe, Sierra Leone and elsewhere. While shortages of SHWs have been cyclical, there is a growing consensus that the present global shortage will not disappear in the foreseeable future.

However, data on the migration of health workers are ultimately imperfect, as the differences between data on emigration flows show. The lack of systematic, comprehensive and comparable data means relying on various sources, with different classifications and measurements, including reports of governments, professional associations and various regulatory bodies (Stilwell et al. 2003; Clemens and Pettersson 2008; Robinson et al. 2008). Moreover, there is even some unwillingness on the part of both sending and receiving countries to acknowledge significant flows of skilled labour (Iredale 2000), even between relatively rich countries (Phillips et al. 2007). Statistics are open to debate and dispute, especially where there is attrition alongside migration, and different forms of measurement produce

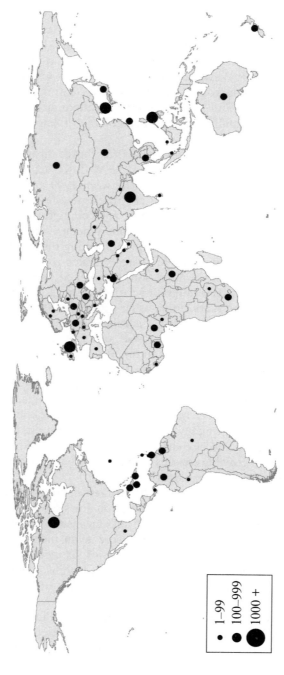

Figure 3.4   National sources of nurses gaining US accreditation, 2001–05

Source: based on Pittman et al. 2007, p. 17.

different outcomes. Thus for SSA the absolute numbers of doctors migrating overseas is greatest for South Africa, the ratio of those overseas to those at home was highest in Malawi and the ratio of the number of those overseas to the population at home was greatest in the Seychelles (Arah 2007). A global need is systematic, comparable data, although the broad perspective is reasonably clear.

Migration is far from the only critical factor influencing the status of health care systems. All the issues that affect health systems and health workers are a function of other issues, above all the adequacy of financial resources, government commitment to health and limited national production of SHWs. This is complicated by rising expectations for the delivery of services and standards of living. An underlying problem in many developing countries is simply a lack of capital. In the midst of so many constraints to the delivery of effective health care, why migration has acquired such recent significance can now be examined further.

4. The scope for migration

A substantial part of the international migration of skilled health workers is from relatively poor countries to relatively rich countries. While migration is only partially demand driven, as many migrants (including health workers) migrate irrespective of any certainties of job acquisition in the destination, increased demand for health workers in developed countries has influenced and directed migration flows, and suggested the greater probability of employment for skilled migrants. This chapter examines why that should be so, and where demand is concentrated. Since employment in health services accounts for about 10 per cent of the total employment in high-income economies, about 6 per cent in the transition economies of Eastern Europe, and rather less in developing countries, social, economic and political changes in the most developed countries have a significant influence on global labour markets.

DEVELOPED-WORLD DEMAND

Growing demand for health workers in relatively rich countries has resulted from ageing populations, high attrition rates (for reasons ranging from patient violence to discontent with wages and working conditions etc.), growing demand for health care, greater specialisation and a rising ability to pay. In most developed countries national policies have increased day-care treatment and encouraged shorter, more intensive hospital stays, discharging patients to residential homes, and significantly increasing the demand for care workers, especially in the private sector. Effective demand is most concentrated in those countries where domestic output of SHWs is inadequate and/or attrition rates are high, but where, seemingly paradoxically, wages are highest. Needs are particularly concentrated in rural areas, and in some inner-city areas, where skilled workers are generally reluctant to live and work.

The outcome of static or reduced local production of health workers and greater attrition is that in most countries the health workforce is ageing and retiring, with several countries increasing their public sector retirement ages simply to enable health workers to stay. Consequently European countries such as Germany, where, without immigration, zero or even negative population growth would have long been established, are becoming more dependent on migration of health workers and others, at least in part because of the ageing of the workforce. In many developed countries (e.g. Australia), widespread retirement is predicted in the near future, which threatens the availability of relatively experienced clinical nurses, academic nurses and nurse managers in both urban and rural areas. Both in developed and developing countries a series of strategies has thus been designed to delay and discourage retirement (Jackson 2008; Chapter 9). Most studies of nurse retention demonstrate that it is either younger nurses who are more likely to leave, often within a year or two of completion of training, or older experienced nurses. Although this has always been the case, it reflects the challenges of employment in the health sector. The attrition of younger health workers, in particular, and the prior challenges of recruiting them, pose substantial future problems. In Canada and the USA the average age of nurses is 45 (compared with 37 in the USA in 1983) and it is gradually increasing (Gordon 2005: 234; Little 2007). Several EU states too have average nurse ages of over 45, and the average age of doctors is also increasing. Some 30 per cent of all doctors in the USA are aged 55 and over (Mullan et al. 2008). Similar trends and situations exist in most developed countries.

Ageing: Will You Still Feed Me . . .?

In most developed countries, health needs have increased, because of the ageing of the population, alongside higher expectations of the extent, sophistication and coverage of medical care. Within the EU region, life expectancies have increased by around 2.5 years per decade since the 1950s; globally, for the first time, the world is about to cross a demographic divide where more of the population are aged over 65 than are younger than 5. Ageing is accompanied by a deterioration of the ratio of taxpayers to health service beneficiaries, and greater challenges in providing health care. At the same time fertility rates have tended to fall, so shifting the focus of health care from paediatrics to geriatrics, and even to palliative care. In many developed countries this transition has recently been emphasised by the first wave of 'baby-boomers', those born between approximately 1946 and 1956, reaching retirement age. As the children of the post-war 'baby-boom' generation have now become adults, still-declining birth rates mean that absolutely fewer school leavers are now entering the workforce. Population projections for Europe, and also Japan and Korea, suggest that population numbers in the age group 15–24 will decline by about 25 per cent between 2005 and 2025, although there will be small increases in countries of immigration, such as Australia (where fertility rates have recently increased) and the USA. The decline means that a growing proportion of young people will have to enter the health profession even to maintain current training rates, which is likely to be a significant problem for the recruitment of nurses (OECD 2008: 20), where the age of trainees is currently increasing.

In countries where there has been significant immigration, such as Canada and Australia, the rate of growth of the population aged over 65 is around three or four times that of the population as a whole, and it is even greater in many European countries, such as Sweden, where immigration has been relatively slight. In Japan, officially the world's oldest country, where fertility has long been low, and immigration is trivial, the impacts of ageing are considerable, resulting in complex policies to meet health care needs without immigration but belated acceptance of its need (Chapter 2). In 11 major countries the population is ageing, while overall numbers decline – an unprecedented combination. There especially, ageing has also slowed economic growth and raised dependency rates – the ratio of working to non-working populations – as countries have exhausted the 'demographic dividend' where age structures were more favourable to workforce participation.

Demographic change has been accompanied by structural changes that have taken substantially more women into the workforce in most developed countries, so reducing the availability of extended household care, since it is women who provide the majority of household elder care. Since there has been little if any gender restructuring of care provision – with men remaining elsewhere in national workforces – a care deficit has appeared. A similar rise in the proportion of single-parent households 'represents both an imperative for workforce participation and a deterioration in the family context of care giving' (Joseph and Martin-Matthews 1994: 171). In most developed countries divorce rates are rising; hence the proportion of people who will have a partner to look after them in old age is declining, while greater mobility has meant that children are less likely to live close to ageing parents (Hugo 2009). At a time when there is growing demand for elder care, at least because there are greater numbers of older people, household support is dwindling, thus putting greater pressure on institutional contexts and non-family workers.

Older populations tend to be characterised by greater incidences of chronic lifestyle diseases, such as diabetes and heart disease, which tend to be time-consuming and costly to manage. More new (and expensive) drugs and procedures are available to deal with health problems, and there has been a proliferation of hip-replacement and other complicated procedures to which patients, quite reasonably, feel entitled as a means of prolonging mobility and enhancing quality of life. Ageing has placed particular demands not only on direct health care (such as the increasing resort to medications and elective surgery for such procedures as hip-replacement and cataract surgery), but also on nursing homes and the provision of home support. Despite predictions that older people may well remain healthy for an increasing proportion of their lives (e.g. Coory 2004), increasing numbers of nursing homes in most developed countries suggest that either this is not so or that other factors influence perceived care needs. Moreover, older people are particularly heavy users of health care; in the USA, despite being only 13 per cent of the population, they account for half of all visits to doctors and half of all hospital stays (Mullan et al. 2008). Migration of SHWs has consequently been invaluable.

Employment Alternatives

Reduced recruitment of health workers has followed declining birth rates in developed countries; hence there are fewer young people and more diverse employment opportunities for women, many of which offer superior wages and working conditions, and greater prestige and respect. The conformity and propriety that ensured post-war numbers have both faded. As demand has increased, fewer school leavers and others apparently wish to take up careers as SHWs. Jobs in the health sector are seen in many developed countries as too demanding, poorly paid and lowly regarded (in line with reduced public sector funding, and disregard for the public sector), and occurring within a context of poor working conditions. While disdain for dirty, dangerous and difficult jobs has long existed, and health work is sometimes seen to be in that category, where alternatives exist, disdain has tended to increase, in both developed and developing countries. As early as the end of the 1940s in the UK, women had become uninterested in nursing, preferring new and better-paid opportunities such as secretarial work, teaching or public service. Nursing, with its long hours, low pay and strict discipline, was less appealing, but choices were still quite restricted (Ryan 2008). Likewise, uniforms, once attractions, became symbols of authoritarian institutions rather than of public success and respectability. The rise of HIV/AIDS and other lifestyle diseases has increased attrition rates of those who are employed (Brown et al. 2002), while co-morbidity (with patients suffering more than one chronic condition) and more older patients undergoing procedures such as dialysis and heart operations, pose new demands. At the same time, shorter, more intensive patient stays in hospital, more complex technology (which may lead to additional procedures such as cochlear ear implants and colonoscopy), alongside ethical issues (involving, for example, euthanasia and new reproductive technologies) have restructured nursing and made it more challenging and demanding, but without parallel improvements in wages and conditions. Indeed a more demanding and regulated bureaucracy (with procedures linked to paper work) has distanced workers from patients. Mechanisation has yet to have any significant impact on employment in the health sector, other than in some administrative areas (Chapter 9).

While medicine, with its relatively better income and prestige, continues to hold more attractions than nursing in most countries, it has also lost some allure. In Australia, for example, high-school leavers have increasingly been

> looking for careers which were less demanding, more lucrative, less dependent on the whims and human failings of their mentors, and free from the demands of an ungrateful public; careers that would give them a better lifestyle, a better balance of public and personal, and would not take fifteen years of penury before they reach their professional goals. (Galak 2009: 31)

Many such 'failings' of the system are, however, only apparent belatedly. It may be that such perceptions partly underpin the global feminisation of medicine as a profession (with France having gone from a 30:70 ratio to a 50:50 ratio in just 20 years, New Zealand from 16:84 to 37:63 in 25 years and Australia having a 55:45 ratio in favour of women).

In contrast, by the 1960s in most developed countries, attractive alternative career opportunities had opened up for women. Social mores changed and women became more acceptable, and more interested, in a range of occupations, especially outside the public sector. No longer was choice broadly restricted to teaching and nursing, where perceptions of long training periods, low pay and understaffing discouraged school leavers. Sex-based occupational discrimination, along with poor working conditions, further resulted in both a shortage of new recruits and a high attrition rate (Whitehead et al. 2007; George 2005: 50). Remarkably, in 2009, more than one Australian hospital was advertising '12-hour shifts' as an inducement to recruitment. Ubiquitously, women acquired more education and increasingly moved into various spheres, including traditionally male-dominated occupations such as military and police service, which offered similar orientations to public service (and also unusual hours and uniforms), and especially private sector business.

In the health sector, however, wages remained relatively low, even in the USA, where in the 1960s the hospitals that employed as many as 70 per cent of all nurses colluded to set low rates (Ong and Azores 1994: 167). That disincentive to local workers was linked to the 1965 Immigration Act, where barriers to migration from developing countries were dramatically lifted and the influx of overseas workers began. During the 1990s nursing wages did no more than keep pace with inflation; hence nurses gained no more purchasing power (Sochalski 2002) compared with most other sectors in the country. Similar situations occurred in other developed countries.

Most nurses are women – 92 per cent in Australia and 95 per cent in Canada – although the proportion of males is very slowly increasing. Efforts to recruit more male nurses have been thwarted in many places by prevailing perceptions of masculinity, and opposition from patients and female nurses (Chapter 9). Ironically, such pressures have directed disproportionately more men into better-paid managerial roles, rather than their being a complement to women.

A final possible deterrent to employment, at least in nursing, is that popular culture has rarely portrayed nurses in a particularly positive light. While doctors are portrayed highly favourably in much of the popular media (Chory-Assad and Tamborini 2001), nurses tend to have no more than bystander roles where little actual health work is undertaken and implicitly doctors are of sole importance (Gordon 2005: 147–72). In the Czech Republic, not only are nursing wages lower than those of bus drivers, and standard shifts are 12 hours, but 'the public still perceives nurses as they were represented in communist-era television shows: as low-level workers who emptied bedpans and cleaned hospital rooms' (Bilefsky 2009: 12). What might have been a source of attraction may be a means of deterrence. For multiple reasons various alternatives to a career in health now exist, particularly in nursing, and especially for women.

The Rise of the Private Sector

In most countries the private sector has grown relative to the public sector. It has usually grown fastest in low- and middle-income countries, although from a smaller base, encouraged by economic restructuring and neo-liberalism. The private sector has also grown because of dissatisfaction with the public sector, and because of the ability to pay, related to the rise of private insurance. Dissatisfaction with the public sector takes a similar form in most places, for example Greece: low-quality services (including doubts over the competence of workers), cleanliness, lack of single, private bedrooms, absence of facilities in some regional areas, long waiting lists for certain specialties, such as cardiac surgery and oncology (Tountas et al. 2005), long waiting times for operations that are not judged to be urgent (Groutsis 2009), and more flexible structures of health insurance. The private sector counteracts such problems, or at least is widely perceived to do so. Its growth has both emphasised the comparative merits of the two systems, and created a greater demand for health workers to supply them. In most countries, for example Australia, the rise of the private sector has also placed added stress on the public sector, where it has become increasingly difficult to retain surgeons and nursing staff, resulting in longer waiting lists and delays in receiving treatment, and challenging notions of equity (*Sydney Morning Herald*, 30 December 2008). A vicious circle has emerged, stimulating further migration of health workers to the private sector (Chapter 2). In turn, such changes reduce the morale and increase the attrition rates of those remaining in the public sector.

JOB SATISFACTION AND ATTRITION

While fewer workers are attracted to a career in health, more of those who have taken up training courses and employment drop out or later leave the professions. Attrition rates, especially of nurses, in most developed countries have risen, and high rates of turnover are disruptive (in terms of morale and productivity) and expensive. Much attrition is for family reasons that have little to do with work contexts, such as the ability to live on partners' wages or the graduation of children from high school. Family responsibilities have also resulted in both a choice of jobs more suited to flexible and more affluent lifestyles, and accelerated attrition. Awkward shift times and long hours are not at all attractive when workers wish to and are able to move towards a superior 'work–life balance'. Night shifts are a primary cause of burnout and attrition (Alimoglu and Donmez 2005). Dissatisfaction and overwork have resulted in nurses retiring early or choosing to work only part time.

For lifestyle reasons many SHWs are said to wish to work shorter hours than their predecessors, which would increase demand for staff. In both Australia and Canada the working hours of doctors have fallen; in Australia doctors worked on average 45 hours per week in 2003 compared with 48 in 1997 (OECD 2008). The growing feminisation of the workforce has probably also reduced average hours worked; without gains in productivity this necessitates more workers. In Australia in 2008, women doctors worked 38 hours per week compared with 46 hours for men. In most other OECD countries, female doctors work shorter hours than men, and have shorter working lives. Male nurses also work longer hours than females.

The reasons for attrition, and to a lesser extent recruitment, in developed countries are remarkably similar to those in developing countries (Chapter 6). They have been reviewed in some detail, emphasising both the extent and significance of job satisfaction, and the growing dissatisfaction experienced by nurses (Lu et al., 2005; Day et al. 2006; Coomber and Barriball 2007; Pillay 2009). Job satisfaction has long been the most important influence on attrition in developed countries (as it has within other organisations outside the health sector). Increasingly higher expectations result in often-reduced chances of achieving job satisfaction, and a greater probability of attrition. Unrealistic expectations have been a significant influence on high turnover rates among newly graduated nurses. However, dissatisfaction with nursing in particular has become widespread. Some 40 per cent of a sample of nurses from five countries expressed dissatisfaction, mainly because of limited autonomy and perceptions of low esteem (Aiken et al. 2001, 2002). While most studies are implicitly about female nurses or make no gender distinctions, male nurses are just as likely to have short careers and drop out for similar reasons (Barron and West 2005). Ward culture and its relationship to patient care is a significant influence on retention, with nurses most likely to leave the busiest, most demanding wards (Chan et al. 2008). Although retention is usually less critical for doctors than for nurses, issues of wages and benefits, working conditions, autonomy and recognition, continuous education and training, job security and collegial relationships, and even the design of facilities are similarly important (Reeves et al. 2005; Janus et al. 2007; Rechel et al. 2009). Where health workers were involved in cooperation and consultation, effective and supportive management processes, with reasonable self-reliance and autonomy, and had what they perceived as meaningful work and were able to achieve positive outcomes with a fair, financial reward, then satisfaction was greatest, resulting not just in lower attrition rates but more punctual committed attendance. Ultimately, individual ability to develop coping strategies enables superior job satisfaction (Golbasi et al. 2008). In management terminology, 'organisational citizenship' rewarded effective workers, and job enrichment (greater responsibility and freedom), job enlargement (a greater diversity and complexity of tasks that reduced monotony) and job rotation all enhanced commitment (Franco et al. 2004). While working conditions are a critical influence on retention, economic incentives also matter. In circumstances where, as in Russia or Poland, doctors earned 80 per cent of the national salary and nurses in Russia earned salaries below the official poverty line (Danishevski 2005; Krajewski-Siuda et al. 2008), it is implausible that incomes, especially relative incomes (see Chapter 6), are not important.

Seemingly intractable hierarchical systems dominate many workplaces. As the policy director of the Royal College of Nursing, Australia has said:

> Nurses have been taught to be able to work in an autonomous way as a health professional, to be working with their colleagues on the same kind of level, to be making critical decisions. They get into a system that doesn't necessarily allow them to be able to do that. There are still the hierarchical structures and so they find they are not being valued for the critical decision-making that they've been prepared educationally to do. (Quoted in *The Australian*, 24 May 2008)

What has been described as 'seagull management', based on 'distance, distrust, destructive criticism, and defensive culture', results in contradictory expectations and pressures, and routinisation, deskilling and work intensification directed towards a 'production line' rather than the more holistic concepts of care preferred by nurses (Cooke 2006; Ho 2008). Authority conflicts with autonomy, and nurses resent the dominance of medicine, in a supposedly more egalitarian and classless era.

Widespread shortages of health workers have placed unusual demands on many existing health workers, extending working hours and shift times, exemplified in one Australian newspaper headline: 'Nurses dead on their feet from too much overtime' (*The Australian*, 20 January 2009). In some American hospitals the more expensive but more experienced senior nurses have been those laid off during financial crises (Gordon 2005: 4). In such circumstances the remaining workers are exhausted, and unable to deliver the quality of care that they would like. Job satisfaction is reduced and attrition may follow. In the USA, as elsewhere, nurses who left tended to be younger, and were more likely to be able to obtain alternative employment, and chose work that had better hours, better pay, was more rewarding and had a more evident career structure (Sochalski 2002). High turnover and attrition pose direct costs in new recruiting and training, and indirect costs in lost productivity (Zurn et al. 2005: 12), resulting in the greater need for migrant workers.

Violence and Racism

Two factors that have resulted in growing rates of attrition – violence and racism – are more significant in rich-world countries. Patient violence towards health workers, especially nurses, has grown in recent decades to become an emerging factor in attrition. In Sweden, health care is the employment sector with the highest rates of violence (OECD 2008: 55), and the prevalence of verbal and physical violence affects as many as 90 per cent of health workers in such diverse contexts as Hong Kong, Turkey and Australia (Kwok et al. 2006; Celik et al. 2007; Hegney et al. 2003). Violence and disruptive behaviour also come from relatives and even, as 'horizontal violence', from other staff (Cembrowicz et al. 2002). A direct relationship has been traced between violence and the limited power and autonomy of nurses at work, and increases in stress, sick leave, burnout and ultimately staff turnover and attrition (Zurn et al. 2005). As health workers work longer hours, and staff-to-patient ratios decline, the ability to provide services to patients suffers and prospects for violence increase.

Many nurses, in particular, are from minority groups within countries, such as African Americans in the USA. Discrimination exists within health systems and racism is expressed by both other workers and patients (Iganski and Mason 2002; Winkelmann-Gleed 2006), to both national and migrant nurses (Chapter 8). Discrimination also prevents upward social mobility, hence discouraging continuity of employment. In the UK at least, black and Asian nurses were more likely to resign than nurses of other ethnicities (Shields and Ward 2001). While racism and discrimination may be little better in other workplaces, they certainly influence attrition.

Domestic Recruitment

Developed countries have sought to meet expanding needs primarily through training programmes, but alongside migration. In many countries there are simply not enough training programmes to produce what is assumed to be adequate numbers of SHWs. Once again, financial issues arise. In countries like the USA and Australia some high-achieving high-school leavers are routinely unable to enter medical schools since too few places are available. In the USA more than 150,000 applicants for entry into nursing schools are also rejected every year, since there is a lack of places, in turn because few people want to be nursing professors, since the salaries of nurses are higher (Garrett 2007). With unwillingness to develop adequate local training facilities, the national shortages of nurses and doctors must be met by migration, even where supply and demand exist simultaneously (OECD 2008).

In some contexts it is not the availability of training programmes but the availability of recruits that poses problems. Only 25 per cent of nurse trainees in Scotland in 2008 were school leavers, and this pattern of late entry into the nursing profession is becoming more general (*Nursing Times*, 14 February 2008; Kingma 2006: 34). For various reasons, including the duration of training, school leavers are less likely to be interested in a health career. Consequently, attempts have been made to draw retirees and former health workers back into the sector. (In 2008 Australia was offering payments of $6000 – after 18 months back in the workforce – to those who chose to return.) Recruitment takes different forms, but in many developed countries is still inadequate to meet needs.

DEMAND IN DEVELOPING COUNTRIES

Longer life expectancies, ageing and growing populations, and the rise of NCDs have placed increased stress on all health care systems, whether in developed or developing countries. In developing countries the same broad changes have therefore occurred. Recruitment can be more difficult (despite the possibility of migration), alternatives greater, and attrition more significant. In the Cook Islands in the 1950s and 1960s, for instance, the health sector was extremely attractive, but by the 1980s the national economic focus had shifted from agriculture towards tourism and business, and health employment and even scholarships were perceived as less prestigious (Connell 2009). In the Seychelles and the Caribbean the same preferences for tourism and business are emerging. In Malawi over 1200 qualified nurses have simply dropped out, switching to better-paid or less stressful employment (Palmer 2006).

More rapidly growing populations and the rise of HIV/AIDS, in particular, have shifted perceptions of the disease burden to one that is more obviously concentrated in developing countries, especially in SSA (Chapter 2). Scaling up the treatment of HIV/AIDS with anti-retrovirals requires an increase of up to 50 per cent of existing workforces, but it has taken its toll of health workers (both directly, in their increased death rates, and indirectly, because of unwillingness to work with HIV/AIDS patients, and thus attrition and migration). Such trends have made global strategies to reduce HIV/AIDS more difficult to achieve. Simultaneously, ageing and the greater incidence of other NCDs have placed new pressures on workforces, while education and access to television have further increased demands for advanced health care as expectations steadily increase among more demanding, socially emancipated populations (Talati and Pappas 2006).

As demand for health care has increased, the discrepancies between needs and responses have become apparent, especially where erstwhile carers have moved away, as they have done in Nigeria (Harper et al. 2008). Ageing in developing countries has tended to be accompanied by the migration of SHWs, at some cost to the well-being of the aged, who experience reduced physical, psychological and emotional support (Chapter 7). The proportions of the elderly are probably growing faster in developing countries, especially where there has been significant economic growth, as in Latin America and South-East and East Asia, whereas in developed countries proportionately ageing populations are more closely associated with declining fertility. In middle-income Thailand, for example, the median age was 19 in 1970 but by 2000 it was 29. In 1990 about 5 per cent of the population were over 60, but by 2008 this had doubled to 10 per cent and was expected to reach 22 per cent by 2025 (*Bangkok Post*, 9 May 2009). Especially in Asia, declining fertility, particularly the 'one-child family' in China, has brought new congruence with OECD countries.

Alongside rather greater participation in the formal sector workforce, and the gradual rise of nuclear rather than extended families, fewer family members are becoming available to look after elderly relatives. This demographic trend has been associated with and paralleled by urbanisation (which has also posed new problems of elder care in rural areas) and individualisation. Numbers of residential homes for the aged are now increasing in developing countries. Hitherto most old people have been cared for at home but, where migration has been considerable, old people have become an increasing burden as the dependency rate increases. One of the first states in the Pacific to have an old people's home was American Samoa, and one of the first to have a hospital wing dedicated to the immobile old was in Niue. Both states are characterised by very high levels of migration and high dependency rates. The availability of SHWs, and also the presence of family, are crucial to the effectiveness of health systems. While demand for health workers may be greatest in developing countries, where disease burdens and inequalities are most severe, the need for increasing numbers of health workers is a global phenomenon.

THINKING MIGRATION?

Just as health workers are less likely to choose to work in rural and regional areas, so they are also less likely to work in particular health fields. In most developed countries need is greatest in aged care, mental health and the broader residential and home care sector – where wages are lowest, workforces least unionised, part time, and fragmented into small, sometimes exploitative, companies. The limited attractiveness of employment in regional areas and domestic care extends upwards to the formal nursing sector partly because of its similar problems (low wages, 'graveyard' shifts, difficult conditions etc.). The outcome for patients is reduced duration and effectiveness of care (Hayes et al. 2006: 245). Simultaneously, some of the most socially important roles in human society – nurturing and care-giving – involving both physical and emotional elements, are gradually being transferred outside the household to the market, community and state, slowly becoming the tasks of migrant workers caring for people's 'most intimate needs: their bodies, their homes and their families' as 'servants of globalisation' (Brush and Vasupuram 2006: 181–2). For many migrants, undertaking these vital tasks means a struggle with low wages, minimum job security, no health benefits of their own, limited, even downwards, occupational mobility and discrimination at work and beyond it (Chapter 8). As migrants dominate such sectors, the attractiveness of those sectors for some local workers may decline further.

Estimates of future demand for health workers are invariably speculative given the multiple variables involved, which relate to the quality of health care and disease burdens, the skill mix required, financial provision, attrition and so on. In mid-2008, Australia, a country of 21 million people with a nursing workforce of about 300,000, was said to have a shortfall of 1300 doctors and 13,000 nurses and to be in line for a nursing shortfall of around 40,000 by 2010, with hospitals in some states having existing vacancies ranging from 60 to 110 (*The Australian*, 24 May 2008, 24 February 2009). Proportionately similar estimates have been made for the USA and the UK (Chapter 2). Even allowing for hyperbole, scaremongering and worst-case scenarios, without any significant increase in national production such figures are indicative of a continued demand for overseas workers. In many contexts, including Canada and Australia, inadequate or conservative human resource planning, fragmented authority and responsibility, between government bodies and between states (where provinces and states are responsible for health care delivery but receive national funding), and limited public funding, have stifled expansion. Despite rising demand for health workers, and the attractions of other forms of employment, the greatest need in most developed countries, which some have been reluctant to face, is that of providing an adequate number of training courses and places for intending health workers. Immigration is the almost inevitable consequence.

Those factors that have made the recruitment and especially the retention of health workers increasingly difficult occur in both developed and developing countries, at the same time as demand has increased. That conjuncture has placed particular pressures on developing countries. Taking up employment in the health sector in most contexts is intrinsically no more attractive – and probably less attractive – than it has been in the past, with the rise of HIV/AIDS, violence, relatively poor wages and alternative sources of employment. The decline, or at least relative withdrawal, of funds from the public sector has also usually made it less attractive (as in other public sector contexts, such as education and transport), so that real wages in the health sector have largely failed to increase in recent decades; relative to many other employment arenas, they have declined. A care deficit has emerged in more developed countries, with work that was once a family and domestic responsibility becoming a commercial activity. A vicious circle has been established: as work in the health sector becomes less attractive, recruitment declines and attrition rises, patient outcomes worsen and morale falls further. Yet, underlying all of this, much like other SHWs, nurses retain a pride in being nurses, and would usually prefer to continue nursing but in somewhat improved circumstances (e.g. Siebens et al. 2006). In such circumstances the rationale for becoming a health worker is highly important, and is examined in the next chapter.

5. An overseas orientation: towards migration?

Migration is primarily a response to global and regional uneven development, but usually explained in terms of such factors as low wages, few incentives, or poor social and working conditions. Quite different scales reflect different ways of thinking about migration – whether in terms of global economic fluctuations and world financial crises, the activities of international recruitment companies, the poverty of developing countries or the particular motives of families (and individual members of these families) – yet all of these interact. Although the migration of skilled health workers occurs for multiple reasons, there is a remarkable uniformity in the factors that influence specific migration moves, even in quite different regions and contexts (Chapter 6). In some part this is because of the emergence of a global care chain and demand-driven migration. Yet even before migration there is often a basic predisposition to mobility, a product of culture, geography and history as much as economics. This chapter therefore examines attitudes towards employment in the health sector: why people become health workers.

Broad influences on employment and migration include incomes, job satisfaction, career opportunities, and social and family reasons. Family reasons, though often neglected, are particularly important since most people only exceptionally make decisions about employment and migration as individuals; rather, they are linked into extended families and wider kinship groups and make decisions in this context. Skilled migrants, however, are more likely than others to be without extended-family ties, because they are more easily able to organise migration opportunities and because they are more likely to come from relatively well-off households for whom remittances are less crucial. But this is less frequently the case in developing countries, and decisions can therefore be complex, even evolving over time towards particular, sometimes catalytic moments. The possibility of migration follows decisions taken earlier in life (about education, training and choice of employment), made by families, especially where a context of migration has been longstanding, and where this is embedded within a culture of migration.

A CULTURE OF MIGRATION

The migration of SHWs, and other skilled workers, is by no means unique, but exists within the context of wider migration flows. This is evidently so in most small island states (including those of the Atlantic, Caribbean and Pacific), Mexico, parts of SSA, and also more developed countries like New Zealand and Ireland, where there have been steady outmigration streams for several decades, with the migration of skilled workers one part of that (Connell 2007b, 2008b; Salmon et al. 2007; Ryan 2008; Conradson and Latham 2005). There is effectively a culture of migration, in which most individuals contemplate migration at some time in their lives. In places where a high proportion of people – citizens and their dependants – are overseas, the balance of life has tilted towards metropolitan states, with migrants becoming key influences on subsequent migration patterns as, in a transnational world, contact between migrants and those at home is easier than ever before. Cultures and economies of migration are shaped by the stories, advice, experiences and incomes of those who have gone before. Migration is neither rupture nor discontinuity in personal and household experiences, but a natural, integral and inescapable part of life, and normative, positive, acceptable and even almost inevitable (Kandel and Massey 2002; Cohen 2004; Connell 2008b) where people consider living and working overseas, at least temporarily, although they also expect never to 'abandon' home or kin, and retain aspirations to return long after it is plausible.

Cultures of migration have emerged where local development opportunities are few, and migration generates a new source of income. Migration thus becomes viewed at different scales as a 'safety-valve', reducing pressures on national governments (and even perhaps households) to provide employment opportunities and welfare services, and on households to be self-reliant. The ensuing paradox is well illustrated in the observations of Kuini Lutua, the General Secretary of the Fiji Nursing Association:

> Global economic changes and the law of supply and demand for skilled health professions is [sic] affecting the retention of skilled health workers in countries that can ill afford losing such category of health personnel. For Fiji and other small Pacific island countries in the region, sending off a relative for a job overseas is considered a great privilege because of the returns that relatives back home would get from such moves. (2002: 1)

This 'safety-valve' effect, and even 'privilege', has resulted in steady and domestically unimpeded outmigration and, as in the Philippines and other contexts, led to the development of labour export policies, which include skilled workers (Chapter 9). In the Caribbean, for example, 'Guyana,

St Vincent and Grenada can be used as base economies for producing nurses for the region [and beyond] as these economies already have a culture of migration' (Hosein and Thomas 2007: 328). At household and national level, migration may be encouraged rather than discouraged, and acceptable rather than problematic.

GETTING A JOB

Multiple reasons account for becoming a health worker. Numerous SHWs have long forgotten the specific reason(s) why they became health workers or simply took up (usually) nursing 'because it was there'. Such statements belie the complexities (Connell 2009). The possibility of migration certainly underlies some decisions to become a health worker, but other factors range from stable, secure employment, with regular wages, to the prestige, even perceived glamour (that smart uniforms once brought) of health work, access to technology, altruism (which may be quite local or even household oriented), the existence of scholarships and training opportunities or because little else was available, especially for women. Nursing brought regular incomes where women might otherwise have contributed relatively little economically, at least in a monetary sense. In many places, nursing (alongside teaching), was one of few opportunities open to women where other job choices might have been ruled out by parents or husbands (e.g. Barclay et al. 1988). Nor were there constraints, since it was even difficult in some colonial and post-colonial contexts to recruit adequate numbers of appropriately educated school leavers.

Nevertheless, there was often some ambivalence about nursing in particular, especially before it became more evidently a route to migration. In India, 'good' families discouraged daughters from working at such unclean activities. At least until the 1980s nursing in Tonga was considered somewhat menial and 'dirty', and not 'ladylike' compared with teaching (James 2003: 316). Much the same was true elsewhere. In Ghana migration was long deemed inappropriate to women and nursing graduates, who had often deferred marriage by entering nursing schools, but were encouraged to marry immediately afterwards to secure their stability (Nowak 2009). In most parts of the Islamic world, including Bangladesh and Malaysia, the status of nursing remains low, because it is perceived as dirty work and women's work (Birks et al. 2009; Hadley et al. 2007). In a patriarchal world, caring may be relatively invisible, devalued and poorly rewarded, and such perspectives, along with concerns over intimate body contact, linger on globally (Mimura et al. 2009).

As nursing (and other professions) have become marketable overseas, nurses became valuable and more respectable. In Fiji, nursing only became a respectable profession for Indo-Fijian women – rather than an unclean and low-status occupation – when it offered qualifications that could be marketed abroad (Leckie 2000: 78), a situation exactly analogous to that in India, where nursing moved from being something of a reviled and impure profession for poor people to a preferred one, and the opportunity for migration became 'an actual strategy' (Percot and Rajan 2007: 320; Percot 2005; see George 2005; Nair 2007; Thomas 2008; Chapter 3). The migratory success of Christian Kerala nurses resulted in Hindus and Muslims taking up nursing as its stigma declined (Percot 2006). Similar perspectives emerged elsewhere in South Asia. It became widely evident, not only that becoming a health worker provided upward social mobility – and incomes – for many women who might otherwise have been unemployed, but that nursing offered job opportunities overseas. So prevalent was this new attitude to nursing that by the 1990s in Tonga 'it became a much discussed stereotype' (Connell 2009). In Ghana (Nowak 2009), Malawi and elsewhere, the transition in rationale was more recent:

> Nurses who graduated before 2000 gave reasons such as their admiration for nurses, pride in having a nurse in the family, and wanting to care for Malawians. However, more recent graduates appear to be less concerned with 'doing good' and more concerned with obtaining qualifications. Competition for higher education is extremely high, and they perceived nursing to be a marketable career that could lead to opportunities for employment with higher paying NGOs or even abroad. (Grigulis et al. 2009: 1196)

The rationale for being an SHW was becoming more narrowly and externally focused. In Tonga at least, where there is no problem recruiting nurses, people do not necessarily enter for the profession itself but often because, as one nurse phrased it, 'it is a job opportunity, where they can go [overseas] on scholarship, and not come back [hence] their hearts are not in it'. As many as one-third of all health workers in the small Pacific island states of Tonga, Samoa and Fiji had the aim of eventual migration in mind when they entered the profession (Connell 2009). Employment in health professions enables migration while also being an instigator of it.

It would be wrong, however, to assume that migration lay behind the majority of decisions to become a health worker. Even in small island states like Tonga, Samoa and Fiji, where migration is common, two-thirds of the workforce became health workers for a rich diversity of reasons. A majority of health workers, especially nurses, most of whom were women, expressed broadly altruistic reasons for becoming health workers. Some of these were generic ('I admired the work done by nurses'; 'I like helping people'), to serve the community ('to help the people in my village who were isolated from a hospital') or one's family ('I decided to take up nursing to help my family'; 'As an eldest child I was responsible for the health of my family'). Family influences, previous family employment histories, a 'tradition of service', and even a sense of religious vocation were all influential. Such broad and generally idealistic perspectives, to 'help people' and 'make a difference', alongside family pressure and tradition, dominate stated decisions to become a nurse in most global contexts (Price 2008: 15–16; Mimura et al. 2009: 2). Some families encouraged health work, even perhaps selfishly, although others discouraged what they perceived as 'dirty work' (Connell 2009: 77–81). If health workers remained at home, they might help their families directly, through income and health care, while overseas they might help indirectly through remittances; hence employment and migration decisions are shaped in a family context.

Duty, reciprocity and vocation thus play key roles in employment and migration, and movement is bound up with social and cultural obligations, going beyond extended families to communities. Individual migrants may be encouraged by extended families with such goals in mind, as in Samoa where individuals are chosen to provide service (*tautua*) to family and the wider community rather than themselves, and migration is part of that role (Macpherson 1994). Migration is rarely an individual decision to meet individual goals, even for the most skilled, but is directed at improving the living standards and incomes of the migrants and their families, at home or abroad. Thus women in the Philippines were often encouraged to become nurses (rather than, for example, engineers) since they could more easily work overseas (Alonso-Garbayo and Maben 2009). As two Filipina nurses in Ireland pointed out: 'I didn't want to become a nurse, for God's sake. That's not the kind of career that I wanted, taking care of patients. But at the end . . . that's the job that sustains you'; and 'If you have one nurse at home, one nurse in the family, then you are better off because that nurse can go out of the country, can earn more, let's say double, triple the amount that we are earning at home and you can send it home and you can help the whole family' (quoted in Humphries et al. 2009a: 9). Even in middle-income countries like Ireland, nursing was perceived as a means of migration 'informed by a sense of ambition, a desire for a better future and an opportunity to earn more money' within a long history of migration to the UK (Ryan 2008: 461). For Samoan households,

> Having young wage earners abroad diversified families' earning streams and reduced their dependence on high-risk activities. Having family members in *several* locations abroad diversified earning sources and reduced risk levels still further. Families, using intelligence from migrants abroad, periodically surveyed risks and returns in various enclaves and encouraged others abroad to relocate in places in which returns were found to be higher and risks lower . . .

[as] risks and returns available in various places were formally canvassed and modeled by families. (Macpherson 2004: 168)

While this may be unusual in its precision, migration does not take place in a knowledge vacuum, although access to knowledge may be limited and tends to flow along post-colonial lines. Even within particular societies, family dynamics vary and potential migration may be both encouraged and discouraged.

Migration decisions are taken within what has been described in Tonga as a 'transnational corporation of kin' (Marcus 1981), where extended families effectively allocate family members, or human resources, to seemingly appropriate destinations for the good of the wider group, to maximise income opportunities, minimise risk, and benefit from the resultant remittance flows. In the Pacific, Kerala, the Philippines and elsewhere, many families are spread over several continents. Such households, usually seen as extended by kinship and over space, were also sometimes deliberately extended into other occupations, as households sought to place family members in other vital arenas of employment, such as banking, education, the police and the army (Connell 2009: 84). Others are anxious to replicate such strategies; as a Nigerian mother of six children in an inner city slum has said

I pray not to die here. I hope to build my own house some day. The important thing is education. I want my children to have an education. I'm hoping one will become a doctor, one will become a pharmacist, one will become a nurse. I'm hoping that my children will move abroad, and when life is good for them, they will say 'Mum, come join us'. (quoted in Meek 2009: 27)

Korean households may likewise 'choose an older son to run the family business, while a middle son is chosen to attend college and (often) medical school abroad, eventually with the idea that he would return with a socially prestigious and high-earning medical degree' (Reynolds 2002: 279). Professional and spatial deployment were carefully combined. Ironically, professions where altruism was at the fore were also those that enabled the greatest prospects of migration, with altruism primarily directed towards extended households.

Health employment continues to offer a degree of certainty that is not always available elsewhere. Even in developed countries, such as Australia, it is sometimes advertised as providing lifetime security, deliberately contrasted with private sector employment. Security comes with a guaranteed income that usually compares reasonably well with much alternative employment, and income has always been a major reason for many taking up health employment. But, significantly, for Fiji, Tonga and

Samoa, where the propensity for international migration was considerable, half of those nurses who had migrated overseas joined the profession for income reasons compared with only 27 per cent of those still working in their home country (Brown and Connell 2004). Attracting workers into health professions is now less easy, where salaries and conditions are less attractive and other options are available. Perceptions of challenging shift work and public sector frustrations are familiar: health workers expect reasonable salaries and reasonable standards. Almost a decade after a series of interviews with Samoan nurses revealed that a religious vocation and impressive uniforms were key motivations for becoming a nurse, a group of senior Samoan nurses ridiculed this notion and stressed that incomes and migration opportunities were now the crucial factors. None the less, at least in the Pacific, most also stressed that entry into nursing especially, but health work more generally, was to help others, a perception that they still valued and indeed helped to define who they were. Decision-making remained shaped within extended-family contexts.

AN OVERSEAS ORIENTATION?

It has become increasingly evident that intentions to migrate may occur even before entry into the health system. For more than 20 years, some people in the Philippines sought to become nurses at least in part, and often primarily, because that provided an obvious means of international migration. By the end of the 1980s the Philippines probably led the way in terms of individuals acquiring health skills with a view to migration (e.g. Ball 1996; Choy 2003). Similarly, by the end of the 1980s, a medical degree at the Fiji School of Medicine was being widely seen as a 'passport to prosperity' and in Kerala 'a nursing diploma is now considered as an actual passport for emigration where "nursing for emigration" is common' (Percot 2006: 172). As one Indian health professional has recently stated, it has been a long time since 'nurses would join the profession for the love of it rather than [to] go abroad, or finance their families' (quoted in Hancock 2008: 259). In 2008, a second-year nursing student in Ghana estimated that half her nursing school class (of 300 students) had 'entered the nursing program as a means of securing an eventual meal ticket abroad' (Millen 2008: 9). Vocation has given way to migration.

As migration and its benefits became more evident, not only did more people seek to become nurses, but they were more likely to express the rationale for becoming a nurse in terms of migration. Thus Kerala women became nurses mainly 'to ease the burden on their families' but also to travel, having seen other nurses return with new fashions, gifts and money

(George 2005: 43–4; Alonso-Garbayo and Maben 2009), and implicitly gain greater status, independence and autonomy in local society. More generally, in India demand for nursing jobs substantially increased because 'communities, which once shunned nursing as a low-grade occupation for subordinate social groups, have now realized that out-migration of women as nurses can open up paths to economic development and even the migration of entire families to more prosperous countries' (Thomas 2008: 103). In Bangladesh, where nursing was traditionally regarded as a low-paid, low-prestige occupation that attracted relatively few entrants, the growing recognition that nursing could lead to emigration, and that graduate salaries in Europe and North America were roughly 15 times local salaries, proved an enormous stimulus to recruitment, as long as emigration opportunities existed (Aminuzaman 2006). Broadly similar situations are evident in several parts of the Pacific, Jamaica, India, Hong Kong, China and elsewhere. Perhaps the supreme irony is that established Asian households in Britain subsequently discouraged daughters from taking up nursing employment for exactly the reasons that previously existed in India (Whitehead et al. 2007). Otherwise, nursing has become a 'portable profession' (Kingma 2006) and becoming a health worker has become a means to migration at least as much as an end in itself.

A more recent phase of this strategic decision-making has involved doctors retraining as nurses for migration in the Philippines, Pakistan and perhaps elsewhere. Specific careers may be chosen that optimise migration opportunities; in the Philippines several hundred male doctors in the public sector have retrained as nurses, and fewer now choose a medical career, since nurses have much superior migration opportunities (Choo 2003; Brush and Sochalski 2007). In Ghana, the number of applications for nursing is increasing, especially from men, and 'better qualified applicants are also going into nursing, seeing it explicitly as an investment in leaving the country' (Mensah 2005: 206). Migration opportunities have overturned the professional and social status of jobs in the health sector, while simultaneously challenging gender stereotypes. In Albania, where nursing was a 'traditional profession' for women, the recent expansion of nursing education was primarily related to migration opportunities, with half the nurses now being men, who had gone to nursing school only so that they could migrate (Chaloff 2008: 17). From the 1970s onwards, in many destinations, from Europe to the Gulf, the migration of nurses was quite distinctive in that it reversed what had been standard migration structures: women no longer migrated as family members and dependants, the 'trailing spouses', but brought their husbands and families after their own migration. Tongans in New Zealand, Filipinos in the Netherlands and Kerala nurses in Austria, the USA and the Gulf, reversed the old social order.

A MEDICAL CULTURE OF MIGRATION

Employment and training as a health worker occur for many reasons, but training may go beyond the requirements of particular positions and their local applicability. Indeed, many people seek to acquire the highest level of skills possible, where incomes are greatest and superior status assured. As in the Pacific, therefore, many health workers

> seek opportunities to have their qualifications recognized by professional bodies and colleagues in developed countries, even though many of them are well trained for the roles they occupy in the home countries. Furthermore training and licensing requirements in destination countries greatly exceed what is needed in their countries of origin. (Pak and Tukuitonga 2006: 34)

Training thus becomes a classic example of the 'diploma disease' (Dore 1976), where credentials are acquired that go beyond local needs, but are evidence of merit and transferability. Education is not simply to get a job, a better job, or even a job in the home country; specialised learning may enable promotion to good positions, but not where such qualifications are necessarily useful. Increased training opens up overseas options, while limited local resources and demand frustrate attempts to use new skills. Such additional training, part of a qualifications spiral, emphasises professionalism, and is widely sought after. An 'important element which has permeated nurse training options in Tonga has been whether the training will be acceptable in New Zealand and Australia rather than [meet] the real needs in Tonga and the Pacific' (World Bank 1994: 227). The more that skills are developed, the more they cannot easily or willingly be applied locally, especially in smaller states or remote locations, where workers need to be more generalist.

Like other professionals in developing countries, SHWs often feel and are isolated from trends in their profession and in the wider world, and are conscious that they may miss out on skills that will enable their professional development (and perhaps future migration). The desire to acquire further training, new skills and extra experience is one of the most significant factors influencing migration in numerous places, as in most Pacific island states (Connell 2009), Pakistan (Syed et al. 2008) and Slovakia (Williams and Balaz 2008). Modern technology and its exponents are powerful attractions, especially for doctors, dentists and allied health workers. Thus Pakistani medical graduates move to developed countries because of 'the long-standing belief of young doctors and their parents that training outside their home country is superior and a mark of achievement [plus] the lure of high-tech training and super-specialization' that will enable higher incomes in a more meritocratic system. Moreover, the 'world's rapid progress excites us, and we want to be involved in the latest medical advances' and avoid 'mundane routine devoid of intellectual stimulus' (Aly and Taj 2008: 6). Often alongside an existing 'culture of migration', a more evidently 'medical culture' of migration exists, which focuses on access to the most contemporary knowledge and technology. The combination of an established socioeconomic context for migration and a newer professional and technological interest has created a dual culture of migration.

External orientation is widely evident. In India, some 80 per cent of trainee nurses in one nursing school applied to overseas recruiters for jobs even before graduation (*The Times of India*, 19 January 2005), while three-quarters of final-year medical students in two Pakistani medical schools intended to go abroad for postgraduate training (Syed et al. 2008). The aspirations of Poles, Lebanese and Ghanaian trainees, among others, are no less externally oriented (Krajewski et al. 2008; Akl et al. 2007; Dovlo and Nyonator 1999; El-Jardali et al. 2009), as are pharmacy students globally (Wuliji et al. 2009). In India, several nursing schools, referred to by one nursing educator as 'shops', target education to the nursing examinations of the USA and the UK, and 'recruitment firms work closely with the academicians to see that post-graduation placements abroad go smoothly' (Mullan 2004: 39). In the early 1990s, the University of the West Indies opened a nursing school in Jamaica because the demand to enter nursing had become substantial, entirely because of a desire to migrate overseas on graduation. In the Philippines, literally hundreds of private nursing schools have opened purely to cater for the demand for overseas employment. Such trends are gradually becoming more widespread. In India, one dean of a medical college has expressed his concern over 'the growing danger of a large number of new doctors who have no commitment to this country or to ethical standards of practice. At least if they go abroad we are rid of them' (quoted in Mullan 2004: 29).

Even between developed countries, valuable knowledge may be gained from experiencing other forms of technology or management. Australian and New Zealand migrants in the USA were drawn by superior technological development, specialist training, research prospects, but also salaries three times those at home (Miller et al. 1998). The more that training occurs overseas, the greater the propensity to become familiar with new places and people, and to remain there afterwards. Countries thus tend to lose the 'best and the brightest': the most able who have received scholarships and grants, undergone more overseas training, and gained valuable skills of sometimes limited local utility (Chapter 7) alongside acquiring new social ties, at times when families are often formed. In order to remain overseas, and perhaps convert a student or short-term visa into permanent residence or even citizenship, a superior education can be essential.

In most developing countries it is axiomatic that superior conditions are elsewhere, both in a broad socioeconomic sense and more specifically in hospital facilities. For some health workers such facilities dominated their own overseas training; others learned of the latest overseas technology from those who had trained or simply travelled abroad, while even mainly US television series offer glimpses of a technology and lifestyle quite out of reach at home (Akl et al. 2007; Chory-Assad and Tamborini 2001). The almost universal desire to experience the best working conditions (including colleagues, medicines, buildings and technology) is implicit, and often explicit, in health care. Aiming for high-quality health care requires access to the best diagnostic and recuperative technology, and that is usually elsewhere.

Access to the most modern knowledge, equipment and experience in the most sophisticated systems is regarded as not just valuable but essential in order to become the best possible health worker. In Nigeria, even senior nurses perceived that a key gain from migration would be the opportunity to work in advanced clinical settings, so gaining superior scientific knowledge. Migration enabled '[us to] acquire more knowledge . . . because they have the instruments . . . things we don't have here . . . knowledge is more over there', and acquisition of that knowledge and experience would bring such nurses 'up to standard with all other colleagues in the nursing profession' that would implicitly give them global competence (quoted in Aboderin 2007: 2242; see also Larsen et al. 2005; Owusu-Daaku et al. 2008). Teaching staff at many national institutions, moreover, not only do not discourage migration but judge their own success as teachers and the success of their students on whether they are able to practise in the more competitive medical environments of countries like the USA and the UK (Hagopian et al. 2005: 1755; Connell 2009: 73–4). The best students and the best teachers simply assumed that some necessary part of their future lay overseas. Such overseas orientation, scholarships and training opportunities may all partly stem from a curative model that perceives doctors and nurses 'as disease fighters (saving individuals) rather than as health promoters (saving communities)' (Finau et al. 2004: 123), and may remain a partial legacy of colonial orientations (Portes 1978) and expatriate instructors. The workplace and tertiary education culture dictated that excellence and the more exciting and complicated aspects of modernity were elsewhere.

Postgraduate training locally, let alone overseas, is seen by many as a stepping-stone to employment overseas. What might otherwise be seen as an almost obsessive demand for superior skills is oriented to the possibility of future migration. Yet even before tertiary training, secondary education is widely seen to provide the human capital that can maximise employment options at home and abroad, with, where possible, children often selectively sent to prestigious urban schools (e.g. Reynolds 2002). Not only is there an outward orientation before training, where people select educational strategies in order to migrate, but in some cases this may also be combined with a desire to move out of the health sector once migration has been achieved. Developing and retaining a valuable national workforce become particularly difficult.

THE TWO CULTURES

Through education, and the social context of education, a more evidently medical culture of migration (but extended into nursing and allied activities) overlays, and has become intertwined with, an existing, more pervasive culture of migration. Both cultures are nurtured by the presence of overseas kin, social expectations of migration, training possibilities and, in some contexts, effectively shared citizenship. Whether migration occurs or not, the acquisition of experience and sophisticated skills at home or overseas keeps dreams and options alive, and boosts incomes.

Multiple reasons explain becoming a health worker even in the midst of alternative options. While conventional and significant reasons include good and reliable incomes, family histories, a sense of altruism, or even the lack of alternative opportunities, more than ever employment in health has become an invaluable means of diversifying, both structurally and spatially, extended family livelihoods across countries and beyond continents. The propensity to take up employment in health begins early, and subsequently epitomises the dual culture of migration. Skilled migrants more effectively open up migration opportunities for others, through their ability to migrate and because of the increasing selectivity of migration and recruitment according to skills (Chapter 6). Becoming a health worker is easier when it follows family tradition. Thus professional Igbo (Nigerian) migrants in the USA 'came from families with professional migratory backgrounds instead of land-bound farming families' (Reynolds 2002: 274). In Peru, although income was a critical factor influencing the propensity to migrate overseas, having relatives in the medical profession was a strong influence on migration, emphasising the significance of existing overseas links and knowledge of opportunities (Mayta-Tristan 2008). As extended families and 'transnational corporations of kin' have extended their beachheads and developed their social and geographical networks, through which information on overseas opportunities can be transmitted instantly, so cultures of migration are better established.

Familiarity with potential destinations, personally or through family members (perhaps accentuated by television, internet and video), language competence, technical ability, and family ties in destinations have all enhanced the socioeconomic culture of migration. Cultures of migration emerged where economic development was relatively slight, and as perceptions of overseas economic success have grown, other parts of the world have acquired similar perspectives. As in so many other places, 'to migrate from Malawi is seen as respectable and admirable' (Grigulis et al. 2009: 1196). The predispositions and preconditions for eventual and successful migration have gradually been enhanced.

Those most easily able to take advantage of distant opportunities have been those with skills, and increasingly so as developed countries impose barriers to family reunion, while encouraging those with skills. Acquiring education and training in the health sector is tantamount to acquiring cultural migratory capital. In many places it may be the most effective means of acquiring a 'passport'; becoming a health worker predisposes individuals to migration opportunities that would be impossible for other occupations. In a sense, therefore, the 'brain-drain is structurally interlaced into cultural norms and higher education' (Reynolds 2002: 280). Overseas training inhibits return migration, despite the formal goal usually being the reverse, and is further constrained by the combination of greater specialisation, credentialism, diploma disease (and the urbanisation of training facilities) as the medical culture of migration gains sway. The two cultures of migration have become entwined around a socioeconomic orientation to migration, accentuated by training and the lure of technology and the modern world, now transformed by the transnationalism of culture and economy. Why migration occurs, and how aspirations are translated into practice, can now be examined in greater detail.

6. Moving out? Rationales for migration

Underlying most migration moves are substantial differences in development status. In 1978, Mejia observed that 'the main factor influencing migration, within and outside the health systems of both the donor and the recipient countries, is the international problem of unequal economic and social development' (1978: 269). That has never changed. While migration takes place in the context of global and regional uneven development, it is usually explained at a local level, and by the migrants themselves, in terms of such proximate factors as low wages or poor working conditions. Perhaps the earliest study of migrant health workers, conducted in 1972 with 147 Filipino nurses in the USA, found that 101 regarded their salaries in the Philippines as inadequate, over 100 complained about the lack of compensation for shift work, holidays and overtime, poor working conditions and nepotism in employment and promotion (Pablico 1972). Inadequate education, lack of leadership and rapid turnover of nurses accentuated these problems (Choy 2003: 113). Remarkably little has changed since then, whether in the Philippines or elsewhere, in terms of uneven development and the rationale for migration, although migrants have reached new destinations, as labour market and other conditions changed and new social networks were created. Promotion limitations, inadequate management support, heavy workloads, limited access to technology, medicines and other supplies have all been regularly and generally cited as 'push factors' and repeatedly documented for 30 years (Mejia et al. 1979; Ojo 1990; Buchan et al. 2004; Bach 2003, 2008; Kingma 2006). Centred on economic circumstances, but strongly influenced by a constellation of social, political and cultural factors, the reasons for migration vary only subtly between social and professional groups and countries. Likewise, the migration of health workers includes contract migration (typified by that from the Philippines to the Middle East), where workers go on fixed contracts, usually negotiated between governments, migration on an individual basis and more broadly based, taking families with health workers towards what becomes permanent settlement. All these flows have common characteristics that are explored in this chapter.

Financial support for health is absolutely crucial in enabling adequate wages and working conditions, since in the broadest sense economic and social development influence the retention of health workers (Stilwell et al. 2004; Pond and McPake 2006). Public sectors especially have struggled in recent decades and nowhere more so than in developing countries. In Africa, the rather richer countries, such as the Seychelles, Mauritius and Tunisia, have a greater ratio of health workers to people, linked to stronger financial support, less poverty and more broadly based development (Arah 2007; Arah et al. 2008). Although migration has occurred, enough resources enable replacements. Elsewhere, economic restructuring has led to reductions in the size of the public sector workforce, restrictions on the hiring of new workers, and a 'pseudo-shortage' of workers alongside the deterioration of working conditions (Chapter 2).

Migration is not the only outcome of problems, and perceived problems, in the health sector. Attrition is common, while 'wastage' – the declining utility or productivity of SHWs (perhaps through ill-health or inadequate access to resources) – occurs in many contexts. Attrition, or early retirement, occurs for multiple reasons, most of which are exactly the same as those that influence migration. Most dramatically, premature death or injury, and marked increases in the death rates of SHWs, have occurred since the 1990s, mainly attributable to the rise in HIV/AIDS. In 1999, death was the main cause of losses from Malawi's health workforce (Aitken and Kemp 2003), while infected workers lose dozens of working days, irrespective of time spent at the funerals of others (Dovlo 2005). Inappropriate skill mixes, absenteeism and even 'ghost workers', invariably absent yet present on payrolls as the beneficiaries of corruption, are further issues in some places. Attrition only rarely results in SHWs transferring into other skilled employment. Some become 'shadow workers', unwilling to work at the prevailing wage rate and in the existing conditions, while others migrate.

STAYING AT HOME

Despite the growing significance of migration, people usually prefer to stay in their home countries, and migration is seen, even by many migrants, as a last resort and not the best solution to their needs. As Ojo long ago noted for SSA doctors, 'the opportunities available at home do not have to equal those available in Saudi Arabia and the Western countries in order to keep people from emigrating. Most physicians, as people everywhere, prefer to remain at home' (1990: 633; Gaidzanwa 1999). The rationale for stability has been well expressed by a Polish nurse:

Even though I see the many problems here (I also earn low wages), I try to look for other solutions instead of thinking about migrating. What influences this decision strongly is the family situation, family stability, the need to stay where I am living, the need to stay beside my family, my parents, my closest family. Really, if I have decent wages, and I have the possibility to support myself, if I have a house or an apartment, there's no need for me to migrate. I'm connected with this country, I'm closely connected with my family. However, if the situation is too difficult, I might have to leave. (Quoted in van Eyck 2004: 17)

Many obvious reasons mean that people want to stay, and they move reluctantly. Home is a familiar place of kin, friends, land and ancestors, of old family and clan histories, of schools, churches, workplaces and burial grounds, where others speak the same language, have similar values, attitudes and lifestyles. Families offer an anchor and a livelihood, however limited and constrictive this may sometimes be. Home poses few surprises and uncertainties. Globally, less than 3 per cent of the world's population have migrated across international borders, indicating both the difficulty of international migration and a widespread preference for stability. Even those with skills cannot always easily cross political borders, or move with families.

A sense of professionalism, autonomy, pride in achievement and the desire to work with 'one's own people' all encouraged workers to remain in Pacific island states rather than migrate. Others had extended kin nearby, a house or partners with good jobs, although the vast majority of those who stayed were there because it was 'home': a largely unquestioned source of stability. Even unhappy workers stayed in Kenya for family reasons and the lack of realistic options (Mwaniki and Dulo 2008). In Lebanon, nurses who wished to stay tended to be female, older, married and less formally skilled, who found their work satisfying and believed it would be difficult to find another job (El-Jardali et al. 2008a). In Ghana, nurses remained because of a reluctance to leave husbands behind, and the effects family separation might have on their children. It was 'unusual' for husbands to migrate in response to women's career aspirations (Ogilvie et al. 2007: 119). Versions of such forms of patriarchy are widespread; hence nurses tend to be more constrained than doctors. More prosaically, many have stayed, fearing that their qualifications and competence would not be recognised abroad, they were 'too old' to make radical adjustments to their lives and those of their families, they feared racism or simply disliked the climate and pace of overseas life (e.g. Connell 2009: 86–90).

Health workers, perhaps proportionately more than in other areas of employment, expressed a sense of vocation, altruism and duty about their work: 'I was a sponsored student. I have a duty to serve the people of Fiji', and 'I wanted to pay back the Niuean people and reduce the language barrier that is associated with expatriates, since we understand local values and conditions' (quoted in Connell 2009: 88, 89; Ogilvie et al. 2007; Oman et al. 2009). The most positive aspects of work usually involved human contact, helping others, meeting new people and working with colleagues, alongside professional satisfaction and recognition (Mathauer and Imhoff 2006). This spilled over into the satisfaction that only a health career could bring: the pleasure in seeing patients recover. Rhetorically expressed by one migrant doctor in Australia:

> Where else could one experience such emotional closeness with a stranger, the drama of a confrontation, the bliss of resolution and the despair of failure multiplied by the confounders of guilt, anger, exhilaration, pathos and the triumph of gifting a life? (Galak 2009: 30)

Interesting situations and altruism, though rarely entirely absent, may better explain why health workers initially took up their positions, rather than remained there. A sense of public worth plays some part in decisions to stay, and health workers are more easily able to stress this, yet pragmatism and inertia have crucial roles.

Health workers have not therefore usually entered the profession solely for the income, but also out of some desire to serve and be of value in the community. In the Philippines, where migration is so often the outcome, nurses argue that nursing is not just a profession, 'but a vocation or calling, and a profession that cares' (quoted in Opiniano 2003). However, such feelings do not sustain a career, as workers become frustrated by poor pay and conditions, especially in remote areas, finding themselves unable to adequately meet the needs of the people they sought to help. As a nursing educator phrased it for the Philippines, 'rendering service without expecting anything in return is quite altruistic. We also overwhelm ourselves with personal pressures . . . I think there is a need to re-evaluate how we perceive nursing and what levels of altruism we are pushing for' (quoted in ibid.). One consequence is the re-evaluation of nursing as a career and consequent attrition or migration. As, increasingly, people do join the health sector for economic reasons, migration becomes even more likely.

Most people would stay if the conditions were right, and many stay regardless. However, in just as many situations, people fear that circumstances will never become more positive. Most migrants leaving African countries thought there would never be an adequate economic and political system (Awases et al. 2004; Chikanda 2008) while over a third of a group of potential migrants from nine countries did not plan to return home to work, although that percentage varied from 5 in Sri Lanka to 55 in Kenya (van Eyck 2004: 22), primarily reflecting their concern over national futures. In

Zimbabwe, migration was loosely tied to 'better living conditions' in the destination but by 2002 to the fact that almost half of a sample of over 230 people could see no future in the country (Chikanda 2004; Oberoi and Lin 2006). A senior Nigerian nurse, working in the UK, effectively summarised such perspectives: 'If the economy were improved in Nigeria we wouldn't leave our country . . . That is why we came here . . . to adapt ourselves to the situation and then to endure. After endurance we go back home' (quoted in Aboderin 2007: 2242). Potential migrants may overwhelmingly want to stay, but may nonetheless move and never return, and skilled workers have particularly high expectations of what a satisfactory lifestyle includes.

INCOMES AND EMPLOYMENT

Income

Income differentials are invariably a key factor explaining migration (in some part because it is assumed to make sense). Income can be a major influence on decisions to join (or not join) the health profession; hence it is not surprising that it also constitutes a reason for leaving it. Income differences between countries have become increasingly well known and sometimes dramatic. Salaries of health workers in American Samoa have been up to ten times those of workers in comparable positions in Samoa, less than 100 km away. A tenfold disparity also separates salaries between Mauritius and Europe, resulting in staff shortages in Mauritius (*Afrol News*, 28 May 2004). Nurses from the Philippines are reported to earn about $4000 per month in the USA, about $180 in urban areas at home and about $100 in rural areas, while doctors earn between $300 and $800 per month. Filipino nurses can earn an average of $45,780 and $41,430 per year in US hospitals and nursing homes respectively, compared to the $2000–2400 annual salary paid in the Philippines – a twentyfold differential (Brush and Vasupuram 2006). A Kenyan nurse in an English nursing home routinely earned 16 times, and with overtime 30 times, what was possible in Kenya (Baird 2005: 10). For doctors, too, income differentials can be significant. Average health worker salaries in Eastern Europe are significantly below those in Western Europe, with health workers sometimes in the lower echelons of the public service. Czech salaries were four to eight times less than in Western Europe; Polish doctors received salaries one-tenth of those in Germany, and were dependent on either a second job or family support (Wiskow 2006: 22). The expansion of the EU thus precipitated significant migration. Between Europe and SSA discrepancies are greater. A family doctor in the UK gets paid more than 13 times an estimated Ghanaian salary, although the real disparity is less when the cost of living is taken into account (McCoy et al. 2008). Jamaican registered nurses with some specialisation were able to earn in the USA 16 times what they could earn at home (Brown 1997: 207). A Nepalese anaesthetist in New York, anticipating a starting salary of between $225,000 and $250,000, compared with the $100 a month she earned at a government hospital in Kathmandu, observed 'you have the answer to why thousands of doctors from the Indian subcontinent end up here' (quoted in Upadhyay 2003). In the late 1990s, junior doctors in Sudan received just 2 per cent of salaries in the Gulf, and one-tenth of that a decade later; unsurprisingly migration was substantial (Ali 2006). Significant differentials are widespread, well known and well documented.

Income differentials have broad implications. By the 1960s, Filipino nurses in the USA had even been criticised for the apparent 'materialism' and 'moral bankruptcy' of their apparent obsession with income gains (Choy 2003: 88). This is partly reflected in a comment from a Kerala nurse: 'Why struggle here and get no money? We can go abroad, make some money, and come back. Staying here, we don't get any respect and we don't get any money' (quoted in George 2005: 54; Nair 2007). Multiple anecdotes, the rationale for strikes, attrition and movement into the private sector all point to the primary significance of income factors (alongside working conditions), especially so for nurses, compared with better-paid doctors, for whom working conditions, experience and career development play a greater role.

An economic rationale in many guises dominates explanations for migration, whether for the personal gain of the migrants or their families (at home or with them), with or without specific goals (e.g. Brown 1997; Astor et al. 2005). Two-thirds of all nurses and almost half of all doctors in nine Pacific island states were primarily motivated to move for income reasons (Connell 2009). For a group of eight nurses who had migrated from lusophone African countries to Portugal, all but one had wages inadequate for basic living costs, since inflation and currency devaluation had depleted the purchasing power of their salaries to the extent that they had taken on second jobs such as selling food, sewing, and engaging in private practice (Luck et al. 2000). In Senegal, too, some 41 per cent of those who sought to migrate had taken up other kinds of employment to supplement their incomes from health work (Awases et al. 2004: 42). Zambian nurses' monthly salaries of $299, although reasonable in comparison with other government staff such as pharmacists, technologists and radiographers with similar durations of training, were low compared with monthly food requirements estimated at $350 for a family of six. Incomes did not meet the additional costs of decent housing, transport and other basic services like water and electricity, so driving them to a 'breaking point' involving movement from the public sector and the search for better-paid jobs at home and abroad (Lusale 2007). A somewhat similar breaking point emerged in Zambia during the 1990s after a long period of inflation caused commodity prices to rise significantly while salary levels failed to compete. In Zimbabwe, the combination of low pay and low status meant that nurses had 'put up with discomfort, uncertainty, frustration and eroded relationships with spouses and children' (Gaidwanza 1999: 54). Migration, as elsewhere, was the outcome.

Employment in the health sector alone has not always been adequate to sustain households. In Peru, where doctors' salaries by 2007 had decreased in real terms to a quarter of 1976 levels, not only did most have two or more jobs to secure a decent income (Jumpa et al. 2007), but 38 per cent of medical students were considering migration to a developed country (Mayta-Tristan et al. 2008). Nurses in Guyana routinely took on second or even third jobs, often moving to higher-paying private institutions before migration, in order to obtain a home or higher education (Anderson and Isaacs 2007: 394), while in countries as otherwise different as Benin and China many public sector workers expected illegal, informal 'gifts' or bribes from patients before they provided treatment. Doctors and nurses in Sierra Leone invariably increased supposedly standard hospital fees since it was 'generally accepted that doctors and other staff have to charge for their services in order to supplement their incomes' (Stevenson 1987: 406). In some countries staff engaged in ethically and legally questionable activities, such as stealing drugs, to survive and achieve what they regarded as adequate wage levels (Muula and Maseko 2006; Brown 1997). Given the degree of corruption in many countries, this is unsurprising. In Cameroon, where salary costs and currency devaluation in the 1990s reduced their living standards, nurses similarly sought 'informal' payments from clients, engaged in 'parallel health sector consulting' and set up small businesses. The need to run such businesses resulted in increased absenteeism from the health centres, and their choice to work there for the number of hours that seemed appropriate to the salaries they received. Even senior Nigerian nurses were often 'forced' to run businesses on the side to supplement public sector earnings (Aboderin 2007: 2240). Moonlighting is thus widespread, and such additional work may affect quality and equality of care. Some workers may become absentees or ultimately 'ghost workers' since the additional 'informal' payments reduce motivation and do not necessarily contribute to retention (Chaudhury and Hammer 2003; Stringhini et al. 2009). No clear relationship therefore exists between migration and public sector wages alone, where health workers can also be involved in private sector employment or other income-generating activities.

Jamaican nurses who went abroad were most likely to be those who had worked outside the capital city where they had less likelihood of acquiring such material assets as a car, home or business (Brown 1997: 205). For South African and Zimbabwean doctors and nurses the main reasons to migrate were overwhelmingly economic, in terms of better wages in destination countries, but emphasised by both economic downturn in Zimbabwe and the desire to buy a car or pay off a home loan (Gaidzanwa 1999; Oberoi and Lin 2006). Similar specific material goals are evident in very many other countries, such as Lebanon and Nigeria, alongside a good education for children. When such objectives could no longer be met at home (and furniture, televisions and even beds were beyond the income of Zimbabwean doctors), migration became the means to these ends (Gaidzanwa 1999; El-Jardali et al. 2008a; Aboderin 2007: 2241). Social mobility is the intended outcome.

Economic issues take several forms. The migration of nurses from Lebanon was stimulated by financial reasons, but combined with professional development (El-Jardali et al. 2008a, 2009). In Cameroon and Uganda respectively, 80 per cent and 72 per cent of health workers intended to migrate for economic reasons, and in Senegal as many as 89 per cent found that public service salaries were inadequate and fully 92 per cent reported that their salaries were not paid on time (Awases et al. 2004), an indication that it is not merely (or always) the actual income that is the most crucial problem. Irregular pay is a remarkably general problem (van Eyck 2004; McCoy et al. 2008), especially outside capital cities. In parts of rural Ethiopia, for example, where 'employees in the government health service are overworked and underpaid', and tend to prefer working in the private sector in urban areas, staff must walk for several days to and from town to collect their salaries (von Massow 2001: 39), which leaves the clinics unattended, and encourages poor performance and low motivation. In Uganda, more than 70 per cent of all nursing students wished to work overseas after graduation, mainly for financial reasons; those who wanted to migrate were more likely to also want to work in urban areas and in the private sector, and those less likely to migrate were those who expressed a sense of professional obligation (Nguyen et al. 2008). In most contexts and combinations, income strongly influences migration.

Migration demonstrates considerable sensitivity to income differences and, in SSA, countries with higher doctors' wages have lower migration rates (Bhargava and Docquier 2008). Migration of doctors to the USA varies with source countries' GDP per capita, with middle-income countries having the highest rates of migration. High-income countries could retain doctors, while the poorest countries produced fewer migrant doctors since they had few medical schools and potential migrants had inadequate resources and skills to migrate and find employment (Hussey 2007). Income differentials within countries are important as health workers balance their lifestyles against those of other skilled workers. Thus Tongan nurses had a greater propensity to migrate than Samoan nurses, partly because the Tongans earned less than the mean Tongan income whereas Samoans earned more than the mean Samoan income, although in real terms their earnings and their potential gains from migration were about the same. Doctors were less likely to migrate than nurses because their wages compared more favourably with other national professional groups (Brown and Connell 2004, 2006). The relative income position of nurses (and other health workers) within their home countries – the basic national salary structure – is thus a critical influence on migration, but this is complicated by the structure of household incomes, since most health workers are married. In Lebanon, nurses resented what they saw as a lack of equivalence with other professional groups (El-Jardali et al. 2008a), while Zambian nurses with degrees resented having the same salary as those without, an implicit lack of recognition of their training (Hansdotter 2007). In Malawi, nurses similarly moved overseas because working conditions and remuneration were the 'poorest in various professions'; hence they 'are leaving the country at enormous cost to themselves, their families and communities . . . it is not so much the "pull factors" that are attracting Malawian nurses to Europe, but rather "push" factors are driving them out of the country' (Muula et al. 2003: 436). In Zimbabwe, strong opposition was expressed to recruited immigrant Cuban doctors, who were paid up to $4000 per month, from national doctors who were paid approximately $200 per month, since they could not afford the houses and cars that the Cubans obtained (Oberoi and Lin 2006: 30). Inequality rankles.

Marginal increases in salaries have little effect in stemming migration. It has been suggested that in Jamaica a 37 per cent increase in public sector salaries would be needed (and presumably enough) to check the outmigration of health personnel (Reid 1999). While there may be reasons to believe such an increase would work in Jamaica, in Ghana a rather higher increase had little effect on reducing the extent of migration (McCoy et al. 2008). A rise of salaries of health workers in Malawi, by between 40 to 60 per cent in the mid-2000s, was similarly expected to do little to reduce incentives to migrate since the remuneration gap between Malawi and the UK (the main destination) remained massive, with salaries still roughly ten times those in Malawi. The main objective of the salary increase was 'to lift Malawi's health workers out of poverty' and reduce attrition, rather than stem migration (Record and Mohiddin 2006). Income grievances also apply to overtime and other special payments (such as regional allowances), which also influenced migration decisions. As one Fijian doctor phrased it in 2002,

> People need to be compensated for their hard work and after hours duty. At present work can be stressful for those who are trying hard to improve the standards of health care. Why would one put in extra hours of work especially when they are underpaid? The 'good Samaritan' and 'Nightingale' days are over. (Quoted in Connell 2009: 92)

Since costs of living in destinations reduce salary gains, 'it is often the relative low pay within a country, in comparison with other sectors, that discourages health workers in their efforts. Considering that the remuneration partly reflects the valuation of the health workforce in the country, the demoralization of health workers is one understandable consequence' (Wiskow 2006: 22). Not surprisingly, therefore, income considerations also influence choice of destination, with doctors from southern Africa who were most concerned about economic benefits being more likely to move to the Gulf and the USA because of the high wages, greater purchasing power and protection against taxation (Oberoi and Lin 2006: 29). In their destinations, too, SHWs may be quite mobile, where alternatives exist, in order to increase economic gains; Romanian nurses in Italy moved frequently to hospitals where incomes were higher and/or to places where living costs were lower (Palese et al. 2008), while most SHWs prefer urban employment.

Relativities constantly change. In India the decline of the Internet boom that reduced overseas demand for IT workers made nursing a more attractive opportunity for overseas employment, so that by 2003 it was said to be 'the next revolution . . . and nurses are already outwitting software programmers by getting paid a lot better . . . Since Indian nurses typically take home monthly salaries of about $84 compared with American salaries of more than $4000 a month it is no wonder that many Indian nurses are eager to work in the United States' (Rai 2003: 4). A similar case has been made in Africa in a rather different context:

> Imagine you're a nurse working in a primary health care clinic in South Africa. A never-ending stream of patients waits for basic medical care, but government financial constraints prevent the clinic from hiring more staff. And now with HIV/AIDS wreaking havoc on the country you find yourself struggling to meet those basic needs and treat people infected with the virus. For all the work and emotional suffering that come with the job the average South African nurse makes about five to seven thousand dollars a year. Now imagine you get an offer from a public hospital in Great Britain, where you can earn $30,000 a year plus benefits like paid vacation and child care. The new job carries a workload that is far less demanding and made even easier by the fully stocked supply cabinet and pharmacy. What would you do? (Parker 2004)

Such reports are emotive, and have limited empirical basis, but neverthe-less point to the substantial differences between health care systems and the primary rationale for migration between them. Yet in the end potential migrants do not simply balance incomes (or even differences in cost of living), but consider a range of other factors.

Not only do wages and incomes influence where health workers work (within countries and internationally), but they also influence the sector in which they work. The private sector usually provides higher wages, and superior working conditions; hence there has been widespread movement from the public to the private sector: a 'perverse' move from a poorly resourced sector, where demand is high, to the converse. The ability to either work part time in private practice, or move entirely into the private sector, significantly boosts income levels, is especially prized in most developing countries, and is a major brake on migration, as it has been in Tonga and Fiji (Connell 2009). In Jamaica, younger doctors took up some of the work left undone by migrating nurses because the prospect of eventually taking up well-paid private practice was alluring enough to discourage migration and keep them within the public sector until they could transfer (Brown 1997: 216). In India, emerging middle-class life-styles partly eroded the satisfaction and altruism of medical employment and income has increased in significance for becoming a doctor, migrating and moving into the private sector (Baru 2005). In Gambia, out of a recent class of 26 doctors, only two remained in the public sector, with the others working for private clinics and NGOs, where salaries were eight times higher, or overseas (*IRIN News*, 11 December 2008). The 'new' NGOs, mainly emerging within international programmes to reduce HIV/AIDS in SSA, have attracted many local SHWs. Such NGOs 'can "rob" local health systems of staff who are attracted by higher wages, better condi-tions and specialist training' (O'Brien and Gostin 2009: 8; Schatz 2008), to the extent that it has been described as an 'internal brain drain' (Larsson et al. 2009). Nurses may also be hired to work in record-keeping and administrative positions in urban rather than rural areas (Gorman and Hohmuth-Lemonick 2009). Where such private sector opportunities are non-existent, for example in Kiribati and in rural Vietnam, there are few incentives to remain (Dieleman et al. 2003: 4). Where additional private incomes are significant, as in Tonga, this is a deterrent to migration.

Employment Conditions

A litany of employment conditions influences migration. Migrants, poten-tial migrants (and many non-migrants, in source and recipient states) frequently complain about the work environment in terms of inadequate support, whether directly through weak management (lack of teamwork, poor leadership, little recognition, limited autonomy and access to promotion and training opportunities) or through the outcome of poor 'housekeeping': meagre access to functioning equipment and supplies, too much paperwork and bureaucracy devolved onto practitioners, poor transport and accommodation, and inadequate security. Managements were never blameless. Technology broke down and maintenance was problematic, replacements and supplies were not ordered, were misplaced or arrived too late. The main causes of dissatisfaction centred on physical working conditions and the lack of career opportunities.

(a) Careers and promotion

SHWs have invariably been strongly critical of the absence of an evident and transparent career structure, and even more so of nepotism. Income is firmly linked to careers and promotion, which many health workers see as being more about 'who you know than what you know': favouritism, linked to region, kinship, ethnicity, class or caste, and longevity in the system, rather than ability. Invariably, SHWs sought to work in a meritocracy where skills, accomplishments and innovations – their own personal social capital – would be rewarded. As one Fijian nurse argued, 'It's hard to make changes here. We try to make changes but other nurses pull you back, because they don't want to change and think you are bigheaded' (quoted in Connell 2009: 99). Classic 'crab antics' defined relationships in some workplaces. Where any one crab appears on the point of escaping from a container – or as one SHW seeks change and innovation – it is pulled back down by others. Escaping the norm, rising above mediocrity, and even seeking to do so, become impossible, even threatening.

Career opportunities were influenced by training. Perhaps unusually, the single greatest concern of nurses in Trinidad was the lack of opportunities for specialisation (Phillips 1996). Half of all Fijian nurses were dissatisfied with the lack of training and mentoring they received, limiting the routine acquisition of new knowledge. Training was not always clearly focused on needs or part of a career structure. As one nurse explained, 'Nurses are sent on training when near retirement. Younger nurses should go as they have more years to serve' (quoted in Connell 2009: 94). Individualism may be necessary and beneficial, and obtaining senior positions does not always result from the acquisition of skills and qualifications, but from kinship connections and nepotism.

Many SHWs simply sought respect and support from management, sometimes lost in a generation gap or a hierarchical system. SHWs were often more concerned about their relationship with the institution, and the extent of support from senior workers – colleagues and management

– than any other factors, including income: loosely, job satisfaction and the ability to work effectively. Equally, many nurses sought support from the doctors with whom they were supposed to collaborate (Nair 2007; Ogilvie et al. 2007; Masango et al. 2008). Korean nurses were overworked in a hierarchical, patriarchal society, where male doctors demanded respect, senior nurses were disrespectful of junior nurses, autonomy was minimal, self-esteem and motivation were eroded, and control extended to the supervision of modes of walking and hairstyles (Chung 2007). Nigerian and Zimbabwean nurses similarly complained of the lack of respect due to them as professionals, rather than as carers, in their relationships with male doctors, and sought migration to enable them to gain 'professional and public respect working in advanced clinical settings' (Aboderin 2007: 2242; Gaidzanwa 1999: 70). Mentoring in any form was often seen to be lacking, when management was weak and information not shared. As a Zimbabwean doctor who had migrated to Australia noted of Zimbabwe, 'Management is very weak, inappropriate work procedures and standards, little orientation of new employees. Also a lack of performance appraisal is evident' (quoted in Oberoi and Lin 2006: 29). The managers themselves had often migrated. Such lack of acknowledgement and assistance was problematic in its own right, but also restricted further education and training opportunities, career development and the possibility of promotion.

Reasonable and equitable opportunities for promotion can be lacking: a somewhat elusive modernity of process, even in modern technological institutions. Such concerns have been raised in many contexts, including SSA and various parts of the Caribbean. One-fifth of nurses leaving Jamaica for the USA cited professional reasons as a key influence on their move; two-thirds of these noted that there was no prospect of promotion and one-third complained of inadequate technology and infrastructure (Brown 1997: 205). In several south African countries the lack of promotion was one of the most commonly expressed reasons for migration, particularly in Cameroon and Uganda, where it was more significant than heavy workloads (Awases et al. 2004: 43). SHWs often feel isolated from trends and innovations in health care, so missing out on skills that would enable professional development and promotion. Where health workers are distant from the main centre(s) the perception that they are being ignored for promotion is even stronger (see below). Inadequate opportunities for promotion – and training – constitute both an incentive to migration and a constraint to morale, productivity and evolution in the health system.

Retention of skilled workers may be particularly difficult in small states, with centralised bureaucracies where many public servants know each other well; hence the task of developing merit-based recruitment and promotion is particularly difficult. The smaller the administration, the fewer the possibilities for a lifetime career within it because of the reduced number of promotion opportunities, which in itself creates frustration. Numbers are few, anonymity is impossible and relationships are more intense, necessitating careful management. Newly trained and hired workers in particular find a variety of ceilings to promotion, and innovations percolate slowly. Yet small administrations tend to have very limited spare capacity, so that the absence of any worker, whether because of training, sickness, leave or migration, places disproportionate pressure on those who remain. Migration, and the culture of migration, is particularly significant in small states.

(b) Work

Long hours of overtime, double shifts, working on overnight 'graveyard' shifts or at weekends, especially without income supplementation, influence migration. Shift work is a universal complaint, particularly in more remote places. Where fewer staff are available, pressures on those remaining are greater and a '24/7' presence may be expected. 'Pay and overtime' were routine responses to queries over dissatisfaction in the Pacific and Trinidad, although many recognised that such problems came with the job: 'Shift work is so inconvenient; I can't participate in community things'; 'I hate the overtime especially since they only pay us time off in lieu – I work for the money'; 'I hate working nights – that's the time to sleep' (quoted in Connell 2009: 92; Phillips 1996). Health care is physically and mentally demanding, with long working hours especially in emergency and intensive care units.

Clean and safe environments are major concerns. Inadequate working conditions may increase the risk of contracting disease. Stress is almost inevitable in a unique working environment where death occurs. The rise of HIV/AIDS has made the nursing profession especially far less attractive than hitherto, although before the rise of HIV/AIDS, malnutrition of SHWs was said to be a greater influence on losses than migration (Ojo 1990). Its rise has substantially reduced recruitment of health workers, especially nurses, and stimulated migration. In SSA, Thailand and PNG, HIV/AIDS has created a working climate that has become more difficult as workloads have increased. As one nurse who had migrated from South Africa to the USA observed, 'Nurses are emotionally exhausted. They are burnt out. If you are dealing with the huge number of people with a disease like HIV/AIDS, it takes its toll on you' (quoted in Parker 2004). In Uganda, as many as 86 per cent of health workers were concerned about contracting HIV/AIDS at work, and in Cameroon and Senegal comparable proportions were 69 per cent and 70 per cent (Awases et al. 2004: 44). More generally in SSA, a major influence on migration is 'fear of infection and the huge stress involved in working in communities that are very badly affected by HIV', notably in Zimbabwe, Uganda and Zambia (WHO 2006b: 7; Ogilvie et al. 2007; Lusale 2007). Nurses have migrated from some countries, including Zimbabwe and Malawi, through concern over inadequate preventive measures against HIV/ AIDS (Chikanda 2004; Palmer 2006) or because they too have HIV/ AIDS (Kober and van Damme 2006). High prevalence rates have been recorded among South African health workers (Shisana et al. 2004), and high mortality rates among Zambian nurses (Buve et al. 1994). Botswana lost 17 per cent of its health workforce to AIDS between 1999 and 2005, and in Lesotho and Malawi death from AIDS is the largest single cause of workforce attrition (WHO 2006b). Mozambique is said to be losing health workers to AIDS – let alone migration – faster than they can be trained (Garrett 2007). Doctors experienced similar perspectives. Every doctor in a group who had migrated from southern Africa to Australia was fearful of contracting HIV/AIDS. As one such migrant from South Africa observed, 'any one of us working in health care could quite easily contract this disease' (quoted in Oberoi and Lin 2006: 29). Such fears now extend beyond SSA.

Other health issues play a part in migration. Korean nurses had multiple sickness problems, due to their irregular work hours, and had a miscarriage rate twice the national average (Chung 2007). In Latin America, where conditions are probably better than in some other regions, working conditions, and the psychological burden of handling critical situations, often push hospital nurses in particular to resign. Nurses are also exposed to biological, chemical and physical risks, experiencing health problems that are osteo-muscular, caused by sharp instruments or result from sleep-pattern disturbances. There was a correlation between those nurses who experienced the most injuries and sickness and those with the heaviest workloads. The specific expression '*malestar de la enfermera*' (discontent of the nurse) reflects the growing difficulty of heavy workloads and demanding hours (Malvarez and Castrillon Agudelo 2005). Paradoxically, particularly in remote places, boredom sometimes created dissatisfaction, through a low or unvarying workload. This resulted in workers dwelling on other frustrations of the workplace, and feeling that they were not usefully contributing, so inhibiting a 'work ethic'. In some more specialised areas there was rarely enough work to enable the maintenance of professional standards: something of a reverse economy of scale. Hence it is not always, or even usually, the 'pull factors' that are attracting health workers to developed countries, but rather 'push factors' are discouraging them from remaining. While this may overestimate the 'push', even without recruitment and overseas blandishments, skilled workers seek to leave health sectors where their needs are unsatisfied.

In many countries, such as Zimbabwe, wide-ranging concerns attend the general decline in the health system, the lack of resources and facilities and the resultant increasing workload (Awases et al. 2004; Chikanda 2004; Oberoi and Lin 2006), or 'work overload' (van Eyck 2004). Migration worsens working conditions further, and places additional stress on those who have stayed. As one doctor at Kenyatta Hospital in Nairobi has pointed out, 'It's like a vicious circle. Our nurses leave the hospitals to go to Europe where they have much better work conditions. Then they come back on holiday and talk to staff here. When our nurses hear about Europe they feel they have been working like slaves and want to move as well.' One nurse at the hospital emphasised similar issues: 'I know it's not good for Kenya but I still want to leave. Here nursing is very hard and we feel we should have a chance to gain more knowledge and nursing skills abroad.' Circumstances are made ever more difficult by continued migration; hence the demand for migration simply increases, and in turn increases the pressure on the system (Mathauer et al. 2004; Volqvartz 2005).

A lack of functioning technology, and contexts where it can be used effectively, and of basic supplies, cause frustration and reduce morale. In Nigeria, where affluent patients pay for their own supplies and other patients receive 'insufficient care', such inadequate clinical conditions stimulate migration. As one nurse observed:

> We don't have enough equipment. You see somebody suffering . . . and you know 'this is what to do'. But where are the things to use? And you just have to watch that person giving up. You feel like crying . . . but you just have to swallow it . . . making one not have that job satisfaction. (Quoted in Aboderin 2007: 2242)

Similar situations recur in various contexts where patients must receive food, bed linen and other necessities from outside, or do without. In lusophone Africa, frustrations emerged from such basic problems as a lack of linen, a changing room for nurses and the removal of hospital wastes (Luck et al. 2000). A global study of nurses simply concluded: 'In many countries employers have failed to address long standing deficiencies related to hours of work, salary, continuing education, staffing levels, security, housing and day-care facilities' (Oulton 1998: 126). While in most workplaces it is normal for some expectations to be unmet, especially where workplaces are small, and workers expected to be flexible, grievances mount without management support.

EDUCATION, EXPERIENCE AND TRAINING

Further education, training and experience are key factors in migration in most countries, and are particularly strong reasons for many movements between countries where economic differentials are not great. Health workers thus move from New Zealand to Australia and onwards to the UK more for experience, lifestyle, variety, new training regimes and different skills, with migration being seen as something of a 'rite of passage', rather than because of superior wages or conditions. Travel and career opportunities dominated the reasons for migration of SHWs, from Australia and South Africa to the UK (Moran et al. 2005). Nurses moving from elsewhere in the EU to the Netherlands went primarily for personal reasons, including marriage and their spouses' employment, followed by the potential to improve knowledge and skills, while income was rarely mentioned (de Veer et al. 2004). Many overseas nurses in the UK resented the perception that they were 'economic migrants' and that they had been 'pushed' into migration, since there were distinctions between nurses from Australia who had come for new experiences and the opportunity to travel and those from the Philippines who sought financial security (Larsen et al. 2005: 356–7). White nurses from countries like Canada or Australia move to the UK, the UAE and elsewhere to pursue a 'working holiday strategy' quite different from the 'life change strategy' or 'working for back home' of black nurses from Nigeria, Filipinos and SHWs from other developing countries (Larsen et al. 2005; Aboderin 2007: 2238). Doctors from developed countries similarly migrate for lifestyle and experience rather than income gains, although unemployment and the lack of specialist positions account for some movement within Europe (Jinks et al. 2000). French doctors migrated to the UK out of a general desire for a lifestyle change, the chance to experience a different culture and develop professionally, alongside frustration with the French health care infrastructure and long hours. Some effectively took salary reductions to move (Ballard et al. 2004). None the less, new experiences, different contexts and mentoring stimulate new skills and potential economic and social mobility.

Training, with its connotations of new knowledge, skills and potential promotion, is eagerly sought after (Chapter 5). Those unable to access continuing education and training programmes at home saw this as a brake on their careers and on their lives. Diminishing finance has usually meant that training programmes are early victims, mentoring is limited and complex procedures less likely to be conducted (Aboderin 2007); hence health workers have sought the missing experiences overseas. The main reason for the migration of doctors in India was said to be to acquire postgraduate training (and prestige), although the initial intention to return often disappeared after a time overseas (Mullan 2006; George et al. 2007). The opportunity to engage in research and experience specialisms stimulated some migration. That superior training will eventually enable superior incomes is an anticipated, but less often stated, intent and outcome.

In a group of African countries the desire for further training and additional experience was a particularly influential factor on migration; in Cameroon as many as 85 per cent of all SHWs sought to go overseas for further training (and this was the single most important reason) and in Uganda and South Africa the relative percentages were 38 and 43. For those who had migrated from Ghana, the need to gain experience and the lack of promotion opportunities were the most important reasons, both listed by 86 per cent of all health workers. In South Africa, the proportion of those seeking to move for international experience varied between professions, with midwives the least likely and pharmacists the most likely to seek to emigrate for this reason (Awases et al. 2004: 46, 41). Limited access to contemporary technology and training is a central concern (Chapter 5).

RURAL AND REGIONAL MALAISE

Almost all the factors that contribute to migration and attrition are multiplied in rural and regional areas, where health workers feel that they and their institutions are too often ignored, victims of institutionalised urban bias in development practice (Dussault and Franceschini 2006). That initially discourages migration to remote areas: urban-trained SHWs are rarely anxious to work in what they perceive as small, remote and backward places (Chapter 2). Wages are usually lower in rural areas, but costs of living may not be, especially where professionals have certain expectations, and some goods are inaccessible. Rural wages, as in Vietnam, are a disincentive to SHWs going or remaining there. Transport costs, lack of information, heavy workloads, lack of support for continued education and training (Dieleman et al. 2003: 4), poor technology and absent supplies, limited interaction with peers and some social isolation, wide-ranging responsibilities, inadequate support for partners' and children's aspirations, and no alternative means of income generation are all disincentives in a range of countries (El-Jardali et al. 2009). SHWs, and other skilled workers, particularly those with higher-level skills, have generally been reluctant to move to outlying areas, especially when posted there, because of the relative absence and inferiority of health care facilities, the lack of other services, such as shops and schools (for their children), language and cultural issues, because they may have to work in administrative positions (for which they are not trained) while practising their clinical skills, and because they may be 'out of sight and out of mind' for salary payments, promotion, training, mentoring, or conference attendance. SHWs are often poorly trained for the particular health needs of rural areas. New, inexperienced recruits may be posted to rural areas, with substantial autonomy and responsibility but minimal monitoring or support, and experience some stress, even in developed countries such as Canada (Hunsberger et al. 2008; LeSergent and Haney 2005). Political instability and insecurity further encourage migration.

Remote areas tend to have poorer service provision, not only in the health sector. As one skilled worker in a small Fijian town said in 2002, 'we always get the rejects from central hospitals' and 'we are already isolated and then to be dumped with outdated equipment you feel more remote' (quoted in Connell 2009: 105). Even where this sort of situation does not hold, it is a widespread perception. Access to modern computer technology and telemedicine, even in rich-world countries, has barely changed that situation in most places. As the evidence from Vietnam and also China indicates, even avowedly socialist states have found it difficult to encourage or direct SHWs to rural areas, despite a range of policies seeking to do just that (Lehmann et al. 2008). Thus, in China, the reasons why many seek to move from rural township health centres (THCs) are much the same as in other parts of the world:

> Some health workers, especially young ones, do not like to stay in THCs, even if the income of health workers is a little bit higher than that in higher level hospitals. This is because the living conditions, including children's education, in the rural towns where the THCs are located are generally poorer than in the county town. (Quoted in Meng et al. 2009: 4)

Over time and place, similar circumstances prevail.

Many health workers in remote areas tend to come from those areas, and accept the disadvantages in favour of a familiar social and cultural context and the ability to work with 'one's people'. Otherwise rural areas were seen as sometimes pleasant, friendly and peaceful, but often stultifying, a place of exile and sometimes even dangerous. (In April 2008, the Ialibu hospital in highlands PNG, serving an area with 200,000 people, closed after frequent attacks on the staff and facilities. A nurse from a different province had lost six front teeth in an attempted rape, the ambulance had been stolen and the doctor had fled after his house was occupied, conditions that readily discouraged health workers from moving to the area.) Without salary or other benefits for working in rural and remote areas, a degree of freedom and autonomy and a greater range of activities and responsibilities, working beyond the cities was hoped to be merely a prelude to social and geographical mobility.

Similar reasons explain migration from the rural areas of both high- and low-income countries. A similar reluctance to work in rural areas exists (albeit intensified in developing countries, because of cultural differences and less adequate service provision). Recruitment and retention of allied health professionals in rural New South Wales (Australia) were affected by lifestyle and personal factors, support for professional development, the size of the team, particularly the need for a 'critical mass' of staff, various management issues, unevenly distributed and limited resources, the need for regular professional supervision and the disincentive of a flat career structure (Denham and Shaddock 2004). In rural Japan, young doctors were least likely to be satisfied with rural lifestyles, because of inadequate access to education for their children, lack of opportunity to continue their own education, and lack of support from local governments (Matsumotu et al. 2004). More generally, heavy workloads, long hours, occupational isolation, poor promotion prospects, limited holidays and low incomes are disincentives to, and disadvantages of, rural employment (Forti et al. 1995; Hays et al. 1997; Pastor et al. 1989; Pathman et al. 1996). These influences on migration, alongside the failure of secondary graduates to remain in, or tertiary graduates to return to, these areas recur in a wide range of contexts, and explain the relative need for rural health workers.

A SOCIAL CONTEXT

In Pacific island states, migrants constantly emphasise that migration is not for their own ends but to improve long-term family prospects, especially their children's education (Connell 2009). African doctors in Portugal and Nigerian nurses in the UK, alongside many others, similarly emphasised the education needs of their children (Luck et al. 2000; Aboderin 2007). Education and the creation of human capital underpin migration, and income is the means of achieving this. Income has social connotations beyond education. The quest for new social status influences migration. Indian nurses from Kerala migrated because their ability to earn and retain significant incomes gave them high status and the consequent ability to find high-status partners in the 'matrimonial market' (Percot and Rajan 2006: 152; 2007: 321). Bangladeshis had similar aspirations (Aminuzaman 2007). Success in the USA gave Indian and Filipino nurses even higher status, downplaying the former relatively high status of their husbands, sometimes pejoratively called 'nurse-husbands' in India, while households subsequently became more egalitarian (George 2005; Espiritu 2005). More recently, many Kerala, Filipino and Pakistani men have taken up nursing careers as a means of emigration. In many contexts gender relations have been restructured following migration.

Somewhat in contrast, many female SHWs face particular constraints related to partners' careers and family obligations, which may make remote postings difficult and overseas migration even more difficult. Individuals rarely make decisions without taking into account wider family considerations. Migration may be discouraged by family circumstances and social norms. As many nurses are married women, and husbands may be more influential decision-makers, even dire personal income and workplace circumstances may not influence migration, but might contribute to attrition. In the Pacific, doctors are almost twice as likely to migrate as nurses, partly because wage differentials are greater but also because men tend to be the decision-makers and most nurses are women (Connell 2009). Marriage itself may be a factor – four of a small group of eight lusophone African nurses in Lisbon had been influenced by marital reasons – two to join a spouse in Portugal and two to escape an unhappy marriage at home (Luck et al. 2000). Several Fijian nurses in the Marshall Islands had similarly moved to escape difficult domestic relationships (Rokoduru 2008). Single workers are more likely to seek to and be able to migrate; in Senegal, typically, the most likely to migrate were young single workers followed by married workers without children (Awases et al. 2004: 42), although those more likely to gain higher incomes overseas were older and more experienced. Social ties may result in pressure to migrate, to support the extended family, but they can also make migration more difficult.

In some parts of SSA, notably Zimbabwe, the economic factors that influence migration have been so immediately overwhelming that social influences and the needs of other generations are less evident or even absent (e.g. Chikanda 2004). In South Africa, however, some 27 per cent of SHWs stated that they would migrate in search of a safer environment for their children, let alone a better educational or economic environment (Awases et al. 2004: 41). While social reasons often account for who migrates, and where and when they migrate, in developing countries, at least, the primarily economic influences on migration are dominant.

POLITICS AND HAZARD

Political factors influence the migration of health workers in usually fairly obvious ways (some of which relate to wages and working conditions), especially if political turmoil reduces funding for the health sector, places new demands on it or marginalises certain groups. Substantial military expenditure, whether as the outcome of violence or the cause of it, reduces resources available for health. Costa Rica, without any military forces, has retained SHWs and constructed an effective health care system. As early as the 1960s, Chinese doctors were leaving Hong Kong, concerned over the future, still distant, reversion of Hong Kong to China, and were leaving Malaysia and Indonesia for other political and cultural reasons (Gish 1971: 90, 98). Instability contributes to migration. In Uganda, Zimbabwe and no doubt elsewhere, the migration of health professionals began or grew under particularly repressive regimes, while the resultant overseas beachhead enabled further migration. Burma, too, has lost many doctors in difficult domestic political circumstances.

Violence, coups, crime, warfare and persistent social unrest predictably hasten migration from countries such as South Africa (Oberoi and Lin 2006), Zimbabwe (Chikanda 2008), Lebanon (Kronfol et al. 1992; El-Jardali et al. 2008a), Iraq (Burnham et al. 2009) and more generally (Clemens and Pettersson 2008). The flow from Hong Kong accelerated again in the aftermath of the 1991 Tiananmen massacre and before the 1997 handover to China (Ho 2008: 149). Emigration from lusophone African countries increased after independence, when funds for the health sector declined, and intensified further during civil wars (Luck et al. 2000). Sierra Leone, where the proportion of health workers to patients was already low, lost many nurses in the aftermath of civil war. Somalia, Eritrea and Mozambique lost many SHWs in war and conflict situations, in parallel with significantly increased needs; Mozambique lost 85 per cent of its doctors during the war of independence that ended in 1974 (Dovlo 2004: 2). In Fiji, the health sector has been repeatedly affected by what has become something of a 'coup culture'. Ethnic tensions and military coups prompted a series of resignations and departures of SHWs, notably after the 1987 coups and again in 2000. The two 1987 coups, construed by many as opposition to the growing political role of Indo-Fijians (some half the population of Fiji), prompted a political, economic and social crisis and very substantial emigration, and not only of Indo-Fijians. In these exceptional circumstances, 100 doctors migrated in a period of 12 months compared with the loss of 67 in the previous five years (Connell 2009). Cultural distinctions have sometimes bred tensions and emphasised migration flows: for over 30 years Tamil doctors have been more likely than majority Sinhalese to migrate from Sri Lanka, Indo-Fijians have been more likely to leave Fiji than ethnic Fijians, and Chinese doctors to leave Malaysia. Coup- and violence-prone countries that have not experienced significant migration include those like the Comoros, where language and skill constraints restrict overseas employment options.

Much more broadly, a worsening political and economic environment has further intensified the desire to migrate. In six African countries, both anglophone and francophone, the majority of health workers were despondent about their future in their home countries and could see little alternative beyond migration. Civil unrest, violence and crime under-pinned intention to migrate in several countries (Awases et al. 2004; Palmer 2006) and correlate with the migration of doctors to the USA (Hussey 2007). Migration from Zimbabwe has intensified in recent years as the economy has experienced a substantial downturn, and one-third of all respondents to a 2002 survey wished to leave because 'the value systems in this country have declined to such an extent that I can no longer see my way clear to remain here' (quoted in Chikanda 2004: 15; Bloch 2005). By 2007, nurses were leaving Zimbabwe for neighbouring states such as Botswana, where salaries were seven times those in Zimbabwe, and the flow was only diminished because of government unwillingness to renew or issue passports. A clear relationship exists between the deterioration of the economy, measured in terms of the inflation rate, and migration and the inability of Zimbabwe to retain health workers in this century relative to other African states: sadly ironic in a country once distinguished from most others in SSA, whereby 'a steady, expanding economy and a sense of national pride combine to keep health personnel at home' (Ojo 1990: 634). Political and economic stability are crucial where middle-class elites are relatively easily able to migrate.

Borders and regulations restrict migration (Chapter 9). Where political circumstances change, as in the case of EU expansion, enabling migration from poorer Eastern states to those in the West, new structures of migra-tion have followed. In this case, for example, there was a substantial and early movement of doctors from the Czech Republic to the West, creating gaps in the Czech health service (Chapter 3). Similarly, emerging points systems, increasingly used to regulate migration in developed countries, have slowed unskilled migration but usually strongly favoured health workers.

RECRUITMENT

In recent years the structure of migration has become increasingly organ-ised and privatised through the expansion of recruitment agencies, and the regular use of these by recipient countries, districts and particular hospitals. Irrespective of any existing intent to migrate, active recruitment has put growing pressure on, and impressive opportunities in front of, potential migrants. Recruitment agencies smooth the way in attending to bureau-cratic issues, such as examinations, visas and work permits, satisfying concerns over different countries and cultures, providing induction training in destinations, and even education and scholarships in source countries. Recruitment both facilitates and stimulates migration, and has increasingly played a vital role, so much so that 42 per cent of all migrant nurses in Britain had come primarily because they had been recruited (Winkelmann-Gleed 2006: 44), just as had 41 per cent of those in the USA (Pittman et al. 2007). A simultaneous study in London found that two-thirds of all overseas nurses had been recruited by agencies (Buchan et al. 2004). In other words, over time migration has become more evidently linked to demand rather than to the volition of health workers themselves.

Recruitment is far from new. By the late 1960s, American hospitals were actively recruiting in the Philippines, utilising rhetoric of travel and adventure alongside income gains (Choy 2003: 100–101). The UK had been recruiting widely from the late 1940s, after the creation of the National Health Service, with campaigns in more than 16 British colonies, but especially in the Caribbean. However, in the 1980s, the direction of Caribbean nurse migration shifted to the USA after aggressive marketing campaigns, using newspaper advertisements and Hilton hotels as interview venues (Phillips 1996). Over time, initially in the Philippines, specific recruitment agencies emerged as intermediaries in the process, and in this century they have proliferated, actively recruiting in most parts of the world, and passively recruiting through websites (accessible in a moment's web search), newsletters (such as that from nurses.co.uk) and advertisements in newspapers, professional magazines and even tourist publications.

In many countries, hospitals prefer the greater certainty of overseas workers, who can be more effectively contracted, compared with agency nurses. In northern Australia, Townsville's main hospital group started advertising overseas in 2006, recruiting mostly from New Zealand and the UK: the chief executive stated, 'We're getting access to well-trained well-experienced nurses and I think it makes the organization a richer place to work. And they're committed to working for the hospital as opposed to our staff having to continually contend with nurses from an agency' (quoted in *The Australian*, 24 May 2008). Recruitment actually emphasises continuity.

Advertisement coverage can be intense. Over a five-year period the *South African Medical Journal* had over 2500 recruitment advertisements for health personnel (Rogerson and Crush 2008), a constant flow of information on overseas possibilities, boosted by Internet sites, that cannot but be tempting. Most were for typical destinations, especially the UK, Australia and New Zealand, but covered more than 20 countries, including other parts of SSA. A high standard of living, with superior wages, better career prospects, good education and a future for children are key themes in recruitment campaigns and advertisements. These may even be verified, sometimes in the advertisements, by migrants already established overseas. Advertisements (in magazines or websites) take similar forms, whether from agencies or from particular employers (regions or hospitals) stressing wages (as in south Australia in 2008 – 'great pay, great clients, immediate start'), friendliness ('register your interest now because we want to work with you'), mentoring and professional support ('support and guidance every step of the way') and external benefits ('subsidized housing'). Many places stress particular local pleasures and activities, with recreational amenities as important as incomes (Kingma 2006: 105; Rogerson and Crush 2008), broadly the same rhetoric employed by the USA in the 1960s.

Little information exists on the actual operations of recruitment agencies, despite their numbers. Indonesia, for example, has 400 and the Philippines some 1200, although the larger recruitment agencies are mainly in recipient countries. The USA has at least 267 international recruitment agencies, a tenfold increase from the late 1990s (Pittman et al. 2007). In the mid-2000s a sample of 85 US agencies were recruiting in 74 countries, and were still extending their operations, although the Philippines, India and Canada were the main sources (Pittman et al. 2007). Simultaneously, dozens of agencies emerged to market Polish doctors in the UK. Most recruitment is still from South Asia and the Philippines to the Gulf and more recently to the USA and parts of Europe, including Ireland and the UK, but the more active processes of recruitment have been instrumental in extending migration beyond post-colonial routes, taking Chinese nurses to the USA and the Gulf, and Korean nurses (once perceived to have a 'language problem') to the USA (Brush 2008). Governments play a key role. In 2006 the St John's Riverside Hospital in New York State signed an agreement with the Human Resources Development Service of Korea (part of the Ministry of Labor), to recruit 10,000 Korean nurses (Chung 2007). Australia has actively recruited Filipino nurses in Ireland. On a smaller scale, in this century, there has been active recruitment of Fijian nurses for the Bahamas and the UAE, countries that few in Fiji would have even heard of until then. Alongside such long-distance international flows there are also intra-regional flows, for example of Filipino nurses to Brunei, and Chinese and Filipino nurses to Singapore and Malaysia. In the Pacific there are similar complex but smaller-scale flows, such as from Fiji to Palau and the Marshall Islands (Rokoduru 2008), none of which would have occurred without active recruitment. For those who had emigrated from Cameroon, the single most important reason was recruitment (Awases et al. 2004), but, like everywhere else, recruitment would not have been successful without other factors.

Recruitment is selective and competitive, even when flows are quite small, as from Fiji to the UAE. In South Asia recruitment has recently intensified (and several states now promote migration) to the extent that, at least in India, 'there is a serious risk of selective depletion of the most qualified nurses in the country' (Khadria 2007: 1434), a situation that is probably already occurring (Thomas 2007). Indeed, recruitment necessarily emphasises selectivity as the very best workers are the most likely to migrate, while some Indian hospitals collude in this process by engaging in 'business process outsourcing' (Khadria 2007), with recruitment agencies themselves financing scholarships and training (Kingma 2006: 89–90).

Many agencies engaged in some forms of exploitation, not least excessive 'placement fees', a more generally reported phenomenon even where unions and industrial legislation exist (Buchan et al. 2009; Goodman 2005; van Eyck 2005; Connell and Stilwell 2006; Pittman et al. 2007; Cuban 2008). Before 1998, hundreds of registered nurses were brought from the Philippines to the USA to work in convalescent homes and other facilities; expecting wages of $13–15 per hour, they earned as little as $5 as nursing assistants, while many had paid up to $7000 for fraudulent visas (Choy 2003: 186–7). Overseas nurses recruited to work in London, especially from the Philippines and SSA, felt underpaid and undergraded, and were subject to exploitative fees and unfair treatment by recruitment agencies (Buchan 2008). The actions of recruitment agencies are resented in various source countries, especially where they appear over-zealous. In Mauritius it was argued by the President of the largest Mauritian nursing union that 'The British send recruitment agents who discreetly make contact with nurses and directly negotiate the contracts. Last week, 26 nurses were lured away by a single recruiter' (quoted in *Afrol News*, 28 May 2004). At its most basic, 'women are increasingly produced as export products and, with the help of recruitment agencies, processed as products that meet the cultural expectations of competing market buyers' (Brush and Vasupuram 2006: 184). Concern over the activities of recruitment agencies has led to attempts to construct and use codes of practice for recruitment, as in the Commonwealth, the Pacific and the UK, but not in major destinations such as the USA and the Gulf (Chapter 9). The success of such codes is ambiguous, since they are voluntary, and they have tended to result in agencies moving the geographical focus of operations rather than modifying practices.

MOVERS AND STAYERS: WHO GOES?

Young, skilled and single migrants, with fewer local ties, are more easily able and more likely to migrate, but they do not always dominate migration streams. The more educated and experienced usually migrate first, and there is a consistent and persistent bias towards the more skilled, especially where distant recruitment is involved. Recruiting agencies lament any decline in the quality of recruits, preferring only the best (and thus their own viability). US hospitals pick particular segments of the workforce, seeking 'people who have been trained to postgraduate level in American health systems in the Philippines. So what we're doing is taking the very best, the next generation of their leadership, out' (Paul Keighley, editor of *Nursing Standard*, quoted in Gordon 2005: 381). Some 79 per cent of SSA doctors working in the USA came from just ten medical schools, mostly in South Africa and Nigeria, the same key sources as in Canada (Labonté et al. 2006: 3). Migrant Indian doctors are disproportionately from the higher-quality training institutions and, even from within these institutions, the better doctors are those more likely to migrate: 'a serious loss of human capital' (Kaushik et al. 2008; Kangasniemi et al. 2007). Pakistani migrant doctors are no less skilled: 'highly motivated, well-educated high performers, deeply interested in improving health parameters and systems and capable of it because of academic strengths and well-developed peer, social and political linkages' (Talati and Pappas 2006: S58).

The same is true of nurses. In Fiji, almost all the nurses recruited for the UAE and Palau were from intensive care units; thus the very best local nurses were being selectively recruited (Connell 2009: 111–12) and few returned, choosing instead to move on to the USA or elsewhere. Nigerian (mainly Yoruba) nurses who had migrated to England were in mid to later life (all but one of a group of 25 being over 40), all had been working for many years, mostly in the public sector, and most had risen to senior positions, an almost identical profile to that of Indian nurses who had worked abroad (Aboderin 2007: 2240; Hawkes et al. 2009). A sample of 67 overseas nurses in the UK, from 18 different countries, had on average 14 years of work experience overseas, and had left senior positions, before starting work in the UK (Larsen et al. 2005: 355). The scale of this selectivity can be considerable; as a Malawian nurse in 2005 reported on her BSc nursing class from the University of Malawi, all 27 of whom were in the UK:

> I think in our hospital if I went back today, I wouldn't know anybody. Everybody is out: the UK, US. The UK has taken quite a few. All the nurses are newly qualified without much experience. I can say that it is being drained of the cream of nurses. More of the senior nurses are here [UK]. Whoever is left in charge is junior. (Quoted in Likupe 2006: 1217)

Scale and selectivity are combined. Universally it has always been the best and brightest who dominate migration flows (Mejia et al. 1979; Ojo 1990).

The consequence is all too predictable, as in Guyana and elsewhere in the Caribbean, that most current nursing positions are held by nurses close to retirement age, while younger workers have gone (Anderson and Isaacs 2007). Skills and experience – implicitly an education bias – characterise migrant health workers.

Almost all studies of the migration of health workers look at influences in the source rather than in the destination, assuming that migrants follow colonial and geographical ties and thus tend to follow others from the same region, or go to areas where obviously superior wages exist. However, most migrants choose between destinations. In India, for example, doctors who go to the USA tend to stay there while those who go to the UK are more likely to return: the USA was seen as a more accepting clinical and social environment than the UK (Mullan 2004: 24). Given that many migrants aspire to higher incomes, it may also be that the ease of access to the private sector is more welcome in the USA. By contrast, fewer migrant nurses choose Italy since wages are relatively low compared with elsewhere in the EU, a language barrier exists and institutional ties are absent (Chaloff 2008: 18). In so many cases, whatever the determinants on the way, the USA remains the ultimate destination (Chapter 3).

MULTIPLE RATIONALES, CONSTRAINTS AND CHOICES

The same broad combination of factors – dominated by low incomes and challenging working conditions – has been recorded for most developing countries, and accounts for attrition, shifts into the private sector, rural–urban migration and international migration. Even social and political factors, from education and experience to coups, are underpinned by economics. Although economic factors play a key role, they do not account for migration. The location of close kin and perceptions of family obligations are major influences, while women are more likely to face constraints. The relative decline of the public sector, lack of financial resources, and uncertainties over national futures reduce the satisfaction of both the working environment and the wider political, social and economic context. Management issues are critical for SHWs, who, perhaps more than most other skilled workers, are rarely motivated by money alone. Long hours, bureaucracy, inadequate technology and even minimal empathy are all significant problems, within sometimes dual cultures of migration (Chapter 5). Migration is multifaceted.

What might once have seemed simply an economic rationale for migration has become more complex and multidimensional. Given the multiple and basic reasons for migration, it may seem surprising that there are not more skilled migrants. Yet even under such worst-case scenarios as Zimbabwe in the mid-2000s, there is no straightforward 'logic' attached to why some people migrate and others stay. Moreover, the factors outlined above are far from ubiquitous; boredom for example does not necessarily accompany a heavy workload. Family connections, a sense of home and duty, partners' employment, the cost of migration, a hope for the future and inertia encourage retention. Poor wages and working conditions are necessary yet insufficient causes for migration. Many SHWs, including migrants, return migrants, potential migrants and probable stayers, demonstrate uncertainty and ambivalence. Relatively few see their present location and position as permanent and most at least contemplate some kind of future change. In the Pacific, health workers can be part of a cycle of circular migration, in response to fluctuating social and economic factors, especially where political boundaries are effectively absent (Hooker and Varcoe 1999: 95). In Jamaica too, nurses 'responded to harsh economic circumstances by establishing a niche in the international labour market as a means of maintaining their position at home' (Brown 1997: 219). Balancing costs and benefits is a function of time periods that relate to the ages of children, the health, age and location of parents, and their own position (and that of partners, and sometimes children) in the workforce. Choices over migration hinge on sometimes quite small changes in these contexts, and by the ease or otherwise of migration. Mobility is a constantly repeated and accessible phenomenon, as migrants balance the changing economic and social objectives of themselves and their kin: 'once you are a migrant you never know where home is ever again' (Bouras 1986: 12). Only death (and not even taxes) can be certain. Yet, one way or another, many skilled workers have left, and migration has often had an enormous impact, in terms of the loss of particularly valuable human resources, whether in the reduced morale of those who have stayed or the very real loss of scarce skills. This has implications for subsequent migration (skilled or otherwise), for the countries, for the households of the migrants, and for their health systems. These impacts can now be examined.

7. Migration and health provision

Migration of skilled health workers has diverse impacts, from more obvious effects on the delivery of health services and the economic consequences of the loss of locally trained workers to more subtle social, political and cultural impacts. Migrants tend to be relatively skilled and experienced, compared with those who stay. They move to improve their own livelihoods, and those of their families, and are usually the key beneficiaries of that migration. Recipient countries benefit from having workers to fill gaps in the health care system. Conversely, source countries and their populations, especially in remote areas, lose valuable skills unless those skills are an 'overflow' or are otherwise compensated for, perhaps through remittances. The provision of health care may be affected in both quality and quantity. Logic, widespread assumptions and vast amounts of anecdotal data suggest strong links between migration and the subsequent reduced performance of health care systems. Actual correlations between migration and malfunctioning health care systems are difficult to make, since it is hard to quantify what is not there, whether midwives or maternity wards, whose loss is often the stuff of journalism rather than academic analysis. Assessing the impact of migration – even indirectly – is difficult, and numerous anecdotes overwhelm reliable data. This chapter examines the direct impacts of migration on health care while the following chapter examines the more complex socioeconomic consequences of migration.

Migration affects both the quality and quantity of health care. While it is axiomatic that lack of workers should disrupt health care provision, clear evidence of this is rare, beyond correlations between health-worker density, sickness and mortality (Chapter 2). In some countries, daily newspapers are replete with articles, headlines, cartoons and photographs of long queues at health centres, accounts of the closure of remote health centres, references to overcrowded waiting rooms, unavailable health personnel, delays in attending emergency cases, lengthy waits and cursory examination and treatment, situations that cause reduced and/or inequitable access to health care. Such loosely anecdotal information often reflects worst-case, perhaps transient and localised, scenarios, which is not to say that problems are absent or trivial. However, in some SSA countries, where problems are reported, pseudo-shortages of health workers also exist.

Even in the earliest years of the migration of SHWs from developing countries, the brain drain was viewed as an almost entirely negative phenomenon, although discussion of actual changes in health care was rarely evident. As early as 1966 the Philippines had conducted an inquiry into the brain drain (Chapter 3) and by 1972 the dean of the Philippine Women's University College of Nursing was observing, 'It is a paradox; we have no shortage of nurses but we lack nurses . . . are we educating the nurses for home consumption or exportation?' (quoted in Choy 2003: 59). The impact of that shortage was unstated. By 1967 it had, however, been calculated that the value of SHW migration to the USA, seen as 'foreign aid', was equal to the total cost of all health programmes provided by the USA to foreign nations (West 1968), while doctors were leaving relatively impoverished states such as Haiti, Lebanon, Nigeria and Paraguay (Mejia 1978: 262–3). That remittances were equivalent to the value of the skilled workers was challenged for the Philippines:

> the argument that emigrants transfer funds back to relatives in their developing country of origin and thus serve as invisible exports was hardly convincing particularly if the funds came back through black markets at unfavourable rates of exchange for the recipient country and thus outside the grasp of the governments, which had paid the original cost of the education. (Abel-Smith 1987: 117; Chapter 8)

In small states such as Fiji the loss of health workers brought references to the brain drain as early as 1974, but negative impacts were implicit rather than evident (Bartsch 1974). However, there was a general perception that, at least until the end of the 1980s, a significant part of all migration was of doctors, and there was an effective oversupply of both doctors and nurses in many countries, so that retaining more doctors would not necessarily be helpful where few people could afford to pay for health care and governments could not cover their health needs (Mejia 1987: 49–53). A decade later attitudes had become less sanguine: doctors were losses, not overspill, nurse migration had become problematic and more appropriate skill mixes and health financing systems were needed.

As migration became more widespread, its effects became more obvious. By 1991, emigration from Samoa had meant that most Samoan doctors practising in the public system were either of retirement age above 60 (15 out of 34) or new graduates (8 of the 34 being aged less than 35), while most of the remainder were United Nations volunteer doctors. Several doctors had been brought back from retirement to cope with the shortage (World Bank 1994: 315). In India, despite the production of thousands of doctors between the mid-1970s and mid-1980s, the overall ratio of population to doctors increased as doctors left government jobs either to emigrate or establish private practices, and the ratio increased fastest in rural areas as doctors moved into the cities (Akhtar and Izhar 1994: 224). In India, Samoa and elsewhere it was implicit that a worsening ratio of doctors and nurses to patients meant inferior health care, but direct evidence of this, for example in higher rates of morbidity or mortality, was absent (and, in any case, would not necessarily correlate with the decline in availability of human resources). The wider global context has witnessed a deteriorating relationship between health-worker density and health status (Anand and Barnighausen 2004). Over time, the impact of migration in source countries has increased, certainly in terms of the number of migrants, but also on health systems. India and the Philippines, both long-term providers of migratory health workers in circumstances initially described as an overflow (Oommen 1989), are more obviously affected, in terms of inadequate and declining nurse:patient ratios, the loss of more experienced nurses, the retraining (and loss) of doctors and the closure of many hospitals (see below). Although the impact of losses has become clearer, it is not much better documented.

CLOSURES AND VACANCY RATES

In certain circumstances the quantitative outcome of migration was fairly obvious, notably in the Philippines (see below). Vacancy rates are extremely high in parts of SSA and the Caribbean, where two states, Trinidad & Tobago, and Jamaica, have nurse vacancy rates of over 50 per cent (Caribbean Commission on Health and Development 2006). In Kenya and Ghana, more than half of nursing positions remain unfilled (Buchan et al. 2004; Volqvartz 2005). In Zimbabwe by 1997, only 29 per cent of all national positions were filled (Chikanda 2004) even before the most rapid international migration. The scale of migration can also be so substantial that it is implausible that there are not significant outcomes. Some 90 per cent of Ghanaian doctors trained between 1985 and 1994 had migrated to the UK within a few years (Dovlo and Nyonator 1999) and 91 per cent trained between 1998 and 2002 also did so (Mensah 2005), while all the 1999 nursing graduates of the University of Malawi had gone within six years (Likupe et al. 2006). A Ugandan doctor observed in 2008: 'I graduated from medical school in 1999. I am the only one of my entire class who has remained in the country. Everyone else now works abroad' (quoted in Millen 2008: 8). In Ghana, 43 per cent of doctors' posts were unfilled in 1999 and 47 per cent by 2002 (Buchan and Dovlo 2004). Where few health workers were left, tasks could not be accomplished. Nurses and midwives in Guyana were too few for new HIV/AIDS prevention programmes since all were needed to work with those who already had HIV/AIDS (Anderson and Isaacs 2007). Lack of staff in many African countries also meant a decreased ability to get medication to patients effectively (Awases et al. 2004: 50). In Malawi, the loss of many nurses to the UK brought the near collapse of maternity services everywhere and meant that only 78 per cent of ministry positions were filled, with 65 per cent of nursing positions being vacant (Palmer 2006). In the Lilongwe Central Hospital ten midwives sought to cope with delivering more than 10,000 babies per year, which meant that many births were not attended (Muula et al. 2003; Dugger 2004; Clark et al. 2006). In Zambia, maternal mortality has increased: 'when doctors and nurses leave a health system the first death marker to skyrocket is the number of women who die in childbirth' (Garrett 2007: 32). In Kenya, staff shortages became so critical that, at Nairobi's public maternity hospital, nurses often cared for 60 to 90 patients in a ten-hour shift (*Afrol News*, 28 May 2004). Even in developed countries such as Australia the lack of specialist obstetricians in rural areas has led to half the rural obstetrics units in New South Wales closing since 1994, resulting in a rise in delivery problems (*Sunday Telegraph*, 14 June 2009).

Surgery often suffers from health-worker shortages, since specialists are more likely to migrate; hence lack of access to surgical care constitutes a public health crisis in developing countries (and it has not benefited from disease-oriented global programmes). In Ghana, 'too many people to recount' are turned away from hospitals where there are insufficient SHWs to perform surgery (Mensah 2005: 209). Operating theatres for cardiac surgery at one of the most expensive hospitals in Malaysia have not been used since 2005 because of a shortage of cardiac-thoracic surgeons and expensive equipment is unused since there are too few specialists (*New Straits Times*, 5 December 2008). A shortage of anaesthetists in Fiji has meant the cancellation of operations. Uganda has an exceptionally low level of operations. The proportion of positions filled is even lower in post-conflict countries like Sierra Leone and Liberia, where migration has been substantial, and resources extremely limited. In Sierra Leone the average age of surgeons was 57 – and most had been brought back from retirement, as others went overseas, were lost 'to an internal brain drain' into NGOs, and there was no 'new generation' of replacements – while hospitals were without basic infrastructure (such as running water) and supplies; hence few could deliver anything beyond very limited surgical capacity (Kingham et al. 2009). While such data are fragmentary, and some may represent worst-case scenarios, but others the tips of icebergs, they point to difficult circumstances in many countries, particularly in SSA.

Closure of facilities may be the sequel to inadequate numbers of workers. The recruitment of several nurses from a cardiovascular unit in a provincial Filipino hospital effectively meant that the unit had to be closed down (Alkire and Chen 2004). At the start of the 1990s the University Hospital of the West Indies had a shortage of nurses, radiographers, pharmacists, lab technicians, dieticians and social workers, and three wards had been closed because of the labour shortage. Fewer patients could be admitted, while the recovery times of patients who were not admitted took longer; although hospital mortality rates had not declined because doctors had taken up some of the slack created by absent nurses and more patients had been 'forced to make greater use of the primary health care system' with unknown consequences (Brown 1997: 212). In Trinidad, wards have been closed, maternity units closed, and male and female units been merged, raising cultural issues, and immunisation coverage and *in situ* training have both declined (Schmid 2003). Research and training facilities have experienced particular problems from labour shortages. The shortage of SHWs in Jamaica meant that the extent of training was reduced, its quality fell (becoming more theoretical than practical) and supervision similarly declined. This resulted in the greater 'incompetence' of new nurses and a breakdown of respect for management structures, resulting in deterioration in the quality of health care and 'disruption of the socialization process of crucial importance in the output of properly trained nurses' (Brown 1997: 210–11, 214). In Nigeria, most medical research institutions have long closed because of earlier emigration of highly skilled doctors (Ojo 1990), and in Thailand migration substantially impeded the development of sustainable research capacity (Sitthi-amorn and Somrongthong 2000). Geriatrics and mental health wards have suffered widely.

The selectivity of migration means that those best able to train, mentor and manage also tend to be migrants. In some cases there have been direct losses from training institutions, such as the Fiji School of Medicine, both overseas and into the private sector. Thailand has experienced a 'brain drain' from public universities, in public health, nursing and medicine, into the private sector where salaries are higher (Bunnag 2008). Migration has both directly reduced the number of qualified supervisors and tutors, and indirectly reduced the amount and quality of guidance. As so many migrants are relatively senior and experienced workers, the loss of both valuable mentoring and more formal training is almost universal, reducing levels of competence and capability. This has also resulted in greater resort being made to technology, and even clinical simulation laboratories (Hancock 2008), but these are not widely available or easily maintained, and nor can they properly simulate 'real-world' situations. Younger nurses have limited opportunities or time to interact informally with more senior nurses. Staff and patients are joint victims of inadequate human resources.

WORKLOADS, WAITING AND MORALE

In most places, neither wards nor hospitals have closed when staff numbers fall, but have continued functioning, perhaps inadequately, with a skeleton staff whose workloads increase and whose morale declines. Greater workloads are less likely to be accomplished successfully, while some previous activities are foregone. In Ghana and Zimbabwe, workloads have increased in parallel with migration, with the workload of midwives doubling in five years (Awases et al. 2004: 35–7). At much the same time the loss of nurses from Taiwan was argued to have reduced ability to care for the elderly (Brush 2008: 21). Maternal health care has been affected in Gambia and Malawi, with increased workloads, waiting and consultation times and poorer infection control (Gerein et al. 2006). Health workers themselves perceive the decline, in such qualitative factors as respect for patients and care-givers, and attention to, and general communication with, patients. A South African nurse in the UK pointed to the dilemma of obtaining benefits for her own family and the social cost to the wider society: 'We are having [a] better opportunity of taking those pounds, money to live and your children can get something. That is why our hospitals are empty at home, they are suffering, our people are suffering. Our parents are suffering, they go to hospital' (quoted in Larsen et al. 2005: 361). Similarly, Nigerian migrant nurses felt guilt and responsibility for lack of health care through their absence (see below), although guilt need not necessarily mean worsened care. In Zimbabwe, staff shortages resulted in patients being turned away from public clinics so that staff could work in their private clinics without an excess workload, with obvious reductions in care and equity (Chikanda 2008).

In recent years, foreign aid programmes have expanded in SSA, to provide drugs to millions affected by tuberculosis and AIDS, yet, ironically, these programmes have been hard to implement, with too few nurses to administer them effectively, so that private sector recruitment has had to be expanded by pushing wages up significantly, with disastrous consequences for the public sector (Volqvartz 2005; Garrett 2007). In Fiji, the emigration of SHWs, alongside internal population migration in response to new economic circumstances, meant that some new clinics had no new staff and fewer SHWs were available to vaccinate children. In the early part of this century the vaccination coverage rate fell from 95 per cent to below 80 per cent and in 2006 Fiji reported many new cases of measles, from which it had been free since 1998. To return the vaccination rate to normal took a massive mobilisation of SHWs with other work being put on hold for three months (Ken 2008). Downward trends in immunisation coverage in the Philippines and some Caribbean states have also been attributed to the migration of nurses (Lorenzo et al. 2007; Yan 2006). Once again it is difficult to distinguish the direct impacts of migration from those of inadequate funding.

Many anecdotal reports emphasise longer waiting times, which raise the opportunity costs of health care, and may result in medical attention coming too late. In Zimbabwe, over a quarter of health workers believed that longer waiting times had resulted in unnecessary deaths that prompt attention could have prevented (Chikanda 2004). Waiting times were problems in Fiji and at least four African countries, and some health facilities had reduced opening times, especially in rural areas (Connell 2009: 130; Awases et al. 2004: 50, 58). Occasionally there is no point waiting; as a village elder in northern Ghana commented:

> When I was a young man people would wait in very long lines to see a nurse or doctor. This was normal back then and we complained . . . But at least we had something to wait for. Today the long lines in so many areas have gone; people simply have no-one to consult. Now we are dying of ailments that used to be so simple to treat. We are sitting here wondering where our health workers have gone. (Quoted in Millen 2008: 8)

Facilities elsewhere may open irregularly, providing no security of care.

The additional workloads imposed on those who remain influence subsequent migration. Decreased morale (albeit subjective), and even fatigue, stress and overwork, create a perception that circumstances can only worsen if more people go. Fatigue may lead to wrong diagnoses and decisions, and may even be manifest in physical symptoms. In 2004, eight Fijian nurses, all aged between 40 and 50, died – a situation partly attributed by the Fijian Nursing Association to the burdens of additional work (Connell 2009: 127). In Palau, increased overtime work alongside restrictions on leave not only caused 'fatigue and a general decline in morale', but overtime payments added $300,000 to the health budget (Miho 2007). Social and economic costs were combined. In Jamaica the loss of nurses meant a significant increase in nurse:patient ratios, so that nurses made decisions to focus on those who were more seriously ill but 'such decisions weigh heavily on the conscience of nurses causing some to suffer acute emotional distress' (Brown 1997: 210). In turn this accentuates migration and may herald an upward spiral of migration, particularly where migrants formally go 'on leave' – an extension of the phenomenon of 'ghost workers' – and cannot easily be replaced until it is clear that they are not returning.

The impact of emigration (and inadequate financial provision) has usually been most evident in remote regions where losses tend to be greater, and where resources were initially least adequate, as rural workers also fill urban vacancies. Negative impacts on the health care system of source countries have fallen particularly on the rural (and urban) poor who are most dependent on public health systems, further emphasising the 'inverse care law'. Health services in many rural and regional areas have declined, while health workers have less time to make visits and work with communities; hence preventive health care, and the poor, receive less attention. Some 'remote' areas may be quite close to urban centres, as in Fiji, where even villages 30 km from the capital city now lack nurses to support primary health care initiatives or even simply monitor particular health needs (Jerety 2008). A further outcome of worsening rural services is that residents have increasingly chosen, or been effectively forced, to bypass their officially designated clinics, to ensure more adequate treatment at regional centres, even for minor health care problems. In a sense rural problems become urban problems, at some economic cost to patients (both directly – transport and even accommodation – and in terms of opportunity costs), resulting in the under-utilisation of rural health centres and congestion and inefficiency in the hospitals (Connell 2009: 131). This emphasises that the more remote and worst facilities are for the rural poor, while under-utilisation suggests that they need no new resources. Migration is a vicious circle for rural and regional areas.

REFERRALS, OVERSEAS TREATMENT AND HEALTH TOURISM

A further consequence of health-worker migration is that some patients travel overseas for health care, or choose other forms of domestic care (see below), either because waiting times are too long, particular specialisations are unavailable or perceived quality at home is too low. Where such referrals are paid by the state, the cost is considerable. Even where they are not, as is usually the case in Asia, resources are nevertheless transferred overseas. In many countries referrals are of elites (who might in any case go overseas), but at considerable cost to national budgets and to equity. Even in countries that are relatively well supplied with health personnel, the cost of referrals is considerable, making the task of financing local health systems and organising more labour-intensive preventive health care more difficult.

Limited specialisation, a lack of funds and migration of SHWs – and a consequent high level of referrals – are particularly significant in small island states (Connell 2009: 31–5). In a group of six African countries referrals increased at the same time as health-worker migration, resulting in 'an unprecedented increase in both expense of care to fewer people and in the use of foreign currency, which could have been used for other development programmes or even for the motivation and retention of the country's health workers' (Awases et al. 2004: 57). Nigerians have been estimated to spend as much as $20 billion per year on health costs outside Nigeria (Neelankantan 2003). With high levels of referrals, national health systems are likely to be regarded as inferior by many of the local population. Lack of SHWs may not be the primary motivation for travelling overseas for treatment, but it none the less contributes to and represents a loss of scarce resources, although it could also allow the domestic health system to focus more on primary health care.

In the past decade health tourism has also resulted in changing structures of transnational migration, as people sought better, cheaper, more rapid or more flexible health care overseas, especially in such Asian states as India, Thailand and Singapore, while mainly coming from the Gulf and the developed world. Again, while not usually primarily a response to the lack of SHWs in the source countries, it has contributed to a dual health care system where rich migrant patients can secure better care than local people, and in the destinations disproportionately more SHWs respond to their needs, accentuating urban bias (Connell 2006, 2008a). A number of Indian doctors have returned to India because of opportunities for earning the salaries that come from practising in the elite private sector hospitals that cater to medical tourists. There, and also in Thailand, doctors have moved away from rural areas to provide more lucrative services for health tourists (Wibulpolrasert et al. 2004), and the distribution of health workers has become more skewed.

THE RISE AND COMPETITION OF THE PRIVATE SECTOR

Remaining in the country rather than migrating may involve health workers moving into the better-resourced private sector, where wages and working conditions are superior (see Chapter 2), in parallel with rural–urban migration, as in the particular case of health tourism (above). Crises in the public sector have resulted in boosts to the private sector; patients lose faith in public health as SHWs cross over, or spend increasing parts of their time in private or NGO realms. Many SHWs, returning from training or employment overseas, have sought to move there. Movement has invariably been in one direction into a sector that often supports a small proportion of the local population, sometimes dominated by expatriates, and provides a model where health care is accessible to the relatively affluent. As a result of stress and heavier workloads, public sector staff have tended 'to neglect public responsibilities' to work in the private sector where wages are significantly higher (Mutizwa-Mangiza 1998). The movement of health workers to the private sector, at the same time as international migration, has disadvantaged the poor, most of whom cannot afford higher private sector costs, alongside growing evidence of less adequate public sector services (Gerein et al. 2006).

In Kenya and Malawi 'large numbers' of health workers have moved into the expanding private sector, including the various NGOs charged with ameliorating HIV/AIDS, where wages are typically three or four times those in the public sector (Palmer 2006). Malaysian nurses have moved into the private sector to avoid poor salaries and long working hours, so that Malaysia has to recruit from other countries (Birks et al. 2009). In Fiji, from the start of the 1980s, the proportion of SHWs in the private sector went from zero to about 20 per cent of all doctors and nurses by the end of the 1990s, almost all in the capital city, posing concerns over health care delivery elsewhere (Connell 2009: 33). In Thailand, the growth of private hospitals in the early 1990s, almost all in Bangkok (and most of which operated considerably below capacity), led to a significant rural–urban migration of doctors, resulting in the difference between the ratio of doctors to people in Bangkok and in the poorest north-east region increasing from 9 to 14 between 1986 and 1997, despite Bangkok's own rapid expansion. Over roughly the same time period the bed-to-doctor ratio in rural district hospitals increased from 7 to 15. Before the Asian economic crisis of 1997, some 21 rural hospitals functioned without a single doctor, and this number increased further after the crisis (Wibulpolprasert et al. 2004). Although medical tourism aggravated the internal drain of SHWs from rural public to urban private facilities 'the bigger causes are the increasing demand for health care among the richer urban Thai population who have higher purchasing power, the social and wealth inequity and the education systems of the qualified health professionals' (Wibulpolprasert and Pachanee 2008: 14). Where middle classes are similarly emerging, notably elsewhere in Asia, as in Singapore, Taiwan and Malaysia, a similar situation of privatisation, migration and diminished equity has also occurred.

REPLACEMENT

Where part of the workforce has migrated, some countries have been able to introduce replacements, either less formally skilled workers, undertaking similar tasks, or skilled workers from abroad. In countries such as Cameroon and Zimbabwe, migration of SHWs resulted in less- or nonqualified people, such as nurse aides, performing tasks that were beyond their expected duties, with the implicit risk of misdiagnosis or inadequate response (Chikanda 2004). Similarly, in several African countries 'young recruits are often left alone to carry out work without supervision, at the risk of making incorrect diagnoses and prescribing inappropriate treatment, while unqualified personnel are left to perform duties that are specialized, and beyond their scope of practice, which may endanger the lives of patients' (Awases et al. 2004: 58).

In several countries patients have turned or reverted to the informal sector with sometimes costly and uncertain outcomes. In Zimbabwe and India, the reduction in numbers of formal medical practitioners has meant that poorer patients especially have resorted more to traditional medical practitioners, especially since in Zimbabwe some claim to cure HIV/AIDS (Chikanda 2004), and to 'amateur doctors' in India (Mullan 2004). While the impact of this on health outcomes was not stated for Zimbabwe, the implication of spurious claims to cure HIV/AIDS suggests that this is unlikely to be beneficial for health outcomes (and in some cases can be expensive). In India, deaths might have been prevented and some patients experienced high costs. A more usual outcome is simply the lack of resort to health care, sometimes until it is too late.

In some Pacific island states, such as Vanuatu, Fiji and the Cook Islands, local workers have been replaced by Bulgarians, Filipinos, Nigerians and Burmese, and most recently by Cubans and Taiwanese (Connell 2009; de Vos et al. 2007), as part of the cascading global care chain. In 2006 as many as 90 (22 per cent) of Fiji's establishment of doctors – with 65 positions unfilled – were expatriates (Oman et al. 2009). Some replacements have been from developed countries under aid agreements. In several countries migrating workers have been replaced by Cubans, in a form of 'medical diplomacy', most going to Spanish-speaking countries in South America, but also to SSA. Cuban doctors were seen to be cheaper, more motivated and more cost-effective than other possible international recruits, and with knowledge of tropical diseases. Many replacements have come at some expense from several states, such as Burma and the Philippines, where health care was inferior to that of the destinations. In the Pacific, the Caribbean and SSA, such replacement SHWs tended to move from places of greater need to places of lesser need: Fijians moved to Nauru, Palau and the Marshall Islands, Guyanans went to Barbados and Bermuda, and Botswanans went to South Africa. Even such small fragments of the global care chain display considerable selectivity in taking health workers to places where salaries are greater and needs are fewer: the inverse care law revisited regionally.

Reliance on expatriates in what are otherwise source countries imposes obvious costs, including salaries, recruitment fees, travel and local subsidies. Salaries are often substantially more than those of local doctors. Replacements may be less effective because of language and cultural differences, which restrict their ability to provide health services, contribute to training and enable sustainability. Immigrant health workers have usually been directed to more remote regions, where needs are greatest, but where English (the language of most migrant health workers) is less likely to be spoken, so creating a basis for confusion. Anglophone Caribbean and Pacific states, such as Antigua and Nauru, experienced language problems following immigration of Cuban doctors and nurses. Japan thus sought to establish language schools in the Philippines before a formal agreement on health-worker migration was in place. In Kiribati, local people believe that Western-trained doctors are too busy, and not adequately emotionally involved with their patients:

> The foreign practitioners do not speak Gilbertese and need a translator. The interaction becomes too complicated and too impersonal, the patient feels insecure, uneasy and becomes too resentful towards the medical practitioner . . . commonly expressed in the attitude of the patient to prescribed drugs, in that patients fail to take the prescribed medication. (Christensen 1995: 103)

While patients and other workers have complained about the difficulty in communicating with some expatriate workers, these claims, like most abstract claims attached to foreign incompetence, cannot easily be verified. Similar problems occur in developed countries. Recruitment of Eastern European doctors in Germany posed language issues for doctor–patient relations and day-to-day dealings with German colleagues, may have caused misdiagnosis and led to 'paperwork' often being done by German colleagues, to their displeasure (Kopetsch 2009). However, language problems have declined, as English has gradually come to dominate not just the world of medicine, although they continue to influence perceptions of failures in practice. Other potential disadvantages are similar everywhere, reflecting varied medical backgrounds, different quality standards and cultural sensitivies (Connell 2009: 135). By contrast, local SHWs tend to be ambivalent about their expatriate colleagues: frustrated over their superior wages, notably so in Zimbabwe (Oberoi and Lin 2006), sometimes finding expatriates to be aloof, but also recognising that many come from different, more modern, technical backgrounds and have useful skills that could be acquired. The supposed failures of migrant replacements are part of a perception that the health system is not providing an adequate service, while demonstrating that health and health care are cultural phenomena.

TRANSNATIONAL CARE LOSSES

Social costs are attached to the migration of SHWs, since the case is often that of women moving as individuals and, in many cases, leaving families at home for some period of time (e.g. van Eyck 2005). Separation of families, across and between countries, usually does little for family harmony, despite the transnational corporation of kin being an accepted basis for migration. There can be social benefits: many Fijian nurses moved to the Marshall Islands to escape unhappy relationships and achieved greater happiness (Rokoduru 2008), but that appears exceptional. Existing relationships may disintegrate over distance.

In the Caribbean, the children of migrant nurses, referred to as 'barrel children' (from the time when parents in the UK or elsewhere sent back goods to them in barrels), tend to be cared for by their grandparents. Universally such children have to make multiple adjustments, experiencing considerable stress, with negative effects on child development and adolescent behaviour, within a 'care deficit', where fathers, children and other kin were left behind (Parrenas 2002; Jones et al. 2004). However, in other contexts, as for Kerala nurses in the Gulf, the women and their families all gained in status through migration and its economic benefits without evident social cost (Percot 2005; Percot and Rajan 2007). Success had broad advantages:

> As nursing opened up a window of opportunity for young women to contribute to the family income, there was a concurrent change in their status both in the family and in wider Kerala society. These young women were transformed from burdens and liabilities into financial assets within the family. (George 2005: 41–2)

While women were rarely 'burdens and liabilities' in other parts of the world, and their contribution to household budgets is unquestionable, doubts remain over the social costs.

Overseas the outcome for many is much like that described by Joyce and Hunt for Filipino workers in the USA a quarter of a century ago:

> though work in the US presented many difficult and unexpected problems for the migrant groups, including the prejudice of other workers, assignments to onerous tasks, and distress from family separation, most migrant nurses were fairly satisfied with life and work in the US. (1982: 1223)

Similarly, Nigerian nurses in the UK resented being seen as merely 'black foreigners' and the racism this entailed, but were willing to endure this and deskilling for economic gains for themselves and their extended families

(Aboderin 2007; see Chapter 9). For most SHWs, migration choices were ultimately voluntary and could be avoided or escaped when wholly negative.

The loss of skilled workers thus affects not only formal institutional settings but is of considerable domestic significance, since health workers are valuable elsewhere than in the workplace. In Nigeria, the migration of nurses has had wide-ranging social consequences:

> The health system is such that necessary care is not easily accessible unless one is close to 'gatekeepers' with connections; nurses prior to migration play such a crucial gatekeeper role for older relatives, and other family members, due to their professional knowledge and contacts. Their absence can mean a serious reduction in older adults' access to adequate routine or critical health care when needed – with sometimes fatal consequences. Nurses expressed a sense of guilt and responsibility for not having been there to help improve their parents' (or other relatives') health or even prevent their deaths. (Harper et al. 2008: 167)

It is not just the loss of health workers that reduces the availability of health care, since many migrants, including of course SHWs, previously played some role in the care of elderly relatives. In Albania, 'remittances flowed back, but in other non-material aspects older people – known as "orphan pensioners" – were left to fend for themselves in an economic and social environment stripped of any meaningful welfare structures' (Vullnetari and King 2008: 142). While over relatively short distances, contact and return increase at times of crisis, and distant care can occur (Baldassar 2007), this is not always possible. Where migration has been significant, a 'care drain', analogous to the brain drain of SHWs, has emerged where demographic changes (declining birth rates, the reduction in family size, and migration) have reduced the number of accessible carers, sometimes at a time of more limited national welfare provision. This gendered care drain is part of the global care chain, where immigrant women fill the care gap in richer countries but 'in migrating to supply care to others, the women – from Albania, the Philippines, Peru and many other poor countries – are depriving their own families and elderly parents of the care they need and expect' (Vullnetari and King 2008: 145, 153). The costs of this emerging care deficit are both emotional, such as the absence of extended family life and loneliness, and physical, as in the inability to be cared for when sick or taken to hospital. There are complex relationships:

> At one level women [migrants] are increasing their agency and power. But there's a cost. A lot of women will have children raised by their own mothers. Their husbands won't be faithful. If nurses send money home to their husband, he usually spends it on commodities. So these women lose intimacy and connectedness of family life, and even if they decide to return home, they find that

all their money has been spent on things like stereo systems or other things – or even other women – and there's nothing left from all their hard work. (Lesley Hawthorne, quoted by Gordon 2005: 381)

Yet, as more general accounts of remittances indicate, this may well be another worst-case scenario. While much depends on the structure and duration of migration, the loss of SHWs is just one part of a global migration context where children and older people can be disadvantaged.

THE COMPLICATIONS OF LOSS

Most data that directly refer to the impacts of the migration of SHWs are either anecdotal or selectively refer to the worst-affected, albeit critically important, contexts. While this chapter is far from comprehensive, it demonstrates the continued need to go from assumptions to evidence since, as various examples indicate, it is extremely difficult to disentangle real outcomes from bias or prejudice, and the impacts of migration from other changes. While assumptions about worsened health outcomes from higher patient:doctor ratios are entirely reasonable, specific data that corroborate this are largely and perhaps necessarily absent; too many variables are involved.

Ultimately, the existence of extreme cases – the closure of wards, the inability to undertake certain procedures, the collapse of morale – emphasises that migration alongside movement into the private sector (especially at the same time as limited financial support) poses obvious problems for health sectors. It is improbable that work is adequately accomplished with fewer SHWs, especially when it is the best, brightest and more experienced, those with 'get up and go', who have tended to leave. Middle management, and technical support too, may also have departed, resulting in substantial problems of organisation (and the devolution of bureaucracy and technical preparation to hard-pressed practitioners). Institutional knowledge disappears. At the very least, the families of health workers suffer from their absence, despite economic gains (Chapter 8). Increased workloads, diminished social support and mentoring, and decreased morale become a small but vicious cycle, while high costs of repeated training, replacement and referrals – where the latter two exist – are additional consequences.

Recent trends in both the Philippines and India indicate that what might once have been seen as an 'overflow' with significant national economic benefits can no longer be seen so positively. Even then, a quarter of a century ago, Goldfarb et al. (1984) asked, 'Why did the Philippines government allow the use of scarce capital for expansion of medical education when so many doctors then chose to leave?' Early fears in the Philippines were ignored as the number of training establishments increased, and remittance flows were substantial. The Philippines went extremely quickly from a situation towards the end of the 1990s when there was unemployment of nurses, so that many worked only in hotels, shops and fast-food outlets (Lipley and Stokes 1998) and migration was logical, to unfilled vacancies a decade later. This occurred at a time when the number of nursing schools went from about 140 in 1970 and 200 in 1998 to about 460 in 2005, most being private and expensive so that graduates had to get jobs overseas to pay off the cost, thus reducing the short-term benefits. Thus education became 'a business not a means of developing skills and competency' (Marilyn Lorenzo, pers. comm., 2005). Sixty per cent of nursing schools focus on 'second-timers', people with professional training who wish to become nurses to work overseas, and have curricula oriented to overseas needs. Despite the increased numbers of schools, the number of nurses produced in the 2000s is less than the number leaving each year, few of whom later return to nursing. In 2006 the recruitment of nurses from the Philippines went up by 65 per cent, 'destroying the core of qualified experienced nurses in many of its hospitals' (Aminuzaman 2006: 9). About 150,000 registered nurses (some 85 per cent of all Filipino nurses) are presently working overseas. 'An attractive offer from a recruiting agency can clean out a ward, a unit or even an entire provincial hospital [to] suck out the workers in busloads and leave their hospitals employee-less' (Manuel Dayrit, Director of WHO Department of Human Resources for Health, quoted in Cheng 2009: 111). The nurses who were most likely to leave were the most skilled, including intensive care unit (ICU) nurses, so depleting the number of managers and trainers. Although turnover has been extremely high, most hospitals remain able to recruit enough poorly trained younger nurses. However, as many as 200 hospitals have closed and many have scaled down their services in recent years, with up to 30,000 nursing vacancies. By 2007, more than 3500 Filipino doctors, many of whom had been doctors for more than ten years and had specialised training, had become 'nurse medics' and 400 more were training to become nurses. Fewer doctors now graduate annually and many choose to work in hospitals in Manila, where salaries are higher. It has been estimated that 70 per cent of Filipinos die without receiving medical attention, especially in regional areas. On some islands, doctors are fearful of operating with inadequate numbers of nurses. About 80 per cent of doctors were seeking to move overseas in 2006. The quality of some nursing schools was so poor that 23 were closed in 2005, while the number of nurses passing graduation exams is falling, indicating the lack of trainers and suggesting that the number of initially qualified recruits may be declining. Limited data exist on the remittances of Filipino health workers (cf. Buchan 2008; Humphries et al. 2009), but they are undoubtedly substantial. Global demand for health workers with proficiency in English may have proved costly to the state but beneficial to households (Kline 2003; Lorenzo 2006; Brush and Sochalski 2007; Lorenzo et al. 2007; Perrin et al. 2007; Cheng 2009). A broadly similar, but less well-documented, situation has occurred in India, where numbers of both migratory nurses and doctors have increased, and inadequate numbers of nurses exist in as many as 38,000 private and public hospitals (Khaliq et al. 2008: 9). Where migration rates are much the same as rates of training, such trends are disturbing.

Health systems require adequate numbers of health workers, and many countries are significantly below that level (Chapter 2), and an appropriate mix of skills, which are not easily substitutable; both of these are affected by migration. The unpredictability of future migration flows challenges human resource planning and extends the duration of what might have been short-term costs because of long training times, and the need for constant repetition if migrants do not return (Chapter 8). The complex social costs of migration are particularly difficult to evaluate – but in most cases migrants themselves make these evaluations (at least for themselves and their families). There are much wider implications for countries. While almost all analyses of the actual migration of health workers – whether international or internal – point to substantial disadvantages for source countries and regions, advantages exist through the flow of remittances and return migration. These can now be examined as a means of making a broader assessment of the costs and benefits of the international migration of health workers.

8. The costs and benefits of skill drain

For half a century there has been concern over the extent to which the migration of SHWs constituted a skill or brain drain, if there was a significant loss or merely an 'overflow', and how costly this might be for the source countries. Despite the obvious significance of such issues, there has been remarkably little detailed analysis. Anecdotes, assumptions and crude estimates have tended to focus on worst-case scenarios, to analyse only part of the situation and to have been confined to a small number of cases. Countries that lose the most skilled migrants have been assumed to bear the heaviest costs, but this is not necessarily so. This chapter therefore seeks to provide a more detailed analysis of the costs, benefits and consequences of the skill drain, at various scales, although this too is necessarily fragmented and incomplete. Migration occurs in very different circumstances.

For 'source countries', where the balance of flows is outwards, there is an overall loss of workers and thus a skill or brain drain. Early on it was argued for countries such as India and the Philippines that the flow was of 'excess' workers – an overflow – since national needs were adequately met. More recently it has been argued, for both India and Pakistan, that since the shortage of doctors was in rural areas and 'most of those doctors who migrate overseas were unlikely to settle in rural areas', it was not a loss (Dalmia 2006: 281; Aly and Taj 2008). In contexts where rural health needs were often inadequately met, as in India, that was always debatable (Engels and Connell 1983). However, exactly how the migration of SHWs might be evaluated has long been open to debate, where there are social and economic costs and benefits, between sectors and between individuals, households, regions and the state.

The extent of migration from the Philippines meant that debate over its impact largely began there. Early on, in the 1960s, while there was some concern over the impact of the migration of SHWs on high vacancy rates, there was ambivalence over the existence of a 'brain drain', not because flows did not exist but because they were seen as reasonable, rational and justifiable, being in response to high levels of national unemployment, low public sector wages and poor working conditions (Choy 2003: 105). It was also argued that migrant health workers generated remittances that made their loss acceptable since this compensated countries even if there was some loss of needed workers. For the Philippines it was calculated, largely theoretically, that the gain from the remittances of overseas doctors was large enough to compensate for other economic losses from migration (Goldfarb et al. 1984). Arguments that this was an overflow could partly be justified, since the number of nursing schools rose from 17 to 140 between 1950 and 1970, to produce more migrant workers (Joyce and Hunt 1982). However, the assumption that at any time there was simply an overflow was questioned, given high nurse and doctor to patient ratios, and high disease burdens. 'Overflows' were at best localised in better-served metropolitan areas. Indeed, in 1973 President Marcos issued a decree that nurses must work for four months in a rural area before they could graduate, in order to relieve rural shortages in the Philippines. At the same time the president of the Philippines Nursing Association was drawing attention to the much better ratios in destination countries like the USA and Canada: 'these are the countries that are importing our nurses yet their ratio is more than we presently have' (quoted in Choy 2003: 114). A broadly similar situation existed in India – a supposedly 'Indian paradox' – and on a much smaller scale elsewhere. By contrast, it was also evident that not all migration was a 'loss' as some workers returned, perhaps with new skills and capital, while most sent remittances.

The earliest studies of the brain drain argued that three types of transfer costs from the source to the recipient country created unfavourable effects: the investment in education and training of migrants (including income tax revenues); the additional jobs that the spending of migrants would otherwise have generated; and the economies that would have emerged from productivity increases (Bhagwati and Hamada 1974); hence migration resulted in slower economic growth and lowered standards of living for the poor. Such perspectives, though only partly applicable to health workers, whose productivity is only indirectly transferred into economic growth, have substantially informed subsequent analyses, but must be extended to take note of return migration and remittance flows. There have, however, been almost as many methodologies as conclusions.

THE ECONOMICS OF MIGRATION

The few economic studies of the 'brain drain' of SHWs have been conducted in Africa. These reveal significant economic losses to sending countries, and considerable cost savings for recipient countries in hiring overseas trained SHWs, rather than training them locally, so that the international migration of SHWs has been described as an inequitable, perverse and unjust subsidy from a relatively poor country to a relatively rich one (Mensah et al. 2005; Mackintosh et al. 2006). Training of health workers is expensive, because of the long duration, costly materials and techniques (and the common need for postgraduate education and training programmes), and is a burden on relatively poor states, whether directly or through scholarship provision. When trained workers migrate, and the process must be repeated for a new cohort, costs mount further. Most estimates have been based almost entirely on the costs of education, rather than additional costs based on foregone health care or lost productivity, or the possible gains from remittances or return migration.

In most SSA countries, governments fully or partially finance education and training for doctors, and usually for nurses; hence the costs of primary, secondary and tertiary education are primarily borne by the state. In middle-income countries, including the Philippines and India, private provision of education – at least at tertiary level – is significant; hence state losses are much reduced. A handful of 'back-of the-envelope' calculations exist, in contexts where almost all education is funded by the state. In the late 1980s it was estimated that the value of a migrant doctor from Nigeria was $30,000, based on all education costs and the value of the service that the doctor would have rendered if remaining in Nigeria (Ojo 1990: 635). The African Union has estimated that, if the cost of training a general practice doctor is estimated at $60,000 and that of other medical auxiliaries at $12,000, then low-income African countries subsidise high-income countries by about $500 million a year through their migration. Another estimate has suggested that there are 3 million health workers from developing countries in developed countries, and since it costs developed countries an estimated $184,000 to train one, the overall cost to developing countries has been $552 billion, about the same as the total overseas debt of these countries (Kimani 2005). It has similarly been estimated that, through migration, Ghana has foregone around £35 million ($55 million) of its training investment in health professionals (Martineau et al. 2002). A more detailed analysis, including primary and secondary education costs, suggested that for each doctor and nurse emigrating from Kenya the lost investment represented $517,931 and $338,868 respectively. This excluded all costs from the reduced effectiveness of health care, while the authors noted the 'relatively meagre remittances' of overseas SHWs and the significant unmet demand for health care, so concluding that 'such continued plunder of investments embodied in human resources contributes to further underdevelopment of Kenya and to keeping a majority of her people in the vicious cycle of ill-health and poverty' (Kirigia et al. 2006: 1). Adopting the same methodology, Mwaniki and Dulo concluded that in the single year 2006 losses to Kenya could be even more than that, dependent on interest rates (2008: 21). Similarly, based on primary, secondary and tertiary education costs, the total cost of training a registered nurse-midwife in Malawi has been estimated at $31,726, with the country losing $71,081 had that income been otherwise invested (Muula et al. 2006). The migration of an average of 40 doctors a year from South Africa to Canada from 1986 to 2000 represented the annual capital transfer of $4 million (Grant 2006). Another estimate suggests that it costs $27,500 to train each doctor in Uganda, but this excludes the costs of training at different educational levels before medical school and the remuneration of those involved in training programmes (Awases et al. 2004: 59). However inaccurate some such estimates are, and some focus only on tertiary education costs, ignore remittances and assume long periods of residence overseas, there is some degree of consistency based on substantial outlays on the training of health workers and recognition that these are largely lost to source countries after migration.

Conversely, as modelling implies (Rutten 2009a), similarly fragmented data from recipient countries show significant cost savings involved in hiring overseas trained SHWs rather than training them locally. By the 1960s it was estimated that training costs in the UK and the USA were respectively four and six times those of India and Africa (Gish 1971: 150). Such discrepancies have subsequently increased. By 1967, doctor migration was such that 'the dollar value of this foreign aid to the United States was already equal to the total cost of all the health care assistance provided by the nation, publicly and privately' (Mejia 1978: 261). A 1980s estimate for the USA justified foreign-nurse recruitment by arguing that hospitals were able to offset the cost of such recruitment in just 13 weeks, versus the cost of temporary staffing and payment for double shifts (Choy 2003). In Phoenix (Arizona), one hospital estimated that at the start of the 2000s hiring 25 foreign nurses saved an annual $1 million on nursing contract labour; hence the hospital was paying a substantial sum to a private recruiter to both recruit and train nurses (*Nurse Week*, 16 April 2003). In comparison to the losses to Ghana (above), Mensah et al. (2005) estimated that the UK had saved £65 million in training costs since 1998 by recruiting from Ghana, based on figures of 293 Ghanaian doctors and 1021 nurses then in the UK, most of whom had migrated relatively recently. Migrant SHWs also seem to contribute more in taxes than they receive in social security (Rutten 2009b), and have multiplier effects on local employment. Not surprisingly, such circumstances have been seen as 'free-riding' on a substantial scale (Padarath et al. 2003), by recipient countries not investing in building, maintaining and running national training and education facilities, a situation already evident in the 1970s, when the expansion of medical schools was faster in source countries than in more affluent recipient countries (Mejia 1978). Ironically, in a number of countries, including the USA and Australia, potential local medical students with very successful high-school records are unable to gain medical school places since too few are available (see Chapter 4). Educational cost savings effectively transfer a proportion of tertiary training overseas.

The economic impact of emigration on reduced productivity following less effective health care is impossible to estimate. Ghana, for example, like many countries, has lost health benefits where staff losses have reduced the level of medical care, and this has been particularly significant in a country where HIV/AIDS is prevalent. There has also been lost productivity and social costs from reduced care in depleted families. Many people have less adequate access to health care, and both infant mortality and inequality of access to health services have been worsening (Dovlo and Nyonator 1999). The UK has had its stock of health workers boosted, enabling better access to, and levels of, health care there – the converse of the impact in Ghana.

There are clearly major discrepancies and variations in calculating training costs, and they do not take into account the costs of any worsened health following the departure of health workers, the costs of finding other workers to take their place, the impact of changes in skill mix and simply the costs of disruption as individuals leave. Most calculations simply estimate the training costs at both ends and neither account for lost productivity by those who are sick, could be cured, and cannot work (let alone social costs) in the source countries nor, conversely, the parallel savings, and the reduced opportunity costs, in the destination. Although such estimates ignore remittances and return migration, and most are little more than guesstimates, they provide a crude dimension to the economic costs.

RETURN MIGRATION

With return migration, the relationship between income losses and the acquisition of human capital becomes more complex (Brown and Connell 2006; Connell and Brown 2004). If significant return occurs, source countries gain returnees with (usually) enhanced skills, knowledge and experience, constituting a positive transfer of technology (unless, as in the first phases of the brain drain, returnees come back with aspirations and demands for technology wholly inappropriate to local needs and budgets), and perhaps also capital and enthusiasm, all within a familiar cultural environment. Yet this may only infrequently be the case, and return migration is not necessarily of the most useful in the right places, so that any compensatory brain gain is slight.

Globally there is remarkably little information on return migration for most source countries, partly because the return of health workers is relatively slight. Not even all students who take up scholarships overseas return, sometimes justified on the grounds that the course was culturally inappropriate to local conditions. Students from Niue who had chosen to stay in New Zealand remained there because of limited opportunities in Niue, low salaries, alongside lack of job challenges, other family members being resident in New Zealand, the lack of a clear future – including the ability to use acquired skills, lack of mentoring and support, no obvious career path and a feeling that the island state was not going forward (Brunt and Morris-Tafatu 2002: 54). These perspectives, shared by many who have returned, and by scholarship holders from other countries, echo the perspectives of those employed in the health sector (Chapter 6). Returnees know only too well what they might be letting themselves in for.

More generally, return has largely been overlooked in research, remaining 'the great unwritten chapter in the history of migration' (King 2000: 7), and a 'compound and complex process', often over an extended period of time, that involves 'the flows of goods and capital as well as the ideas, attitudes, and skills of the migrants themselves' (Thomas-Hope 1985: 157, 172). The few studies that exist suggest that few (or, implausibly, even no) migrant health workers wish to return (e.g. Troy et al. 2007) and that many health workers prefer to move onwards, through a hierarchy that culminates in the USA, rather than return to their home countries (Chapter 3). None of 500 Albanian nurses who had migrated to Italy had gone back (Chaloff 2008); however, 20 per cent of nurses in one Indian hospital had gone back, after working overseas for periods of two to 15 years (Hawkes et al. 2009). None the less, the return migration of nurses has been perceived to be so slight that Kingma (2006: 201) has referred to the 'myth of return'. Recent studies have recognised limited return, and the diversity of both returnees and their rationales (Maron and Connell 2008). On balance, migrants are unlikely to be tempted back by a system that they left, at least in part because of its perceived shortcomings, although they may return for reasons that have nothing to do with employment in the health sector.

For all the problems of health services in developing countries there is still a considerable will to return, and also to stay. Although most Ghanaian pharmacists sought to migrate overseas, all expressed a wish to return (Owusu-Daaku et al. 2008). Nigerian nurses invariably sought to return to families at home: 'Nigeria is sweet if you have the money' but without money, life had become bitter hence many endured long stays in the UK (Aboderin 2007). In a diverse group of countries, some 66 per cent of health workers stated that they would return, but only 14 per cent actually planned to return home, but that too was uncertain (van Eyck 2004: 27). By contrast, none of a small group of lusophone African nurses in Lisbon wanted to return to their home countries, despite all failing to find employment in the health sector and experiencing difficult employment circumstances, stressing the problems of economic instability that had caused them to migrate in the first place. Even in adversity, the closest any came to an expression of any intent to return was one who might return 'some day' (Luck et al. 2000). Only 29 per cent of Jamaican nurses in the USA intended to return, although 70 per cent sent remittances. The rationale for Jamaican nurses returning, although most intended not to, was primarily family, followed by a nebulous 'love of country' and some dislike of the American way of life. Half of those who had returned enjoyed practising nursing more in Jamaica than abroad, despite the 'bad working conditions' since nursing abroad was seen to be much more impersonal and stressful (Brown 1997: 206–7). Jamaican nurses also returned, like others elsewhere, because they were refused extensions to their visas. The majority of overseas Lebanese nurses had no wish to return, since return would depend on significantly improved wages, best practice in health care, greater autonomy and access to higher education opportunities in a context of political stability (El-Jardali et al. 2008a: 1498). Again in contrast, potential Ghanaian nurses, like so many more, did intend to return, perceiving international migration as a means of accumulating the capital to buy a car and a house, and then perhaps start a business (Dovlo 2006). Nurses tended to be both more geographically conservative and more family-centred than doctors, but they also wished to return if they had achieved the socioeconomic mobility through which they could move beyond nursing.

In developing countries the return of doctors is less frequent than that of nurses (Dovlo 2006), but is highly likely between developed countries, since migration has usually been for professional development rather than income acquisition (Williams and Balaz 2008: 1927). The return of just 40 out of 900 medical graduates from one Pakistani university who undertook postgraduate training in the USA (from a total graduating group of 1100) was regarded as positive (Aly and Taj 2008). Few Bangladeshi doctors, especially those in North America, plan to return, and consequently sent relatively few remittances (see below), preferring to use their resources to finance family reunification in North America (Rahman and Khan 2007: 140). Similarly, few Nigerian doctors in either the UK or the USA intended to return (Healy and Oikelome 2007). Between 10 and 15 per cent of an annual loss of between 100 and 1500 doctors do return to Pakistan (Talati and Pappas 2006: S56). Not only are there significant variations in the intent, extent and rationale for return, between doctors and nurses and across regions, but intent is never reality. Most migrants stay overseas significantly longer than they initially intended.

The growth of overseas migrant communities as the demographic balance shifts, significant income differentials between origin and destination, education overseas (for migrants, spouses and their children) and perceptions of limited opportunities and uncertain futures in home countries have slowed return migration. Superior salaries, facilities and working conditions contribute to new and more congenial workplaces. Where SHWs have migrated with families, children of migrants have been educated in the destination and lost some degree of contact with 'home' societies, including linguistic skills, with both parents and children embarrassed by the prospect of returning 'home' unable to speak the language. Southern African doctors in Australia tended to remain longer than they expected as their children settled in schools, further education enabled them to pursue more specialised careers and they developed friendship networks (Oberoi and Lin 2006: 30). Not untypically, one South African nurse, who had worked for five years in the UK, before working for five years in an oncology clinic for Aramco in Saudi Arabia, and who had originally intended to stay there just two years, stated: 'The longer I stay here the more comfortable I feel. It's more home than home now. I like the weather, the salary is tax-free and life is much better than back home' (quoted in *Nursing Times*, 12 February 2008: 38). Intentions to return, most evident before migration, are diluted after departure. While migrants may proclaim anticipated return, that is often the public face of private stability (Macpherson 1994; van Eyck 2004: 27). Duality and ambivalence are central to notions of return migration.

In Pacific island states, although many SHWs had returned, less than 20 per cent of them had worked overseas before return. Most returned, often with some degree of reluctance, because they were bonded to do so. Where return migration was not dictated by bonds and contracts, it has often occurred for social reasons, as in both the Caribbean and Pacific (and no doubt elsewhere), where 'it's my country' or 'family reasons' were recurrent themes. For a significant proportion, return was a duty as much as an act of free will. Migrants tended to return at key moments in the life cycle – after training or before marriage, for example – but often when ageing parents experienced particular needs. Return was invariably little to do with economics or employment, but in response to household needs; thus many returned not necessarily at times of their own choosing or of their own volition (Brown 1997: 206–9; Connell 2009: 139). Many who have returned, including the earliest Filipino nurses (Choy 2003: 86), often sought to go back overseas as soon as they could.

If health systems improve, then return migration occurs. Indian doctors returned to India after new technology was introduced, but the overall number of return migrant doctors has been modest. Most tend to return to senior positions in medical education or private practice, and their numbers increased with the emergence of corporate hospitals and high-tech centres catering to medical tourism, where overseas credentials are important, rather than work in the public sector with local people (Connell 2006, 2008a). However, many found reintegration difficult because of corruption, poor regulation of hospitals, lack of credentialing and a poorly coordinated health system (Mullan 2004: 30–31). For Indian nurses from Kerala, working again as a nurse is 'understood as a sign of failure' or misfortune, such as divorce, the death of a spouse or commercial bankruptcy, and only those who can get a superior position as a matron or teacher work again after return (Percot and Rajan 2007: 322; Percot 2006). Returning SHWs, at least in Pacific island states and the Philippines, were particularly likely to establish a business on their return, having accumulated enough savings overseas. In the Philippines that was the primary goal of migration (Ball 1996; Alonso-Garbayo and Maben 2009). In the Pacific, some who had returned to the health sector also sought to get into private business or simply 'be a part-time shopkeeper in addition to nursing to earn some extra dollars', or 'set up my own used clothing business' (quoted in Connell 2009: 139). Although three-quarters of Jamaican nurses did return to work in the health sector, the more qualified with the most to contribute rejected this because of poor salary and working conditions, and a lack of official support: 'this sense of an uncaring and even indifferent Jamaican government repeated itself in all the categories of nurses . . . and did much to fuel their sense of alienation' (Brown 1997: 206–9). Similar problems explain why few return to work in health sectors elsewhere. The economic rationale for return migration was therefore largely outside the health sector, with other sectors providing greater income and a degree of individualism, independence and autonomy. Moreover, the Jamaican nurses most likely to return were those whose husbands had high-status occupations hence their own incomes were less important (Brown 1997: 219). Returning Filipinos, Pacific islanders and many Indians too became part of multi-income households. This was both truer and more necessary when returnees were sometimes asked to restart at the bottom of the hierarchy.

The pleasures of return were usually detached from any workplace. Returning was often socially successful, being with family and friends, in a familiar place. But that could also be stultifying. A smaller world may make what was once home seem more constricting, bereft of opportunities and excitement, and hemmed in by petty restrictions and social controls. Jamaican nurses who had returned and who had a partner in a high-status occupation that was economically secure 'expressed a strong sense of belonging and love for Jamaica that overrode the allure of life abroad'

(Brown 1997: 219). Their own incomes were not enough to allow this. One Pacific returnee concluded that returning was good 'for her people and country' but not for her and her family, believing that she could have done better for her extended family had she remained overseas (Connell 2009: 140). Private and public gains may not be correlated (so emphasising the rationale for migration).

While public health strategy favours the employment of those with new skills, not everyone welcomes nationals returning and filling coveted posts (just as expatriates may also be resented). In the 1960s, Sri Lankan doctors wishing to return as specialists were challenged by the local Medical Association, who saw them as queue-jumpers (Gish 1971: 82). In Botswana there is hostility towards returnees even though it is conceded that they are 'more experienced and patriotic' (Sheila Tlou, pers. comm., 2007). Public statements express the need for return but actual practice may discourage and militate against it. Returnees have sometimes lacked support to put their new skills into operation, received poor wages and been forced to resume a health career at the foot of the ladder, where salaries did not match their expectations of appropriate standards of living. Some experienced resentment, in the tension between new skills, loyalty and local experience. Others found difficulty in getting work when they returned, faced nepotism and favouritism, or a lack of welcome, encouraging attrition and discouraging other potential returnees.

Limited evidence exists for the effective transfer of skills and experience acquired overseas, as technology often differs, resources are lacking, conservatism prevails, few return and some have worked overseas in areas that failed to significantly enhance their previous competence (see below). Countries may lack adequate absorptive capacity to receive return migrants, and especially to benefit from new skills and the ability to work with new technology, that their return might entail. Conversely, increasing technological convergence, especially between developed countries, has resulted in fewer technological benefits (Williams and Balaz 2008: 1928). Equally significant constraints to using new skills, and innovation, rest in rigid hierarchies and uncomprehending, suspicious and uninterested superiors. Managerial and organisational skills can be resented; hence they can often be more useful outside the sector (where there are obvious entrepreneurial gains). Return migrants may be 'agents of change' but conformity is often more appreciated than change, in workplaces and in local society. None the less, half the Jamaican nurses who had returned claimed to have gained additional skills and two-thirds of this group were able to use them locally; those who could not cited a lack of equipment or stated that they worked in areas where these skills were not required (Brown 1997: 209). Doctors were more likely to express the benefits of migration. All

Slovakian return migrant doctors gained something, ranging from specific techniques they had sought to learn (such as spinal fusion in the USA and immunisation chemistry in Germany) to a more general understanding of more complex and sophisticated management and clinical systems, attitudes to learning or cultures of patient care, in addition to personal development. Moreover, two-thirds of the returnees believed they had been able to share their enriched experience and knowledge with Slovakian colleagues, although constraints existed because of cultural differences, for example in attitudes to patients and in health service funding models. This broadly positive situation was partly a function of somewhat similar health care systems (Williams and Balaz 2008). By contrast, in small states particularly, where multi-skilling is valuable, some highly skilled returnees no longer had an appropriate or amenable place in the system, nor were new specialisms necessarily valuable in different epidemiological contexts (Connell 2009: 142–4). The benefits to the health sector from return migration may therefore be quite limited, and tend to accrue to individuals rather than the health system, with benefits more visible in wider society. Yet bonding ensures that new skills and young graduates do return, while return is not merely of failures and retirees.

REMITTANCES

A key reason for migration is the wish to help families remaining in home countries, and the most obvious, anticipated and effective way of doing so is through remittances. While relatively few SHWs may return, they and other skilled migrants make a substantial contribution to the economic well-being of those who remain at home. Creating that income informs many family migration decisions, and its use within home communities provides social insurance for return migration. The flow and use of remittances are central to wider debates on their contemporary role: notably whether they are used for production or consumption, if they contribute to inequality and ultimately whether they offset the loss of skills.

Although migrant remittances are considerable in many contexts, few studies differentiate the remittances of health workers from those of other occupational groups, and little is known about the remittances of doctors. While limited global evidence suggests that skilled migrants may be less likely to generate remittances than unskilled migrants, Pacific islander nurse households in Australia remitted proportionately greater sums than unskilled migrants. Where households have invested in human capital and the choice of occupation was linked to the possibility of migration, then individuals are more generous and reliable remitters (Brown and Connell

2004, 2006). In this case at least, the remittances of health workers very substantially exceeded training costs. However, they were almost entirely directed to households and thus benefited the private sector, and did not contribute to greater equity, new training programmes or improved health care provision (Connell and Brown 2004; Brown and Connell 2006). Most remittances combine altruism with self-interest to support the extended families of migrants, result in improved welfare (for example through house extension and construction), the creation of additional human capital (through education expenditure) and some investment in small-scale business. Limited evidence suggests that the extent and use of the remittances of SHWs are much like that of other migrant workers, with some bias towards investment, as a function of higher incomes and aspirations. Remittances may also go to social groups, such as churches, and some village projects, but never to governments; hence they do not directly compensate for the loss of skills that have been produced mainly in the public sector (through education, training and scholarships). However, the prominent use of remittances for consumption, and high purchase and other taxes in some countries, ensures that some proportion of remittances does eventually reach the public sector. At the same time, multiplier effects introduce more jobs into the economy, primarily in the service sector (notably retailing and construction).

The volume of remittances is usually considerable. A quarter of Jamaican nurses in the USA saved more than half their salaries and two-thirds sent remittances home, constituting around $2000 per year (the equivalent of three months' salary in Jamaica), while most also sent goods (and a quarter brought home a motor vehicle). Remittances mainly supported their families, and enabled nurse households to become home owners, but over one-third used remittances for investment (Brown 1997: 208). Rather similarly, Tongan and Samoan nurse households in Australia sent over $2000 per year – more than 10 per cent of their income – and sustained this level over periods of 20 years (Brown and Connell 2006). Some 57 per cent of recently recruited overseas nurses in London sent remittances home (with the highest percentages being sent by African nurses, suggesting some relationship to need) and 20 per cent of all nurses were sending home more than a quarter of their incomes (Buchan 2008: 57–8). Some 87 per cent of Indian and Filipino migrant nurses in Ireland sent remittances home at least monthly, mainly for education, health care needs and as forms of pension and unemployment payments, making sacrifices, including foregoing training, to ensure these flows (Humphries et al. 2009a). Nurses are more likely than doctors to remit and to return, and the two are related.

The objectives of doctors were often different. In India, it is generally believed that because doctors come from relatively wealthy backgrounds, and remittances go to family members, they do not send much money home. However, in recent years, many Indian doctors have sent money back as investments in commercial medical enterprises, such as hospitals, medical schools and medical equipment firms (Mullan 2004: 31). Bangladeshi doctors have largely sent remittances for investment in real estate, or to finance the educational and professional education of family members, but in the absence of significant return migration remittances have been limited (Rahman and Khan 2007: 140). Similarly, some 45 per cent of a sample of migrant doctors in the UK sent remittances, on average amounting to 16 per cent of their income in the UK, and ranging from 8 per cent for those from middle-income countries to 22 per cent for low-income countries (Kangasniemi et al. 2007). In Ghana, remitting money and investing in property were the key goals of migratory nurses, whereas doctors were more likely to emphasise training rather than direct material objectives (Mensah et al. 2005: 28). And for Pakistani migrant doctors, 'repatriation of foreign exchange is insignificant in comparison with large flows from low-skill émigrés' (Talati and Pappas 2006: S58). Overall, therefore, doctors are less likely to send remittances than nurses, and less likely to send significant amounts, supporting the global evidence that the more skilled remit proportionately less (Faini 2007; Adams 2009) and that women value social ties more strongly and are more conscientious remitters than men.

Remittances are particularly important in smaller states and SSA, where they play an increasingly important role in household economies, and indirectly in national economies, as a significant part of disposable income. Since they are potentially countercyclical, they can act as a cushion during economic recessions and after natural hazards; however, at least for Indian and Filipino nurses in Ireland, there was some reduction in flows after the 2008 financial crisis (Humphries et al. 2009a). Remittances are primarily used for consumption and welfare objectives; they stimulate human resource development, maintain social networks and create social capital. Education is highly valued, both generally and to create human capital for potential migration. Filipino and Indian nurses in Ireland specifically targeted their remittances at the education of kin (Humphries et al. 2009a). Even with imperfect knowledge, households consciously make decisions in favour of the quantity and quality of education of children that boost their chances for migration. Successful development of small businesses provides incentives for those who have sent remittances to return home. In overseas Polynesian households that include nurses, the greatest propensity to return came from those with business investments at home (Brown and Connell 2004). Migration and remittances thus stem from and contribute both directly and indirectly to human capital formation.

Overall, remittances are positive and satisfying for households but usually insufficient to significantly influence national development. Education (including scholarships) is mainly in the public sector; remittances return to households and the private sector. Remittances lead to greater out-of-pocket expenditure on health services, take some pressure off the public sector, and boost household incomes, enabling some SHWs to stay, but that cannot easily be demonstrated. They may also enhance inequality. Although remittances from SHWs may be substantially greater than training costs, they do not directly compensate for skill loss. None the less, over time, as economies have struggled, there has been a shift in national policy directions in many source countries towards support for the migration and remittances of skilled workers (Chapter 9).

DESTINATIONS: SKILL LOSS AND BRAIN WASTE?

What happens to SHWs in their destinations is of considerable consequence. Many have used their skills effectively, received salaries much greater than available at home, and contributed enormously to health systems, and to the welfare and economic success of their own extended families. Other individuals and households have found real difficulties in becoming established overseas. Not all migrants have made smooth, satisfying transitions between places and social contexts, in the face of racism, unanticipated high costs of living, homesickness and family concerns. Beyond the brain drain, a further outcome of migration can be a 'skill loss' or 'brain waste' when migrants with specific skills do not exercise them. This may result from unrecognised qualifications (or language ability), discrimination, a preference for other jobs with better wages and conditions, family formation or the failure to gain employment. Moreover, there is a pecking order of geography, specialisms, hospitals and care homes, and migrants are rarely well placed.

Migrant health workers may experience difficult circumstances, especially where cultures are at variance with those at home. Numerous examples exist of their experiencing racism (including institutionalised racism) in developed countries, and of being ignored or experiencing reprisals when complaining of such problems; being denied parity with local workers, promotion or wage gains; experiencing non-recognition or much-delayed recognition of qualifications; lack of respect from patients, colleagues and managers, and pressures to perform poorly paid unqualified work especially in the independent nursing home sector (Culley et al. 1999; Hardill and Macdonald 2000; Robinson and Carey 2000; Yi and Jezewski 2000; Hagey et al. 2001; Hawthorne 2001; Foner 2001; Turrittin et al. 2002; diCicco-Bloom 2004; van Eyck 2004; Larsen et al. 2005; Kingma 2006; Likupe 2006; O'Brien-Pallas and Wang 2006; Percot and Rajan 2007; Aboderin 2007; Pittman et al. 2007; Cuban 2008; Blythe et al. 2009). Migrant workers routinely work long hours, and longer hours than local workers, because they are encouraged or requested to do so, they have yet to establish social worlds or they wish to pay off debts or earn larger incomes to support kin. Many choose to work evening and weekend shifts to that end, and can thus be characterised as extremely flexible and hard-working (George 2005: 60). Nigerian doctors in the UK worked longer hours, had less autonomy and lower morale than their local colleagues, and believed that their skills, experience and hard work were inadequately rewarded (Healy and Oikelome 2007: 1926). Many migrants received minimal cultural orientation in their new countries, and most were disappointed in their goal of working at a higher level, appropriate to their education, training and experience in their home country (van Eyck 2004). Reviews of the experiences of African nurses in the UK, and Asian nurses in a range of developing countries, concluded that 'most' have a negative experience in terms of salaries and working conditions, minimal recognition of skills, challenging cultural and linguistic contexts, reduced access to training and promotion, deskilling and racism, that pose threats to their identity and raise issues of social justice (Likupe 2006; Xu 2007; Xu et al. 2008). Fewer accounts exist of migrant SHWs from other regions and in other destinations.

In some cases largely negative experiences have led to attrition or return. Some nurses were victims of crime, or simply lonely, but unable to return home because their families depended on them for income. Most found housing costs higher and ability to save lower than they had expected, hence spending less on themselves (van Eyck 2004: 25). Filipino and other nurses in the UK found the work more arduous than they anticipated, since patients' relatives were not there to provide support, while shift systems and the variety of English accents made adjustment difficult (Daniel et al. 2001; Dyer et al. 2008). Overseas doctors in the USA faced routine discrimination (Balon et al. 1997) and even doctors migrating within Europe experienced problems, ranging from high costs of living and inadequate accommodation to hostility and discrimination in the workplace, and long, unpaid overtime hours, while they themselves recognised language difficulties (Williams and Balaz 2008: 1929). Such migrant Slovakian doctors faced difficulties despite being mainly on short-term training visits in neighbouring countries of similar ethnicity, rather than long-term potentially rival workers from a distinct ethnic minority. Finnish nurses in Norway experienced similar problems (Kingma 2006: 71–2) and Irish nurses in the UK experienced deskilling and discrimination

(Ryan 2007). Compared with local health workers, migrants are much less likely to be unionised and organised, and in a position to know and maintain their rights, and so more likely to have reduced autonomy and authority (Percot 2006; Rokoduru 2008). In the case of Indian doctors in the UK, this migration perhaps even 'bears closer comparison with the migration of Indian peasants' (Robinson and Carey 2000), at least in terms of their rights and access to social support.

The circumstances of migrant nurses are invariably more difficult than those of migrant doctors, partly because of gender differences. All non-white migrant nurses in southern England, from the Caribbean, Asia and Africa, experienced a lack of opportunities to exercise their abilities (especially in management), the allocation of roles incompatible with their previous experience, discrimination and lack of equal opportunities (especially for promotion), being ignored and thus feeling invisible and conscious of a lack of trust placed in them. Language and accent issues, and certainly colour, may partly underlie discrimination. That even led some to self-blame. African migrant nurses in the UK were more likely than those from South Asia and the Philippines to believe they had been passed over for promotion for racial reasons, while nurses in regional areas were more likely to complain that equal opportunity policies were ineffective there compared with London (Alexis and Vydelingum 2009). Ghanaian nurses and midwives in the UK also experienced relatively limited promotion, because of cultural differences and some real gaps in knowledge. Such constraints could become institutionalised and entrenched by practices in wards, particularly by unequal patronage, creating informal and non-transparent systems of promotion (Henry 2007). Such experiences are by no means confined to the UK. Indeed, institutionalised racism and entrenched hierarchies are much worse in the Gulf, in a context where wider society is similarly structured but where health workers are more acquiescent, being primarily there to earn incomes and gain experience rather than become settlers. Nurses, often from Catholic regions, such as the Philippines and Kerala, left in search of greater personal and religious freedom, when they were able (Alonso-Garbayo and Maben 2009).

Such experiences were usually set in a context where most were fearful of speaking out, conscious that they might be asked to leave, or believing that complaining by powerless people would be pointless. A male South African nurse in the UK thus pointed out: 'we are temporary nurses here and if we say something they don't like we may be thrown out of the country', and a Ghanaian noted, 'we have an extended family' that must be supported (quoted in Alexis et al. 2007: 2226; Henry 2007: 2202). Recruiting overseas workers can thus be a useful strategy since local employers 'do not have to provide training . . . and they could secure a non-threatening workforce who could work overtime, under pressured conditions, without questioning British labour laws and their rights as workers' (Cuban 2008: 90; McGregor 2007). Recent migrants, irrespective of cultural differences, are unlikely to be particularly assertive. In a wider sense nurses may also be less willing to challenge hierarchical and inequitable structures because of a sense of altruism, vocation and feelings of duty towards patients: the 'prisoner of love' dilemma (Folbre and Nelson 2000). Careers can be stunted, out of frustration and withdrawal. Workplace issues thus exist in a wider societal context where similar issues of racism, invisibility and discrimination exist. Migrant SHWs may well experience not just 'double jeopardy' in the work context, by being female and migrant, compounded by being of minority ethnicity (Dyer et al. 2008), but a quadruple jeopardy, where many such women migrate alone and face parallel problems outside the workplace.

Where recruitment and regulation may demand no more than that nurses be 'fit for duty [and] communicate in English' (Brush and Vasupuram 2006: 182), it is unsurprising that many migrant SHWs work in positions below their previous capacity in their home countries. Routine temporary periods of 'training' or familiarisation may turn out to take years, and language differences and national accreditation procedures slow access to equivalent positions. Nurses may therefore be underpaid, certainly with respect to their expectations (George 2005: 59). In the UK, overseas nurses often worked for up to a year as low-paid domestic workers or nursing assistants, before even commencing training, and then often as enrolled rather than registered nurses. They failed to gain new experiences and when they already had superior skills, such as in ICU nursing, feared they would lose them (Smith and Mackintosh 2007). From a sample of 67 nurses in the UK, who had been there for an average of 3.8 years, more than half had a status lower than when they left their home country (Larsen et al. 2005: 355), a situation indicating systematic downgrading. In both Australia and Canada migrant nurses were assigned responsibilities far below their skills and experience, and directed into long-term care responsibilities, while national nurses gained specialisms aligned to their experience and preferences (Omeri and Atkins 2002; Hagey et al. 2001). Many senior Nigerian nurses worked in UK nursing homes, although none had sought to do so, and found the work routine, tedious and restricted, while also experiencing racist, discourteous, domineering treatment by white carers and management that challenged and ignored their professional and social status (Aboderin 2007: 2243). Deskilling and disempowerment are thus widespread, ironically especially where overseas workers are recruited because of their skills (Allan 2007; O'Brien 2007; Dyer et al. 2008), but also where their migrant status is insecure (McGregor 2007). Migrant doctors in Canada, Australia, Israel and elsewhere were directed into general practice rather than enabled to take up their previous specialisms (Shuval 1998; Labonté et al. 2006). Although rather less likely to be deskilled than nurses, almost half of a sample of doctors in the UK had experienced a reduction in their grades after migration, and this proportion was as high as 63 per cent for Indian doctors; some 27 per cent had also experienced periods of unemployment (Kangasniemi et al. 2007). Where migrant doctors are routinely directed to rural areas, where multi-skilling rather than specialism is required, as in Australia (Chapter 2), a broadly similar situation occurs.

The most significant skill loss comes when SHWs cannot gain registration overseas, because their qualifications are deemed inadequate, or they cannot afford registration or the necessary local courses. In Canada as many as 40 per cent of international nurses never complete the application process: a massive waste (Kolawole 2009). Doctors, too, are often discouraged from registration by high costs and challenging procedures (e.g. Lillis et al. 2006). How many SHWs are lost in this way cannot be measured. A secondary skill loss occurs when nurses are employed as care-givers in nursing homes rather than working in hospitals, a widely reported situation, sometimes where unscrupulous employers have taken advantage of nurses as a source of cheap labour (Hawthorne 2001; Buchan 2008). From a large sample of Pacific islands nurses in New Zealand, most of whom were Samoan or Tongan, a significant proportion were working in rest homes and residential care, having failed to have their qualifications recognised or registered, and so earned lower incomes. Not only were nursing skills, albeit unrecognised, effectively discarded, but if nurses again took up nursing they tended to be in the least skilled areas. Pacific islander nurses in New Zealand consequently tended to work in continuing care, particularly of the elderly, and very few were in management; compared with nurses as a whole they were disproportionately likely to be employed in public hospitals, rest homes or residential care (Koloto 2003). Filipino nurses in Japan routinely found themselves undertaking lower-status work, for lower levels of pay, in care homes (Iredale 2001). Many Micronesians, Fijians and others work as poorly paid, unskilled care-givers in Australian, New Zealand and US nursing homes (Scott 2003; Marshall 2004; Connell and Voigt-Graf 2006). In some cases this follows duplicity. Filipino nurses, some of whom were university graduates, were brought to Greece under the 'nursing aide permit', officially to be employed as nursing aides by specific employers, but found themselves working as maids (Lazaridis 2000), while there was similar downward mobility of Filipino nurses in Spain (Ribas-Mateos 2000) and South American and Eastern European nurses in Italy (Chaloff 2008). In Greece even doctors and midwives from

Eastern Europe, with years of work experience, routinely found work as carers and nurse aides. Higher incomes somewhat compensated for downward mobility and many were grateful to have found any job in the health sector (Groutsis 2009). Deskilling is effectively reinforced by substantial flows of women into this somewhat precarious and unregulated part of the labour market. In all these circumstances expensive training is almost completely lost, incomes are lower than anticipated, and neither health systems, nor migrants or their kin at home, who wait for remittances, may make significant gains. Migration is no great success story in the short term here, other than in keeping low-cost health care structures of developed countries functional.

Health workers are often recruited for, and directed into, positions and locations that are unattractive to local health workers, especially when there is relatively full employment in the health sector. As far back as the 1960s it was evident that migrant doctors 'for the most part fill the less desirable posts, which often means that already deprived social and ethnic groups get a lower standard of health care' (Mejia 1978: 264; Gish 1971). Peripheral geographical placement is common and is effectively demanded of many migrant health workers. Usually this is in remote areas, but in the USA may be in 'difficult' inner-city areas. This often displaces and isolates migrant SHWs far beyond fellow migrants, who are more likely to be in large urban areas, where cultures may be quite different and common languages few.

Migration incurs unanticipated problems, especially where migrants must work in skilled teams. From the perception of existing workers, adaptation of newcomers may be difficult. As a Polish nurse observed, 'if we have to adapt to quite a new person, a stranger, with unknown qualifications and unknown reactions, this is a terrible risk and is difficult . . . especially because our work is based in trust – every member of the team has to trust another person' (quoted in van Eyck 2004: 20). Consequently new migrants are unlikely to be involved in specialist activities, despite previous experience, and at least initially may be placed in the least attractive fields of specialisation, in a parallel to outlying parts of the country. The social marginalisation of migrant SHWs, their direction into areas (geographical and clinical) where they are probably of less value than in their home countries, and discrimination suggest that their contributions to health care are less than optimal, despite being in regions of need.

Numerous migrant workers have left the health sector, or never even entered it, either out of frustration or because better opportunities became available. Filipino nurses in Vancouver routinely became nannies and care-givers to secure migration opportunities, and had limited subsequent chance of regaining their old status (Pratt 1999). None of eight nurses from Portuguese-speaking Africa in Lisbon had initially been able to find a nursing job, citing racism and the non-recognition of qualifications as the main reasons. All had therefore first obtained unskilled work as nursing aides or cleaners, without either social security or long-term job security (Luck et al. 2000). Such brain waste is not unusual. Nurses in particular have sometimes migrated as partners rather than as workers, and taken up 'temporary' unskilled work to support families before eventually seeking to get their qualifications recognised and take up nursing positions. Some, in every destination, never succeeded. A substantial number of Tongan nurses in Australia gave up nursing partly because their qualifications were not recognised (and they needed jobs immediately to pay off debts and rent etc.), thus 'finding work was often a matter of subsistence and the fact that many "fell into" nursing again, a function of familiarity rather than vocational passion' (Fusitu'a 2000: 60). Health work was sometimes distant from homes, new family structures posed different demands and jobs such as taxi-driving allowed necessary flexibility. Moving out of the health sector may of course have advantages, with evidence of former health workers achieving greater success in other spheres, but these too are rarely documented. The first South Indian restaurant in Vienna was opened in 1996 by one of the first Indian nurses to have gone to Vienna in 1972, and her husband (Hintermann and Reeger 2005). How widespread success may be beyond the health sector is impossible to know.

Despite the multiple difficulties and challenges of new working and living environments, most migrants none the less gained valuable experiences and new skills, alongside financial gains for themselves and their families, that supported positive social and economic change. This was particularly true of doctors. Many nurses also gained 'soft' (non-monetary) rewards in caring for appreciative patients, and chose to endure any problems for the sake of their families (Dyer et al. 2008; Aboderin 2007). For many, deskilling may be a temporary phenomenon – though it may be 'temporary' for many years – and most SHWs do move up through the hierarchy after a period where they 'learn the ropes', achieve language fluency, cope with discrimination, manage to access support structures such as unions and demonstrate competence. Most migrant nurses, for example, have a strong commitment to their own professional development (Winkelmann-Gleed 2006; Xu and Kwak 2006), preferring 'reskilling' rather than deskilling, and many stay for lengthy periods, despite initial short-term intentions, not merely to generate income for return, but because they have made a successful transition. Moreover, in recent years this has taken place in a context of unstable labour markets, and widespread deskilling, especially of nursing and similar occupations (Carey 2009), within increasingly competitive states (Chapter 10).

The outcome of balancing economic gains with some social costs varies considerably over place and time. As more migrant workers from a particular country or region become resident in a single city, social costs tend to decline. Greater numbers of Fijian nurses in the Marshall Islands meant that they could assert workplace rights more effectively, collectively support nurses with problems, share CDs, DVDs and other goods from Fiji, organise weekly Christian meetings (which helped strengthen social ties and provided spiritual support), and even organise their own fishing trips (Rokoduru 2008). No more than 15 nurses, all without families, in a country where there were few other Fijian migrants, had established a supportive community. In contexts where there are many more migrant health workers, with families and within a wider migrant community, social support is much greater and becoming established somewhat more easily.

Most literature on the migration of SHWs examines their role in the health systems they have left or joined, but not their role as members of households and broader social communities. Some SHWs moved away from difficult political and cultural contexts, and weak economic systems, and, for the first time, had significant spending power, especially if they travelled alone, as was the situation for the early Filipino migrants in the USA, a fact they were proud to discuss in the Philippines, so stimulating further migration flows (Choy 2003). Overseas, Kerala nurses escaped gender stigma based on patriarchal control over the mobility and sexuality of young women (George 2005: 34–5). Some Tongans and Samoans became nurses to experience similar freedom and independence, absent in their patriarchal hierarchical societies. Becoming a health worker and being able to achieve mobility offered new freedom of movement, and an autonomy rarely accessible in other contexts (Connell 2009: 84). That new autonomy may, however, be a partial explanation of why so many health workers who eventually returned to their home countries sought new careers in business.

While migration is a loss to sending countries, mitigated by significant incomes and the flow of remittances, individual gains in destinations may be muted. Some SHWs simply failed to practise at all, and others held positions below those at home. Not only do SHWs, especially nurses, migrate internationally within the context of the 'inverse care law', but some are deskilled through that process, and reskilling takes time. Migration thus tends to feed into and sustain nursing workforces in particular, which are already highly structured on class, gender and racial lines, and built on international hierarchies of disadvantage. Such hierarchies have strong historical roots in colonialism and empire in Europe and America (Smith and Mackintosh 2007: 2217), representing the social configurations of an established 'empire of care' (Choy 2003). More recently, similar 'empires' have emerged in the Gulf, replicating old hierarchies of race and class. Quite simply many migrants are routinely expected to fill gaps in places, positions and conditions that are unacceptable to local workers, and thus be relatively disadvantaged by specialisms, grades and geography. Both discrimination and the regulation of educational and professional qualifications exclude many skilled migrants from higher-status and higher-income positions, wasting skills, dampening morale, and reducing incomes and thus remittances.

Deskilling emphasises what has been seen as something of a 'race to the bottom' (Cuban 2008: 83), where SHWs are in the contradictory position of being well-educated but low-cost labour: a form of 'contradictory class mobility' (Parrenas 2001). Migrant status and ethnicity reinforce nursing and labour market hierarchies, so that race, class and gender remain divisive, with migrants long-time strangers in a strange land. Nurses, and other SHWs, travel thousands of kilometres to look after the relatives of others: the quintessential emotional labour, that is 'the induction or suppression of feeling in order to sustain an outward appearance that produces in others a sense of being cared for in a convivial, safe place' (Hochschild 1983: 7), but at the expense of the suspension of direct emotion for their own relatives. Thus carers in Cumbria (UK) achieved little social mobility but had become a 'hidden, silenced group' despite their crucial role in providing care and reducing costs within an increasingly liberalised and privatised 'audit culture' (Cuban 2008). Essential work is ultimately undervalued, and not only for migrants.

A BALANCING ACT

The migration of SHWs has been widely seen as harmful for source countries since it leads to gaps in essential services, lost investment in expensive professional education and training, loss of future tax revenues and, less directly, reduced economic growth, and declining morale and health status among those who remain (whether health workers or relatives). Because of the necessity for appropriate training, it is more difficult to substitute for (or transfer from elsewhere in the public service) absent skills in the health workforce. Remittances flow in the opposite direction to SHWs. Yet the 'brain drain' is much more complicated than even the most complex social and economic balancing sheets suggest, especially since it is a constant work in progress. The duration and outcome of migration are never fixed. In the end, substantial flows of remittances, with their often positive transformative role, and the replacement of departed workers by others, alongside technology and knowledge transfer, cannot easily be balanced against the 'failure' of so many skilled workers to return effectively, 'brain waste' and, more dramatically, even the 'sense of guilt and responsibility' (Harper et al. 2008: 167) of those who have gone away and whose relatives have died in their absence. Equally dramatically, based on an analysis of the remittances of Ghanaian nurses, Quartey concluded that despite significant flows of remittances, 'the net benefit will be negative if one could cost it in terms of deaths due to staff shortage' (quoted in *Poverty News Blog*, 13 July 2006). How such deaths could be costed was not stated.

The transnational migration of SHWs can be exceptionally positive. Despite almost universal social costs, such as discrimination and deskilling, migrant health workers tend to remain overseas longer than they had originally intended, and are often joined by their families, if they can sponsor them, or they may move onwards to other overseas destinations (notably the USA). When SHWs do return, many are reluctant to work in the health sector – especially in public health – preferring a more entrepreneurial future, a new status, and greater independence. Consequently much literature on this kind of migration 'paints it as empowering, democratic and liberating, particularly in the light of other global trends towards the concentration of wealth and power' (Mahler 1998: 92). And so it is for many socially mobile migrant SHWs. The costs largely lie elsewhere, in the countries and societies from which the migrants come. Individuals and households have gained from migration, rather more than wider source country society and economy. Remote areas particularly have lost, ultimately worsening their welfare and bargaining positions, and their economic productivity.

An additional layer of complexity derives from the argument that, although the emigration of SHWs obviously directly reduces their numbers (and reduces the overall stock, where migration exceeds training rates, as, for example, in the case of nurses from Malawi), a high emigration rate might none the less increase the stock of skilled workers. Successful migration increases returns to education so that individual (and household) incentives for training in particular skills in overseas demand should also increase significantly. Migration generates remittances, while not all those additional trainees would emigrate. In such circumstances the human capital losses to emigration would be offset by gains in investments in the home society (Stark 2004; Record and Mohiddin 2006; Robinson 2007; Chand and Clemens 2008; Clemens 2007). A brain drain would benefit all if the possibility of migration greatly increased the incentive to acquire education: the so-called 'beneficial brain drain' hypothesis (Mountford 1997). In this context the potential for enhanced incomes from overseas migration would be a powerful driver to increased enrolments in education for health work (see Chapter 5), as occurred in India and the

Philippines. Hosein and Thomas have thus argued that the additional mobility of nurses within an expanded Caribbean community labour market 'may attract a larger number of trainees into the field, because of the greater sense of job security the expanded labour market will now provide' (2007: 329). This broad assumption, alongside recognition of the apparent inevitability of migration, is the basis for strategies of 'managed migration' (Chapter 9) where larger numbers of workers are trained by Caribbean countries for migration to the USA.

Education for migration is important in many contexts, while remittances are widely directed into the acquisition of education by kin, and the creation of further human capital. Clemens (2007) has argued that the migration of doctors from SSA potentially constitutes such a case, since the possibility of emigration contributes to the production of increased numbers of doctors, so that stocks of doctors have not fallen, while poor health status in SSA is independent of the migration of doctors, being a function of other factors such as the geographical distribution of health workers, their public and private sector distribution, skill mixes and performance incentives. This internationalist perspective has been particularly strongly formulated in the context of proposals to constrain the recruitment of SHWs by developed countries:

> A ban on recruitment of skilled professionals by rich nations from poor countries will dissuade training for emigration, and thus reduce the pool of medical professionals available for the globe as a whole. Any proposal to train and then 'trap' skilled workers in poor nations will only discourage schooling, and therefore run the risk of trashing the hopes and aspirations of many poor people to improve their wellbeing through emigration . . . The train and trap proposal, therefore will create losses for all – the potential trainee, and residents of the source and destination nations. (Chand 2008b: 1576)

In Fiji there is good evidence that over a decade the demand for tertiary education has increased in response to migration opportunities (Chand and Clemens 2008), as would be expected, especially in a context of a declining economy and civil strife, but simultaneously there are wide-ranging skill shortages. This investment in education may not have been enough to offset declining stocks of human capital over a longer period than ten years.

An alternative perspective on SSA has argued that the loss of doctors is correlated with higher death rates, especially from AIDS, resulting in a 'vicious circle of higher HIV prevalence rates leading to increased emigration of physicians, which in turn lowers the quality and quantity of care for AIDS patients, increasing death rates and the number of orphaned children' (Bhargava and Docquier 2008: 364). Both lower wages and high

HIV rates are predictors of high emigration rates, suggesting that worsening health status is both a cause and a consequence of migration and that both trends reinforce each other. This therefore challenges the internationalist position. However, in each of these three analyses (Clemens 2007; Chand and Clemens 2008; Bhargava and Docquier 2008), time periods were quite short – never more than 15 years – so that correlations, and their absence, are somewhat speculative. Different data sets were used and neither of the two SSA health analyses considered nurses, who may well be more critical for health care. Moreover, in many SSA countries, especially in rural areas, health care is not provided by doctors or even nurses, but by other categories of health workers (Kruk et al. 2009; Daviaud and Chopra 2008), so that the migration and density of doctors may have limited relationship to health outcomes. Quantitative analyses are necessarily limited by a focus on what is measurable rather than a more qualitative appraisal of performance.

In the case of Indian migrant doctors in the UK, there was a weak link between training and migration possibilities. Only the very best doctors got through the screening procedures for migration while those with more limited education and training did not, and even some of those who succeeded found employment problems in the UK; hence returns to education in terms of a successful migration outcome were small (Kangasniemi et al. 2007). However, it may be that for nurses, where demand is greater and training regimes less demanding, thresholds are reduced, migration is more probable, remittances are greater and the returns to education higher (also accounting for some doctors retraining as nurses).

Rapid loss of SHWs does pose challenges to organisational structures, especially for smaller countries, where training capacity is weakest and managers and trainers are also prone to migrate. Even proponents of the greater migration of SHWs, as in Bangladesh, recognise that constraints to the production of SHWs are the high cost and small number of training opportunities (Rahman and Khan 2007: 139). Selectivity of migration by skill and education is thus problematic, with a probable distortionary effect on secondary and tertiary education systems in source countries. Over a longer time period there is likely to be a reduction in the local skilled workforce (as in Malawi, and more recently the Philippines) since there is a very high level of migration of those who are qualified, limited training capacity and no inexhaustible supply of appropriate graduates from high schools, especially if teachers also migrate. For small states, there are both limits to the numbers of high-school leavers who may be appropriate as SHWs and possibilities of geographically uneven labour markets (Connell 2007a). The migration of teachers is significant in many developing countries, especially in SSA and small states (e.g. Voigt-Graf

2003), to the extent that the only code of practice for recruiting a migratory skilled group, other than health workers, is for teachers (Chapter 9). Moreover, the emigration of even a few SHWs can entail significant adjustment costs (in teams and skill mixes) and possible sharp rises in salaries (especially in the private sector), while SHWs provide valuable social roles beyond their clinical expertise, generate taxation and create additional employment (Robinson 2007: 16–17). More intangible losses of leadership and institutional capacity follow the selective migration of the most skilled, raising concerns over 'managed migration' and challenging the possibility of a 'beneficial brain drain'.

Where financial resources for health are very small, and SHWs are unemployed (so appearing to enable an 'overflow', as opportunity costs to migration appear close to zero), this is not actually 'market failure'; although the benefits of migration are primarily reserved for household members, the costs are borne by the state (despite the secondary impacts of remittances), by the wider population (who pay for training through the taxation system) (Record and Mohiddin 2006) and by inadequately served regional populations. The argument that migration constitutes an 'overflow' is still reiterated, for example in South Asia, where most emigration comes from relatively well-supplied metropolitan areas. In Bangladesh it may well be that 'it is hard to make a case that preventing out-migration would materially affect access to health services' (Rahman and Khan 2007: 139), but the country has a very low ratio of SHWs to a population with a high disease burden, even though migration is not primarily responsible for unfilled vacancies. 'Overflow' only appears to exist alongside considerable urban bias. Losses in the Philippines and India now extend beyond mere overflow (Chapter 7). There is neither a good 'overflow model' (except perhaps in the unique case of Cuba) nor any real empirical basis for a beneficial brain drain.

The intensifying global structure of demand and recruitment ensures that relatively poor states continue to experience a steady migration of SHWs, and therefore continued high training and replacement costs. This skill drain provides some gains through human capital transfers (with return migration), new knowledge of health practices and procedures, new experiences, social mobility, remittances and the investments of returnees. The evidence that exists, fragmented and superficial though it often is, suggests that source countries are at the losing end of a global care chain that primarily benefits metropolitan recipient countries. Global economic welfare may benefit from the free flow of skilled workers, as do many workers and the households of which they are part. Source countries largely do not and losses of SHWs may be compounded, rather than absorbed, over time. While remittances go to households, and the extended households of SHWs are rarely the relatively poor, they only subsequently go to states (via taxation etc.), and finally trickle down to the health sector. Remittances are short-term gains, while health systems fade more slowly, where migration exceeds production of SHWs. However, as the costs of education and training are increasingly borne by the private sector (as with so much nursing training in India and the Philippines), the legitimacy of that critique of the role of remittances has weakened somewhat. None the less, many of the beneficiaries of migration are in the private sector (including recruitment agencies), while losses are mainly experienced in the public sector.

Even in this critical area, it sometimes remains difficult to go much beyond anecdote and speculation in any analysis of the consequences of migration. There is simply inadequate data for a cost–benefit analysis that elegantly balances education costs, remittances, social costs and so on. Health resources in many primarily source countries seem stretched, sometimes alarmingly, in downward spirals and vicious circles. It is not mere 'populist suspicion' (Rahman and Khan 2007: 139) to express concern over the emigration of SHWs, and of the beneficial brain drain hypothesis, but indicative of the need to recognise the widespread 'Fijian paradox' (Chapter 5), where migration may benefit individuals and households but not necessarily nations, and apply precautionary principles. Indeed, it is unsurprising that policies and practices to remedy the impact of migration have been urgently and widely sought, and these are examined in the next chapter.

9.   Policy implications

Well-established structures of migration exist in many developing countries, influencing both skilled and unskilled workers. SHWs have moved to take advantage of superior wages and salaries, training and research opportunities and working conditions for themselves, and to better the lifestyles of their children and extended families, through education, social change and remittances. Without significant changes, migration is likely to continue, where such aspirations remain, and kin are increasingly overseas. Policies that redress issues of supply and demand have proved difficult for most countries. Not only has the rationale for migration been more or less similar for 30 years and in a multitude of countries, but many policies for slowing and reducing the negative effects of migration are similarly longstanding (Mejia et al. 1979; Gish 1971), indicating the problems attached to developing and implementing retention policies. Moreover, governments in source countries have infrequently sought to discourage international migration, and have been less likely to do so in the present century. While the rationale for migration ultimately relates to entrenched issues of global uneven development and national financial support, most migrants assert that they do not want to migrate. Policy initiatives are therefore plausible.

At a relatively high level of abstraction it is implicit that in order to achieve the United Nations Millennium Development Goals by 2015, with their particular focus on health issues, a situation that already seems unlikely for SSA (WHO 2006a), better access to health care interventions and thus to SHWs is necessary. That requires more effective recruitment, retention and slowing of migration. Such notions have been translated into events, such as World Health Day, and principles, for example in the Ottawa Charter of 1986, a precursor to the Commission on Social Determinants of Health (WHO 2008b) and, more specifically in the present context, the London Declaration of 2005, the last endorsing four principles: all countries must strive to achieve self-sufficiency in their health workforce; developed countries must assist developing countries to train and retain doctors and nurses; all countries must ensure that health workers are educated, funded and supported; and action to combat the skills drain must be linked to the right to health and other individual human rights (Labonté et al. 2006: 9). How exactly such broad principles might be translated into policy and implemented raises many questions, and multiple responses (Global Health Workforce Alliance 2008), but 'train, retain and sustain' has become a mantra.

A perceived shortage of SHWs is common to most countries. Yet defining shortage is challenging: vacancy rates are basic, but even calculating the staffing establishment is difficult, where nurses may undertake the more 'invasive therapy' of drips and drains, and bed-making and store maintenance are devolved to others. Politicians, bureaucrats, SHWs and patients differ in their assessments of needs, and unions invariably claim that their members are overworked (and underpaid), while the most appropriate skill mix varies and changes. In an ideal world, national and regional training facilities would produce appropriate numbers of skilled people, who would deliver effective services. But in many states, failures of governance, broadly the inadequate delivery of services (whether health, education, transport etc.), have been key constraints to development.

Mobility is a basic human right (and indeed it is central to the United Nations Convention on Human Rights, and often enshrined in national constitutions, at least for internal migration) and should not be constrained. It is sometimes argued that this is particularly so for professionals, who have globally valuable skills. An open international market is said to offer efficiency and economic gains. However, while there are aggregate gains in economic efficiency, they are localised in receiving countries and the largest cities. As the evidence of costs to national health systems has mounted, there has been repeated interest in developing policies and mechanisms to diminish and mitigate the impacts of migration.

Not all countries have sought to prevent migration, and some, such as India, Cuba, Egypt, China, Spain and the Philippines, purposefully export workers, including health workers. Bangladesh, Pakistan, Solomon Islands, and more recently Vietnam and Indonesia (Yeates 2009), have begun to develop similar perspectives, primarily for economic reasons. In several countries, from Tonga to the Philippines, there are even tensions between government departments, where migration is perceived as a valuable economic policy but an inappropriate health policy. In 1973, when President Marcos decreed that nurses must work in rural areas, to relieve regional shortages and reduce rural–urban maldistribution, he also pursued a policy of accumulating scarce foreign exchange through remittances from overseas workers, including nurses (Choy 2003: 115–16). None the less, even in countries where migration may be perceived to be a right there is concern over excessive migration and interest in preventing, or compensating for, this.

Tensions in the Philippines (and elsewhere) demonstrate that it is not only ministries of health (or their equivalents) that are the key decision-makers for health policy, especially where that affects workforces. Regional organisations (state and urban governments) are involved, and critical decisions are made by public service commissions and finance ministries. Policy formation is also influenced by NGOs, unions and professional organisations, broadly the 'medical establishment'. Supra-national organisations, such as the EU, play some part within a context of globalisation. Growing attention to finance in health care has meant that, at all scales, there may be more concern for the management of costs than the management of care, so that staff numbers are reduced and skill mixes emphasise lesser skills (e.g. Gordon 2005: 252–7). Ministries of health may be both policy-takers and policy-makers – especially in a human resource context – and, at the very least, are curtailed and constrained in their ability to garner resources and construct effective policy.

Not only may ministries of health have only limited planning ability, but in some countries there is very little national planning at all. In the USA the private sector plays a critical role in medical education, hence there is no national planning or formal quotas or other restrictions within medical schools, although the various states do fund medical education. The outcome is that 'dependence on migration is almost explicit in medical education policy' (OECD 2008: 26). OECD countries as a whole 'favour long term policies of national self-sufficiency to sustain their physician workforce [but] such policies usually co-exist with short-term or medium term policies to attract foreign physicians' (Forcier et al. 2004: 1). Even where ministries have the capacity to develop policy, the length of time required to train SHWs emphasises how farsighted policies must be, while seemingly unrelated national policies – for example on working hours or occupational health and safety (OHS) – may have complex consequences.

The widespread health care crisis, especially in SSA, extended and intensified by the accelerated migration of health workers, requires both national policies and an integrated global approach to mitigate the nega-tive effects of migration and reinforce its positive effects. Thirty years ago Mejia et al. (1979) argued, first, that the lack of good data should not be used to justify inaction, and, second, that the failure of workforce plan-ning could be attributed to a lack of political will to deal with the critical problems. Both conclusions remain valid (Bach 2004), in a context of even greater need, where the brain drain has flourished. Given the pressures on public sectors in less developed countries, and the limited room for manoeuvre that exists where national economies are weak, the onus for achieving a more equitable distribution of SHWs has gradually shifted on to recipient countries, where demand and recruitment occur. Continued migration has thus led to renewed calls for national self-sufficiency, ethical codes of practice on recruitment and compensation for countries experiencing losses, yet political and practical realities confront ethical arguments. No easy solutions exist.

EARLY DAYS

By the end of the 1960s, and initial concerns over the brain drain, policies were already being directed towards a more equitable system of skilled migration. Recommendations made by Gish in 1971, that centred on the need for adequate and transparent promotion opportunities, remain remarkably valid. His overall conclusion for Ireland, then experiencing substantial losses, was that

> Countries like Ireland would appear to have two unattractive choices open to them. The first is to allow an international free market in 'human capital' to operate, and the second is to control rigidly both emigration and wages and produce only that number of physicians equivalent to the planned absorptive capacity of the country. A third more attractive choice would be an appropriate educational, manpower and employment strategy . . . which would lead to the output of a combination of different types of medical manpower, perhaps with more nurses and fewer physicians . . . [and] an employment policy which would combine carefully thought out income incentives and prospects of promotion . . . [and] include higher levels of support from the state. (1971: 22)

More detailed recommendations on rural health services emphasised themes that remain familiar and crucial: the need for medical auxiliaries, proper infrastructure, more rapid promotion, better access to training courses for those undertaking rural work, more flexible salary scales, bonding, and a bar on foreign recruiters (ibid.: 122–8). Similar contemporaneous recommendations stressed the need for a focus on paramedics rather than expensively trained doctors, the construction of health posts rather than expensive hospitals, a more appropriate locally based training programme, tighter bonding and bonuses for those working in remote areas (Sharpston 1972).

A decade later however global concern shifted towards an oversupply of doctors in particular, and policy prescriptions went into reverse. In what was described as the 'late pathogenic' stage of overproduction, policies were advocated to cut student numbers, discourage return migration, reduce the workload of doctors, encourage and compel early retirement and introduce job-sharing (Mejia 1987). In various countries fragments of such policies – notably the reduction in training places – have frequently resurfaced, often supported by professional associations. Despite this particular cyclical shift, it is indicative of the problems of policy implementation (much more than policy formulation) that most recommendations to reduce the extent of migration and develop a sustainable and appropriate workforce largely remain valid. Since then policies have been debated, and occasionally implemented, but their essence has barely changed.

For almost half a century, policy formation has stressed the need for an integrated package of policies that span economic and social issues, often extend beyond the confines of the health sector and operate in both source and destination countries (e.g. Wibulpolprasert and Pengpaibon 2003; Yumkella 2006; Connell et al. 2007; Lehmann et al. 2008; Masango et al. 2008). Various possibilities exist for more effective production and retention of SHWs, ranging from diverse financial incentives (inside and outside the health system), strengthening work autonomy and improving the status of health workers, increasing recruitment capacity, introducing intermediate categories of workers, such as nurse practitioners, and ensuring effective financial support for health services. Where 'packages' have been implemented that include some or all of such policies, as in Thailand, Malawi and Swaziland, a combination of social and economic components, including continuing education, provision of housing, and establishment of a clear career structure, seemed to result in improved job satisfaction and retention (Mathauer et al. 2004; Noree et al. 2005; Kober and van Damme 2006). Indeed, it is implausible that they would not. Where such packages are absent, as in Ethiopia and Nepal, retention is particularly difficult (von Massow 2001; Butterworth et al. 2008). Most countries have implemented particular measures, some with a degree of success, but there has rarely been a concerted approach to the implementation and monitoring of policy packages, that would multiply single-policy benefits. Such implementation demands effective management, yet these skills may also have been lost through migration.

FINANCING THE HEALTH SECTOR?

Different national priorities and ceilings on public health spending have been a constraint to the development of adequate workforce policies, as they have always been (Alubo 1990; Chapter 2). Economic restructuring has sometimes meant the deterioration of conditions rather than the intended greater efficiency. In many SSA countries, funding for the public health sector has been shrinking in real and relative terms. No African countries have reached the 2001 target of the Organisation of African Unity for 15 per cent of public budgets to be spent on health, and tax revenues in low income countries amount to an average of only 15 per cent of GDP compared with 30–40 per cent in high-income countries. This has stimulated complex and wide-ranging debates about the role of development assistance for health funding, including that of the 'new philanthropists', such as the Global Fund to Fight AIDS, Tuberculosis and Malaria, PEPFAR and the Bill and Melinda Gates Foundation, some of whose programmes have a disease focus rather than a health systems and workforce approach, and have pushed up wage rates (Drager et al. 2006; Garrett 2007; McCoy et al. 2008; Cavagnero et al. 2008; Birch 2009; O'Brien and Gostin 2009). With low budgetary allocations, some public sector institutions experience shortages of protective clothing, basic equipment and drugs, and uncompetitive salaries, since governments have sought to reduce public expenditure, and especially wages. That has sometimes led to simultaneous high unemployment and high vacancy rates: real incentives to migration. Quite simply, 'low-income developing countries need to substantially increase expenditure to meet universal coverage goals for essential health services and to achieve significant improvements in public health' (Cavagnero et al. 2008: 864). But most such countries are unlikely to achieve a level of economic growth that would make this possible without external development assistance, while retaining a growing health workforce would still require parallel movements towards sustainability in rich-world countries.

Adequate finance is crucial for recruitment and training in the public sector, where demand is greatest and equity best served. That is partly contingent on international agencies, aid donors and governments recognising that health constitutes a 'special case', central to the MDGs, and nations require a productive workforce. In itself that would provide a positive climate, strengthen morale and increase the likelihood of better management. Most developing countries have primarily rural populations, and because most national economies in developing countries strongly depend on the productivity of the rural sector, effective decentralisation and infrastructural support for rural and regional development are at the neglected core of national development. Absolutely crucial to providing an effective health care system is an 'improved economic performance, a stable political situation and a peaceful working environment' (Awases et al. 2004: 54). That might be obvious, and is true both nationally and regionally, yet it is hard to be sanguine about positive changes after decades of invocations to change (Ojo 1990) and where stable economies and committed, conscientious political systems are unusual.

Increasing Recruitment Capacity

Fewer people are now being attracted to health careers, as other employment arenas seem more attractive. Potential employees witness the frustrations of health workers, and a career in health has less prestige and fewer income benefits than it once had, whereas 'business' is the place of income generation, progress and action, in some part a function of declining community consciousness (Chapter 4). In a number of countries, especially relatively poor countries in SSA like Mali, there is a 'paradox of overproduction' where trained doctors, unable to find positions or adequate wages in the public service, have become taxi-drivers, or in Indonesia, where nurses, despite having inadequate skills or English-language capability for working overseas, refuse to work at the prevailing salaries. In these circumstances of 'pseudo-shortage', only a combination of vacancies and superior wages and conditions is likely to retain in or attract SHWs into the health sector.

Assuming that some health workers will migrate or resign, additional recruitment is essential, but school leavers now have more options than in the past, and several countries lack the capacity to train much larger numbers. A standard bureaucratic response has been 'train more' and 'train them here', but recruitment of adequate numbers, and creating more places, is not straightforward. Failures of recruitment may reflect education in high schools, which may be inadequate for high-school graduates to be confident of a career in the health system (or for the health system to take them on). In the Marshall Islands, Malawi and elsewhere, most high-school graduates lack the basic literacy and numeracy (and commitment) to become SHWs (Gorman and Hohmuth-Lemonick 2009). In Vanuatu, for example, there are simply inadequate resources or training capacity to train and then employ the increasing numbers of nurses, and other SHWs (notably those who require scholarships), required to meet the needs of a growing population. In Malawi, nursing schools have a low annual intake 'because of a lack of hostel accommodation, inadequate classroom space, too few tutors, insufficient teaching and learning materials and poor finance' (Muula et al. 2003: 435). Similarly, Cape Verde can only afford to accept a new intake of nurses every three years, while both Malawi's and Swaziland's annual output of nurses is below the migration rate (Record and Mohiddin 2006; Kober and van Damme 2006). Higher priority, and greater finance, for the education of health workers, alongside related accommodation, facilities and faculty are crucial but, where migration is significant and economies stagnant, that is much easier said than done.

Some countries have thus sought to 'throw the net' much more widely. Most countries have, at least in some part, a 'pseudo-shortage', where former SHWs are unwilling to work at the prevailing conditions (for personal or professional reasons). That has partly meant turning to older workers, to return or train. In Ghana and Samoa, nurses and doctors are the only public servants who are allowed to go beyond the compulsory retirement age as long as they are functioning effectively. Caribbean governments have sought to extend the retirement age of 55 to 60 or 65 (Yan 2006) and Guyana has successfully recruited retired nurses to work with HIV/AIDS patients (Morgan 2005). Conventionally, the health workforce has been recruited from immediate school and tertiary education leavers, but Tonga has both sought to recruit previously trained staff who have had families and are ready to return to the workforce, while also training mature students up to the age of 45. The Fiji School of Nursing has abandoned its policy of recruiting only up to an age limit of 25. Such 'established' residents, with families, are less likely to be interested in migration. In developed countries too, like the UK, older graduate nurses are more likely to remain; hence their training has proved invaluable (Robinson et al. 2008). For community posts, especially, local people have been involved in the selection of others who are likely to remain or return; West Bengal villages have selected resident, married women for training since they are almost certain to return, and in Ethiopia community health workers must be women voted for by the community.

Most nurses are women. Many countries have not begun to go beyond these gender stereotypes and consider the more active recruitment of men, as there has been considerable cultural and economic opposition, sometimes a legacy of colonial contexts where men were considered productive and women nurturing and domestic. Some 46 per cent of Fijian nurses, 97 per cent of whom were female, opposed increasing the intake of males, despite a nursing shortage, because the few male nurses climbed the career structure more quickly (Fong 2003). In Niger, serious consideration has been given to changing the gender bias in nursing schools towards men, to improve both the retention and national distribution of nurses, since the objective of most women who enter nursing schools is to make a good social investment, through which they can 'marry upwards' and neither return nor move to rural areas (C. Lemiere, pers. comm., 2009). The low wages paid to nurses are at least partly a result of the gendered division of labour and concentration of women in these professions, within a loosely male sphere of curing and a female sphere of caring (Leckie 2000); hence a shift towards the recruitment of male nurses might even enhance the possibility of better earnings, and higher retention rates. Men are, however, usually more likely than women to migrate.

Local Training

Locally trained SHWs are more likely to stay (and may have more appropriate skills) than those trained overseas; hence training programmes have increasingly been located within countries, and upgrading of skills has been done by migrant educators rather than learned by migrant SHWs.

Countries have usually sought to adapt medical curricula to local needs, because of the obvious relevance and because this potentially reduces the employability of graduates elsewhere. 'International' curricula increase the probability of subsequent migration (Dovlo 2003). Local training implies a local curriculum. Tanzania achieved early success in the 1970s but even then there was opposition to the 'devaluing' of courses (Mejia 1978: 271). In many places there have been pressures, often from potential SHWs, for an internationally recognised common curriculum, as in the Caribbean, ASEAN and Pacific regions, specifically to enable at least the regional accreditation and wider mobility of health workers. It is still possible to argue that 'much of the curriculum for training nurses in Africa is inappropriate', as in Gambia, where it is oriented towards NCDs rather than the still more prevalent diarrhoea, malaria and acute respiratory infections, where PHC is involved (Hancock 2008: 260). Increasingly, however, as global health trends have tended to converge, for example with the rise of NCDs in developing countries, the appropriateness of a distinct curriculum has declined. Moreover, as public policy has moved away from nationalist positions, constraining mobility through a place-specific curriculum is less likely to be acceptable.

Since the early 1990s in Samoa there has been some slowing of the migration of doctors, partly as a result of a decision to have all training of medical officers done in nearby Fiji, because of the perception that training there was more appropriate and cheaper than in metropolitan New Zealand, and 'there was a lower propensity for graduates to emigrate to [Pacific] rim countries relative to graduates of rim country institutions' (World Bank 1994: 322). In Thailand the emigration of health professionals was reduced once training was entirely conducted in Thai and graduates were less fluent in English (Dovlo 2003). In-country training is invaluable for the retention of SHWs, but is not always possible and is inadequate without other changes in health systems.

Some states have sought preferential recruitment of nurses especially from rural areas and outlying islands, since they are more likely to stay or return and work there (Matsumotu et al. 2005; Playford et al. 2006). This has sometimes proved difficult since such potential recruits are often initially locationally disadvantaged by poorer education levels. However, while health workers in rural and regional areas are, at least in part, motivated and sustained by their work, their partners are unlikely to be, nor are their children. Attracting SHWs to such areas may therefore depend at least as much on what is available to family members, especially for the education of children. In Indonesia and the Pacific island states, those who are most likely to work in regional areas are those who originally came from there (Chomitz et al. 1998; Connell 2009); hence it makes sense to train more such people. Globally, Cuba provides international scholarships for those willing to return to 'humble communities' and 'marginalised areas' (Huish 2009), as has Australia at a smaller scale (Muula and Broadhead 2001). Several countries, including the USA, Australia, Norway, Indonesia and Thailand, have made particular efforts to develop distinct training programmes, deliver adequate PHC, enable the retention of health workers in remote areas, and give some priority or special scholarship provision to students from such areas (Ross 2007; Smith et al. 2008; Humphreys et al. 2008; Pong 2008). Such distinct programmes are less evident in developing countries where resources are limited and trainers reluctant to work in regional areas.

Training in relatively remote states and provinces, such as Nebraska, Newfoundland and Finnmark, of people from these regions, slows migration to larger centres and overseas (Baer et al. 2000; Mathews et al. 2006; Kristiansen and Forde 1992; Wilson et al. 2009). None the less, in Norway at least, doctors, who devoted much of their time and effort to their medical practice 'gave concessions to their spouses' by allowing their choice of geographical location (Kristiansen and Forde 1992). In the USA, doctors were most likely to stay in rural areas when they could be integrated into the community in terms of a security and identity outside the medical practice (Cutchin 1997). In Mexico, local training discourages the migration of doctors to metropolitan centres or richer provinces, but provinces without medical schools are the most deficient in doctors (Harrison 1998). Similarly, in Mexico, Newfoundland and India, female doctors were more likely to remain in regional areas, and less likely to migrate internationally (Harrison 1998; Mathews et al. 2006; Kaushik et al. 2008). Even so, in many remote areas, such as inland Australia, the lack of training facilities has been a constraint on the ability to train local people, especially indigenous Aborigines. And, as the evidence from Fiji indicates (Oman et al. 2009), even the existence of local high-quality training may not prevent the perception that superior training and facilities may be elsewhere. Relativities and the perception of them are crucial.

Retaining Existing Health Workforces

Most SHWs cite wages, multiple workplace problems (often centred on uncertain career progression), inadequate support (in a personal and technical sense) and a simple lack of appreciation as sources of dissatisfaction. Both financial and non-financial incentives are important motivators for health workers to work effectively and to remain in the public sector (Awases et al. 2004; Mathauer and Imhoff 2006; Masango et al. 2008). Financial incentives, including wages and salaries, bonuses, pensions, insurance, allowances (for clothing or overtime), fellowships, loans and tuition reimbursement, are the most common approaches to improved recruitment and retention. Adequate and timely remuneration, and wage structures that offer opportunities for significant salary progression, are crucial.

Improving salaries, however, is particularly difficult where budgets are small, and relativities within the public sector constrain increases. Marginally improving wages could never be enough to significantly reduce the demand for migration, given the substantial wage and salary differences between source and recipient countries. Where at least two-thirds of most health budgets are already absorbed by labour costs, it is impossible to pay international 'market' salaries (of health or other skilled workers) without a financial crisis. Even doubling local salaries has not reduced migration (Vujicic et al. 2004; Vujicic and Zurn 2006; Chapter 6). In Peru, medical students had salary expectations four times those of the average doctor's salary; since such expectations could not be met, over one-third were contemplating migration (Mayta-Tristan et al. 2008). The ability to work in the usually better-resourced and -remunerated private sector deters migration, although enabling such opportunities has been resisted where it is seen to divert doctors away from public responsibilities and areas of particular need. Private practice meant that migration of Kenyan psychiatrists was negligible between 1997 and 2007 (Ndetei 2008). Tonga, where additional private practice is permitted for public sector doctors, has retained them more successfully than neighbouring Samoa, where this is not possible.

Similar salary issues occur within countries. To achieve even a 60 per cent probability that doctors would move from the capital of Niger, Niamey, to rural areas would require a 70 per cent boost in salary, otherwise they preferred to remain and develop private practices (C. Lemiere, pers. comm., 2009). In Benin, as also in Tonga and Kenya, 'it is much more attractive and profitable to stay in urban areas' because of alternative income-generating activities (Mathauer and Imhoff 2006: 5). In Indonesia, too, 'moderately remote' regions could be staffed using 'modest' cash incentives, but financial incentives would have to be prohibitively expensive to staff remote facilities, particularly in West Papua, the most remote, culturally distinct province with challenging geographical conditions (Chomitz et al. 1998). While health workers usually argue that the single strongest influence on their remaining would be better wages (Awases et al. 2004: 58), improved wages alone would not cover all needs. Other factors are involved. The motivation of final-year Ethiopian nursing and medical students to work in remote areas was influenced by extended household incomes, not solely that of the SHW, and also by their intrinsic motivations, specifically their 'willingness to help the poor' (Serneels et al. 2005: 19). Not only is a combination of incomes important, but altruism also plays a part. Wages alone have only some bearing on migration rates, and it is implicit for skilled migration that it is not the poorest who move but those who have managed to acquire enough capital, skills (and connections). It is impossible to make simple calculations that suggest that a particular wage rise would stem migration, since too many other factors and relativities are involved.

None the less, many countries have sought to raise salaries for SHWs and have used particular strategies involving overtime and similar payments to achieve more effective recruitment, retention, geographical distribution and skill mixes. Since relative income levels influence migration, doctors' wages must be demonstrably above those of others; increasing skill levels (and thus salaries) may drive up wages and salaries or prompt migration; hence the need to avoid salary compression. Some marginal shifts have been achieved. Cape Verde has selectively given rural doctors a 30 per cent salary increase. South Africa introduced a 'rural and scarce skill' allowance in 2003 to attempt to curtail migration from rural areas. Ghana implemented an additional duty hours allowance to discourage migration of doctors, and Zambia (with the assistance of the Global Fund) has subsidised the salaries of doctors and nurses in order to tackle the growing incidence of HIV/AIDS (Yumkella 2006). Exactly how successful, and for how long, such marginal interventions have been is unclear, yet in both South Africa and Ghana greater retention of SHWs appears to have occurred, despite tension between doctors and nurses, whose allowances were less than those of doctors (Kingma 2006: 27). Better salaries are necessary but insufficient.

Non-financial incentives are also crucial. Strengthening work autonomy, encouraging career development, providing opportunities for training, adapting working time and shift work (for nurses), reducing violence in the workplace, open leadership, study leave, working in a team and support and feedback from supervisors, alongside issues beyond the working environment, such as adequate housing and transport, all potentially reduce migration (WHO 2006a; Wilson et al. 2009). Trust, sensitive management, and a degree of autonomy are crucial; ultimately, as a senior Tongan health manager stressed, 'flat management must come from the heart'. Flexibility has not always been present for work practices. However, with realignment of career structures and promotion based on ability rather than nepotism, as Zimbabwe achieved in the 1990s, migration slowed (Awases et al. 2004).

Promotion opportunities are few, especially in small states, which cannot simply create posts for the sake of promotions (Ramo 1991: 270);

hence a transparent promotion structure is invaluable to ensure that health workers are not doubly disadvantaged. Annual review of salaries, a clear career structure with opportunities for ongoing training, and delegation of responsibilities at least boost the morale of those for whom opportunities of promotion are poor (Bakeea 1991: 256). Relativities are invariably important; both Swaziland and Malawi have responded to concerns that career opportunities favoured doctors rather than nurses by restructuring the latter's career pathways to increase meritocracy.

Outside the workplace other factors are important. For more than half of Ghanaian health workers something as seemingly straightforward as better day care for their children was a priority (Awases et al. 2004). Malawi has provided low-cost housing facilities to doctors and Ghana has given them cars at no cost. Sudan has gone even further, providing housing, a car and free admission to university for the children of returning doctors (Badr 2005). Jamaica has provided health insurance, paid vacations and free transportation for nurses, and St Vincent has sought to offer nurses low-interest loans for securing a home and car (Hosein and Thomas 2007), two of the typical objectives of many SHWs. Czech incentives (Epigraphs) are, thus far, unique. Diverse support structures, within a package, are invaluable.

SCALING UP AND TASK SHIFTING: NURSE PRACTITIONERS AND OTHERS

Within a wider context of 'scaling up' recruitment and training of SHWs, certain categories of health workers may be particularly valuable. It is no accident that poorly paid, low-status nurses are usually more likely to migrate than doctors. Introducing or expanding the role of nurse practitioners, intermediate between nurses and doctors, offers nurses new status, fresh challenges and better salaries, as in more developed countries where nurse practitioners have proved cost-effective and safe (Thornley 2003; Venning et al. 2000; Jones 2008). Upgrading nursing skills, or 'task shifting', so that nurses undertake a series of tasks hitherto undertaken by doctors, has been successful in various places, with the dual advantage of relieving hard-pressed doctors and giving greater job satisfaction to nurses, especially where they provide some curative services, and receive additional prestige and salaries. In resource-constrained settings nurse practitioners can effectively bridge gaps in primary care services.

Variously called physician assistants, health officers or clinical officers, alongside nurse practitioners, such non-physician clinicians (NPCs) trace a legacy from nineteenth-century French *officiers de santé* to more low-key twentieth-century *doktabois* in PNG and Chinese barefoot doctors (Fendall 1972; Flahault 1978; Mullan and Frehywot 2007; O'Connor and Hooker 2007). They have recently gained greater prominence in both developed countries, such as Canada and Scotland, and in developing countries. Half of all SSA countries, especially anglophone states, have active NPCs; nine even have more NPCs than doctors. In some countries this was a direct response to structural adjustment, which required reduced salary expenditures, or the accelerated loss of SHWs to the private sector (Dovlo 2004; McCourt and Awases 2007). In countries like Mozambique, Uganda, Kenya and Malawi, they have become the core of the health system, doing surgical procedures and giving anaesthetics (e.g. Cumbi et al. 2007), having prescriptive authority, and playing prominent roles in HIV/AIDS treatment, with several countries basing their anti-retroviral treatment strategies around NPCs (Record and Mohiddin 2006). Such strategies make better use of the time and skills of both doctors and nurses; within SSA, and globally, there were minimal differences in patient outcomes whether they were attended by doctors or nurse practitioners (Buchan and dal Poz 2002; Dovlo 2004; Laurant et al. 2009). Many NPCs came from poor rural areas, with lower levels of education than doctors, and trained closer to their homes and eventual places of work than most SHWs, at less expense and over a shorter time period. In the Pacific and in SSA, their presence had been particularly valuable in rural and remote areas, where they also reduced travel costs for patients; in Fiji at least it was a requirement that they be based in rural areas (Usher and Lindsay 2003; Dovlo 2004; Mullan and Frehywot 2007). Superior training improves the status of nurses, but it also makes their qualifications more transferable.

Similarly, community health workers (CHWs) in rural areas and nursing auxiliaries in urban areas can support nurses. Indeed, the lack of SHWs in most rural areas has meant instituting CHWs (health assistants or nurse aides), with limited training, for work at the local level. Here too this has also been of significance in developed countries, especially those with remote indigenous communities, such as Australia and Canada (Roach et al. 2007). This also confers prestige on participants, and contributes to bridging the gap between hospitals and villages. However, poor management and mentoring, weak education standards, inadequate supplies, misdiagnosis and patient preferences for 'superior' skills have blunted their effectiveness, and seen them bypassed. In many places where village-level CHWs have been introduced, such as Nigeria (Iyun 1989), they have tended to seek to practise curative medicine rather than preventive care, yet their presence remains invaluable. Malawi introduced a category of mainly male nursing auxiliaries (medical assistants) to support nurses, with preference given to 'those already employed as hospital attendants, cleaners, and people who can demonstrate that, after their training, they will remain in the same district' (Muula et al. 2003: 435). This gave opportunities to those who might not have otherwise contemplated semi-skilled employment, and, without recognised international qualifications, unlike nurses, almost none migrated (Palmer 2006). At the same time such strategies effectively boost primary and preventive health care and more effectively meet the needs of rural and regional areas.

It is also possible to raise the status, and increase the knowledge, of workers outside the formal sector, such as traditional birth attendants. While TBAs usually have high status in local society, they have often been derided and ignored by modern health care systems. In Sierra Leone, recognising their value and providing brief training courses had mutual benefits: 'The TBA who has a good relationship with the hospital does not want to keep to herself the woman who would be likely to die in childbirth in the village. And the hospital could not cope if everyone went there for delivery' (Stevenson 1987: 409). Mexico has raised the status of TBAs by giving them additional training and bringing them into formal medical settings to work with doctors; this has been particularly valuable in poorer provinces such as Chiapas and Oaxaca, where 60 per cent of births are attended by midwives, and has reduced demands on doctors and nurses (Braine 2008). How traditional health workers may or may not be incorporated into contemporary care systems is highly variable.

The growing incidence of HIV/AIDS, especially in SSA, has brought renewed focus on 'task shifting': moving appropriate tasks to less specialised workers. Doctors were not needed to prescribe and dispense anti-retroviral therapy when that could be done by nurses, and CHWs could deliver a range of services that freed up nurses. In Malawi and Uganda a 'basic care package' for people living with HIV was designed to be delivered by non-specialist doctors, nurses, nursing assistants and CHWs, and also by those people living with HIV. Somewhat differently, this scaling up may be particularly valuable in specialised areas, such as psychiatry, where specialists are relatively rare, and there is a strong case for nurses being able to prescribe psychotropic medicines in rural and regional areas of countries such as the Solomon Islands, Fiji and Ethiopia, where doctors are scarce (WHO 2007: 46–8).

The rise of nurse practitioners and CHWs, with a role and status below that of doctors and nurses respectively, has however been resented by some, notably doctors, who see this as an erosion of their privileges and authority. Demarcation disputes, prestige and privilege hamper innovation, and have a colonial legacy. In SSA, professional associations have resisted task shifting unless better wages and working conditions were also implemented. It has been argued there that

> Nurses have to jealously guard their boundaries and professional image. It is important to carefully delineate the roles and titles of these new cadres, and avoid use of 'nurse' or 'nursing' in their titles. These cadres often assist other health professionals with menial work. Thus their training and titles should reflect the nature of their job. (Seboni 2009: 1036)

This does not only occur in developing countries; in Australia, doctors' associations have resisted additional roles being given to midwives and nurse practitioners. In Canada, migrant SHWs, alongside other SHWs, opposed new roles in developing countries, arguing that it would result in overall deskilling and a less trained medical workforce, which could be detrimental to national health, with one migrant SHW believing that the training of auxiliary workers was inherently racist, with developed countries continuing to receive SHWs but source countries left with inferior health care workers for their own needs (Labonté et al. 2006: 11), a similar position to that of the Nigerian Medical Association (Mullan and Frehywot 2007: 5). In Ghana, Malawi, Zambia and Kenya, nurses' lobbies succeeded in banning the training of enrolled nurses, despite increased migration and shortages of registered nurses.

In the Cook Islands, from the 1990s, nurse practitioners were trained for work in the remote northern islands, a system that worked well (assisted by salary bonuses) until doctors were sent there for political reasons. The migrant doctors who went there (from India and later Burma) were less effective and more costly than the nurse practitioners, who had then been redeployed as nurses and could not use their additional skills. When Tonga developed a new category of health officer, trained in a limited two-year course within Tonga, and who largely ran rural health centres or worked in hospital outpatient wards, their replacement of doctors produced controversy: 'public perceptions of their competence have been less than fully favorable' (World Bank 1994: 322). When the Samoan Ministry of Health similarly sought to create a new 'medical assistant', intermediate between a doctor and nurse, members of parliament who had hospitals in their districts resisted this and demanded fully certified doctors (Hoadley 1980: 452). It took 30 years for Samoa to try again. Some have therefore seen, or chosen to see, the term 'health care assistants' as an oxymoron, with such people being pressurised to go beyond their levels of competence, without supervision or accountability (McKenna et al. 2007; Mullan and Frehywot 2007). The mirage of 'quality medicine' – favoured by doctors and politicians – tends to displace the need for simple but competent and readily available service delivery, especially in rural areas. Overcoming such perceptions and responses is as difficult as providing adequate services and staff in the regions.

Trading on privilege and general problems of vested self-interest (even in what are sometimes seen as altruistic and vocational arenas) within power-ful professional establishments hinder change. Moreover, there is some-thing of a paradox. Task shifting and scaling up tend to be accompanied by pressures to improve the working conditions of those who undertake additional and more skilled tasks, so making them increasingly similar to those they are replacing. Even in the 1960s a process of creep was evident, as auxiliaries sought longer periods of training to make themselves com-parable with professionals, alongside 'rumblings of discontent and a desire to have training incorporated within a university' (Fendall 1972: 173). In Surinam it has proved almost impossible to upgrade health assistants in rural areas since as soon as they acquired 'superior' qualifications they sought to move to the capital city. That kind of shift, or 'role drift', is not unique to nursing, but occurs among allied health professionals, pharma-cists and dentists, and challenges the production and maintenance of an appropriate skill mix.

A TECHNOLOGICAL SHIFT?

Technological change characterises medical practice yet almost all techno-logical innovation is directed at diagnosis and cure rather than supporting or replacing labour. For over a decade attempts have been made to create 'nursebots', mechanised robots that would perform basic hospital tasks such as cleaning, mopping up spillages, taking messages and guiding visi-tors to hospital beds. Robots would free up hospital staff to do important tasks, they would be immune to disease and would work long hours unless they malfunctioned. However, robots remain largely in an experimental phase, they are expensive, and require considerable monitoring and inter-vention. Technology cannot easily replace workers (Folbre 2006; Bower and McCullough 2004). Technology may potentially free up labour, reduces the need for some radiologists, and there has been 'talk of trans-Atlantic video night nurse monitoring of the elderly' (Sinclair-Jones 2000: 28), but no obvious labour replacement has occurred.

Similarly, despite the promise of telemedicine, especially for rural and remote areas, even in developed countries the uptake of new technology has been marred by poor planning, an emphasis on hardware rather than on teaching staff how to use the software, and conservatism. Expensive machinery tends to be under-utilised while doctors continue to use expen-sive referrals, despite significant potential cost savings, support for exist-ing diagnostic processes, increased equity, and the probability of greater recruitment and retention of doctors in regional areas (Smith and Gray 2009). In inland Australia, telehealth services reduced feelings of isolation, lessened meeting times, improved diagnostic capacity and improved quality of life; while both doctors and nurses in such isolated areas raised familiar concerns about work problems, and barely half had been there for more than a year, technology may have had a marginal impact on increasing retention rates (Windeyer 2002). In some countries telemedicine is inhibited by insurance policies but also by attitudes where, like NPCs, it appears 'second-best'. In developing countries, where telemedicine is more obviously seen as a response to shortages of SHWs, limited finance, inadequate technical support, isolation and fragmentation, both for distance learning and diagnosis, have slowed acquisition (Smith 2004). However, in Pohnpei State (Federated States of Micronesia) Internet diagnosis has significantly reduced some health care costs, where international referrals represent 10 per cent of the state's health budget and serve 1 per cent of the population (Hedson 2000). In the Cook Islands some of the southern group of islands are linked to the main island of Rarotonga for health assessments, basic management and ease of access to laboratory results. Technical complexities mean that skilled labour is required in places where it is least likely to exist, while telemedicine has largely been beneficial in diagnostics (notably radiology) rather than in reducing labour needs. Health care remains labour-intensive.

RURAL, REGIONAL AND REMOTE

Securing and retaining a workforce in rural and regional areas have been particularly difficult. Attempts to encourage or bond recent graduates to work in rural and regional areas have had a long and frustrating history. As long ago as the 1960s the West Bengal government made promotion easier for those who had served longest in rural areas, and also banned private practice in the capital, Calcutta, while Indonesia required new medical graduates to serve three years in a rural area before they were permitted employment in Jakarta (Gish 1971: 77, 97). The most obvious consequence of this was that rural employment was seen as 'some form of forced labour . . . as a preliminary to a "proper" medical career in the city' (ibid.: 122), akin to China's rustification programme; hence the impact on rural health care was slight. Kiribati, Mongolia, Ecuador and Thailand have sought to bond doctors to work in rural areas, but there has been massive reluctance; Thai doctors have bought themselves out of schemes reasonably cheaply, Ecuadorians experienced a range of problems both practical and cultural, but felt they benefited in the one year they were there (Cavender and Alban 1998), while Mongolians went only because they would otherwise have been unable to graduate.

Three problems reduce the value of bonding within countries. Rural bonding is for a short time period, and is neither continuous nor sustainable; people may pay their way out and 'punishments' are too trivial to deter breaches. In Thailand, bonding was linked to compulsory rural service, underpinned by heavy fines, but the scheme suffered from corruption and favouritism and well-connected or better-off individuals were able to bypass the scheme, undermining its utility. Moreover, while compulsory transfers of doctors between provinces were enforced, this was the single most important reason for resignations (Wibulpolprasert and Pengpaibon 2003). More positive inducements include training priority: Nepal, India and Myanmar all give priority in postgraduate programmes to doctors serving in rural areas. Bangladesh offers accelerated promotion.

Most developed countries have difficulties in developing and devolving a health workforce for rural areas, and even relatively wealthy countries such as Australia and Canada experience sustained problems. Many have established special scholarship schemes for those who wish to stay and/ or work in rural and remote areas (above). Bonding and scholarships retain policy potential. Some developing countries have adopted similar strategies; Tonga has long had regional nurse training quotas, effectively ensuring a regional nurse workforce. In Australia, achieving a reasonable rural health workforce has only been partly accomplished by a concerted battery of policies, including training local workers in local institutions, and a range of incentive payments and bonding, in a context where regional doctors were supported by their own semi-political organisations (such as the Rural Doctors' Association). Even then, overseas doctors and nurses, directed to regional areas, have been crucial to propping up the system and 'without them, the private and public health system as we know it would collapse' (McEwin and Cameron 2007: 45; Gardiner et al. 2006). In Canada, notably northern Ontario, some 42 programmes, ranging from telemedicine to financial incentives, have been developed over a 35-year period to encourage training and retention; they have become more sophisticated over time, and loosely shifted from a focus on recruitment to retention, but problems of retention remain (Pong 2008). Financial incentives alone are inadequate (Barnighausen and Bloom 2009a, 2009b). While the vast size, climatic and logistic challenges of thinly populated Australia and Canada make the achievement of an adequate health workforce in remote areas particularly difficult, institutional and financial resources are far beyond those of many developing countries, indicating the great challenge where resources are much scarcer, and health workers and problems more likely to be ignored. Meanwhile, most isolated regional workers are unlikely to be effectively organised to raise their status and concerns at the centre.

In remote areas, more than anywhere else, an integrated package of measures is needed to attract, train and retain new (or indeed any) SHWs, and many such measures may lie outside the health sector. Such packages are necessarily dependent on both finance and effective management capability. Even in developed countries such as Australia, management, alongside support and mentoring, is frequently identified as critical for retention of health workers (e.g. Han and Humphreys 2005; Stagnitti et al. 2005). One evaluation of health care in Ethiopia concluded

> The health policy includes plans to develop an attractive career structure, with appropriate remuneration and incentives for all employees. There are no signs of this being put in place. There is a serious need to strengthen the planning and management capacity of the local government officials who are responsible for overseeing the implementation of the policy, and to strengthen the lines of accountability between local government, the health services, and the community. In fact few health-service providers have even seen the health policy. (Von Massow 2001: 25)

Financial support, effective, appropriate and sensitive policy formation, management and implementation – a political and practical will – are at the core of all policies for the recruitment and retention of SHWs at national and regional levels. While Ethiopia has particularly challenging problems, lack of success there is indicative of comparable failures elsewhere.

BANS, BONDS AND TAXES

The most obvious means of preventing international migration of SHWs is simply to ban migration, and refuse to recognise or issue passports, and this has been a persistent theme in discussions of international regulation, despite its denial of rights (Kingma 2006: 137–9). In 1998, Bangladesh introduced a ban on women wishing to work abroad, nominally because they were vulnerable to abuse and mistreatment, but the ban had been lifted by 2003. Sri Lanka briefly imposed a ban on the emigration of mothers of children younger than five. Such bans, invariably focused on women, are generally ineffective, and encourage clandestine migration, as they did from Bangladesh. Outright bans on the emigration of SHWs, and others, are increasingly implausible for ethical, political and, above all, economic reasons.

The single most important policy to have slowed migration, especially where smaller countries depend on overseas education and training, and a rare direct approach, has been bonding, which has had considerable success in bringing people back to their home countries after training overseas. Both Tonga and Samoa bond nurses on a 'year-for-year' basis, according to the duration of training, issuing certificates only after completion. The Ghana Nurses and Midwives Council required two years' national experience before certification as a nurse, but there was poor compliance on the part of both nurses and the Council, hence new procedures were introduced to bond nurses to the Ministry of Health for five years (Bump 2006; Buchan et al. 2009). Bonding has been less valuable within countries, both geographically (to remote areas) or for retention within the public sector (see below). It has also been suggested, in the form of 'conditional scholarships', as a means of retaining health workers for SSA countries of high HIV prevalence (Barnighausen and Bloom 2009a). Like training, bonding occurs at a significant time in the life cycle, coinciding for some with the start of family life and the possibility of establishing local family roots. Bonding implies a sense of duty, and emphasises costs, even though skilled workers have tended to leave at the end of bond periods (usually equivalent to the two or three years that have been spent overseas). In many developing countries, however, bonding has been of limited value because of poor administrative efficiency in management systems and lack of agreement between the education and health sectors (Dovlo 2003). Graduates resist its structures, and fail to return or, as in SSA, escape legal consequences by taking up employment in the Gulf, after five years of training but before their licences are granted. While it has been detested and resisted, when few if any other skilled workers are similarly directed (and rather similar military service is now infrequent), and regulations are often broken, it has been invaluable, as much for the practice of return as in the inculcation of notions of duty and loyalty. Taking bonding from being punitive to pleasurable would be a major challenge.

Initial responses to perceptions of a brain drain became attempts to encourage or force recipient countries to compensate source countries that had financed their education through some form of taxation (see below). Only rarely have some countries, like Malawi, contemplated the direct taxation of overseas workers, a 'brain-drain migration tax' (Record and Mohiddin 2006). Multiple problems are attached to this and parallel those involving direct compensation from developed countries (see below), but with a greater private reluctance to pay such taxes. Eritrea requires external citizens to pay a 2 per cent income tax to the home government, which is said to generate a high proportion of development aid (Dovlo 2005), but this is widely resented by migrants, whose migration expressed some measure of discontent with Eritrea and who distrust government policies. Any such 'brain drain tax' penalises migrants by subjecting them to double taxation. Similarly, more formalised transfers of remittances, enabling their more effective use as temporary capital, have been suggested (Brown et al. 1995; Dodani and LaPorte 2005; Record and Mohiddin 2006), but these too are resisted by migrants seeking to maximise the household utility of remittances. Attempts to encourage financial investment from overseas Bangladeshi doctors largely failed because of their lack of trust in the government, bureaucracy and the lack of an attractive investment climate (Rahman and Khan 2007: 140). The outcome was private investment rather than investment that directly benefited national development. In many countries various policies have been implemented to encourage greater investment by overseas nationals and the more productive use of remittances (Gamlen 2008: 850), but none have been directly targeted at SHWs.

OPTIONS FOR RECIPIENT COUNTRIES

Given the pressures on public sectors in source countries, and the very limited scope for policy implementation, the onus for a more equitable global distribution of SHWs has gradually shifted on to recipient countries, where demand is created. Without that demand only a fraction of the contemporary migration of SHWs would remain. Continued migration has resulted in increased calls for ethical recruitment guidelines, adequate codes of practice constraining recruitment and/or compensation to countries experiencing losses. While source countries have sought, however imperfectly, to put in place policies to stimulate recruitment and retention, recipient countries have been rather more reluctant to develop policies for greater self-reliance and reduced international recruitment and migration. Bluntly, in the long term, self-reliance is 'the only viable solution to resolving the shortage of health workers' (Rutten 2009b: 312). Beyond a crucial shift towards greater self-reliance, and increased and better targeted aid delivery (Ravishankar et al. 2009), there are relatively few policy choices in recipient countries, and little movement towards a multilateral framework for regulating migration at the international level.

Raising Recruitment and Reducing Attrition

Few recipient countries have taken sustained, effective measures to increase recruitment and reduce attrition of skilled health workers, at a time of greater demand, either by increasing the number of training places or improving wages and working conditions (Pond and McPake 2006), despite recent shifts in Norway and the UK towards greater national recruitment (Buchan and Seccombe 2005; Norwegian Directorate of

Health 2009). Neither the USA nor the Gulf states, all major recipients, have moved towards national self-sufficiency. Indeed, US health workforce 'policy' has been wholly derided: 'There is probably no example of a more poorly-conducted or more deliberately distorted planning activity in the history of the world' (Cooper 2008: 27). France has maintained a long-established policy of restricting medical practice to those with French qualifications, and little has changed elsewhere. Without expanded national training capacity in developed countries, demand will continue to exceed supply, but in most recipient countries there are weak prospects of domestic supply increasing significantly, and national gaps between supply and demand have tended to widen rather than contract (Chaguturu and Vallabhaneni 2005). At the same time the age of nationals recruited into nursing in developed countries has increased considerably. In most primarily recipient countries the same kind of package of policies is required to increase local recruitment, reduce attrition rates, and improve the status of health employment. Here, too, this demands a significant increase in economic support.

If demand for SHWs were to fall in developed countries, that would lead to reduced migration, although migrants, as many already do, may choose to work outside the health sector. Falling demand might also lead to a reduction in the number of trainees in developing countries if migration opportunities declined, especially where migration and health employment are linked, notably in Kerala, the Philippines and parts of the Caribbean and Pacific. As has been suggested for Jamaica, 'a reduction in the demand in the United States may well represent one less allure associated with the practice of nursing. This may contribute to reduced numbers or persons of less calibre entering the profession locally' (Brown 1997: 222). None the less, greater self-reliance in recipient countries would almost certainly enable greater self-reliance in source countries. The prospects of this being imminent are, however, minimal.

Compensation

The economic costs to sending countries, and the recognition that recruitment is accelerating, have renewed interest in compensation for the loss of investment in training and more generally of human capital. During the 1970s there was considerable discussion of the possibility of compensating source countries (Bhagwati 1976; Gish and Godfrey 1979; Bohning 1982) but no action was taken and the issue soon disappeared. Even the most simple formulation raises obvious questions of whether there should be compensation from countries that benefit from migrant health workers but do not actively recruit, what is the situation of migrant health workers in private sector employment (as is common), how an appropriate sum might be calculated and who should pay whom. Recipient countries and hospital systems have no interest in putting in place compensatory mechanisms in countries supplying skilled labour, arguing that markets operate in this way (and migrants gain from it) and there is no means of knowing how long migrants will stay, despite strong ethical arguments in favour of restitution (Labonté et al. 2006; Mackintosh et al. 2006; Connell et al. 2007; Agwu and Llewelyn 2009). Notions of compensation also founder on migrants' agency, and their ability to overcome structural impediments to development through migration, while health-worker labour markets are part of an increasingly global economy, beyond the restrictions of national borders (Raghuram 2009a). The possibility of financial compensation to source countries for losses of workers has thus proved impossible to implement, because of rejection of the specificity of health-worker migration, the impossibility of estimating costs, shifts of workers between the private and public sectors, uncertainty over the duration of employment and the migration of health workers between several countries, and within countries (in federal systems). Previous considerations of this, more than a quarter of a century ago, were rejected as too idealistic and impractical. They probably remain so.

RETURN MIGRATION AND THE DIASPORA

The growing extent of international migration in recent years, and especially skilled migration, has resulted in particular attention being given to the potential for utilising the skills of overseas migrants, even on a temporary basis, and encouraging return migration. As greater numbers of migrants settle overseas, diasporas and remittances have assumed a new importance (Faist 2008; Gamlen 2008). Many source countries, even those where the migration of skilled workers has been significant, have no strategies or policies for benefiting from such migrants, although almost all the evidence on overseas workers and migrants suggests that they are at least rhetorically anxious to support their home countries (Bloch 2005). Most countries, and health ministries, have no obvious data on how to contact overseas migrants, despite the growth of homeland associations. A number of countries have even dissociated themselves from overseas migrants, on the grounds that they have 'voted with their feet' and abandoned their home countries (even if they send remittances), and national policies should be directed towards benefiting those who remain. Resentment of return migration, where promotions and other 'privileges' may be hard won (Chapter 8), is not uncommon. While developing countries have lost disproportionate amounts of skilled labour, ironically the greatest recent interest in harnessing the skills of the diaspora has come from rich-world countries like the USA and Australia (e.g. Fullilove 2008; Gamlen 2008). Indeed, for over a century, Italy has constructed a vision of an 'international' nation consisting of a transnational network of loyalty, support and shared culture (Choate 2008). Most initiatives, such as enabling dual citizenship or stimulating remittance flows, must come from source countries.

Developing countries and international institutions have none the less emphasised the potential role of the diaspora in assisting home countries in ways that go beyond remittances, and include the transfer of skills, knowledge and technology. Given the limited interest in more permanent return migration (Chapter 8), temporary return is increasingly held out as offering more development potential. One such expatriate programme is the Ghana–Netherlands Healthcare Project, managed by the International Organization for Migration, whose objectives are to transfer knowledge, skills and experiences through short-term assignments and projects in Ghana. Over a two-year period, 20 Ghanaians, the majority of whom were doctors, returned briefly to Ghana. Numbers were few, the impact was limited, since many returnees were psychiatrists and needs were elsewhere, costs were high, but their role as cultural interpreters was important (Long and Mensah 2007). Return migrants can thus play some role in health care. Diverse Pacific islands overseas migrants intermittently return 'home' in association with aid projects to provide short-term surgical assistance in specialised areas, and may also contribute to skill transfer (Connell 2009). Nigerians and Bangladeshis in the USA have expressed similar wishes but without obvious outcomes (Healy and Oikelome 2007; Rahman and Khan 2007). Other recipient countries might stimulate such cooperative projects.

CODES OF PRACTICE AND MOUs

With growing awareness of the adverse effects of health-worker migration on health systems in source countries, the demand for ethical recruitment strategies has increased, as other forms of 'control' have been lacking, impractical or inadequate. The approach to some form of more 'managed migration', negotiated and regulated between countries and regions, has been contingent on both the growing realisation that source countries cannot prevent migration, while accommodation to it might provide benefits, notably through remittances.

Complaints from developing countries over increasingly aggressive recruitment resulted in a subtle shift towards 'ethical international recruitment'. From 1999 onwards, codes were formulated in different regions to guide international recruitment. The UK introduced various codes after 1999, which sought to discourage direct government recruitment of health professionals from developing countries, but the code did not apply to private recruitment agencies or prevent the public sector from hiring SHWs who applied independently. The Pacific Code of 2007 focused on similar principles of transparency, fairness and mutuality of benefits, established in an earlier Commonwealth Code, where, for example, recruiters should not seek to recruit health workers with an 'outstanding obligation to their own country' (Commonwealth Secretariat 2004). Codes have usually had a tripartite rationale: protecting the migrant workers; supporting them in the workplace; and preventing any disruption of health services in source countries. Those emerging from the UK focused on the first two objectives, while the Commonwealth and Pacific Codes shifted the balance to the third. Only the Pacific Code mentioned any notion of compensation.

While codes have led to some greater consciousness of issues, it proved difficult to agree on what constituted 'aggressive' recruiting, or how any negative impact on source countries might be measured. Moreover, codes are voluntary; moral sanctions alone have been possible and they are of limited effectiveness even where the public sector is prominent (Bach 2003; Buchan et al. 2009). None the less recruiting within most developing countries for employment in the UK was scaled down, although it partly shifted towards the USA and the Gulf, which were not covered by any code, while individuals could continue to migrate freely, but often taking up employment in nursing homes rather than hospitals (Chapter 7). Nursing homes thus became a 'back-door entrance' to the public sector, while migration became more complex, for example resulting in new flows of nurses from Zimbabwe to Australia. One outcome has been pressure for movement towards a more comprehensive global code.

Bilateral agreements and Memoranda of Understanding (MOUs) enable more effective regulated and managed migration. MOUs, such as that between Spain and the UK, and between the Philippines and the UK, have sought to organise the formal placement of workers from 'surplus' countries or regions to where there is a shortage. MOUs are more specific by countries, time periods and numbers, and tailored to particular country needs (both recipient and source), and exclude intermediary, private recruiting agencies. Thus in 2002 the Philippines, through its Philippine Overseas Employment Administration, recruited and supplied nearly 200 nurses to work for at least a year in the UK (Buchan 2008). Several Italian regions have developed bilateral agreements with

Romanian provinces and nurse training institutes, with Italian institutions providing training courses in languages and clinical skills in Romania (Chaloff 2008). Limited numbers of SHWs work for established periods under appropriate and monitored conditions, and should return with enhanced skills, experience and capital. MOUs can even be envisaged as a form of organised working holiday, which may enable promotion on return. However, not all those on temporary schemes do return home, as with Polish health workers in the UK, and human rights would be violated in demanding this. MOUs also lack short-term flexibility where situations change quickly. More effective regulation, and more ethical recruitment, alongside bilateral relationships, suggest some partial solutions, despite continued concern over the ethics of recruitment (Connell and Stilwell 2006; Rogerson and Crush 2008). Indeed, the movement towards codes and MOUs has been a necessary attempt to harmonise and regulate flows, and something of a prelude to both the formal legalities of migration under GATS and a shift towards more complex forms of managed migration.

GATS and intra-regional migration

The emergence of regional trading blocs and agreements in different parts of the world, loosely modelled on the experiences of NAFTA (the North American Free Trade Agreement) and the EU, will result in greater regional migration, as it has done in Europe, especially within the post-2004 and post-2007 extended Europe, which increased migration from the relatively poor Eastern European countries into Western Europe (Chapter 3). Professional qualifications have tended to become harmonised in these large regions, with, for example, NAFTA urging Canada, Mexico and the USA to establish mutually acceptable criteria for licensing and certification (Oulton 1998; Bach 2003). Within the EU, registered nurses and midwives can move freely between member states. Japan and the Philippines have negotiated a bilateral free trade agreement enabling Filipino SHWs to move to Japan. These are all likely to be precedents for further bilateral and regional agreements, based on structural differences, notably intra-regional wage differentials, between member states within particular regional groups.

More generally, international migration of SHWs is linked to the General Agreement on Trade in Services, established in 1995 through the World Trade Organization (WTO) to liberalise international trade in services, including the movement of so-called 'natural persons' (under Mode 4 of GATS). It also covers other evolving trans-border linkages, such as telediagnosis, medical tourism and international hospital chains.

GATS is a complex, multilateral agreement covering all WTO members, but few have been signatories to all its components, ultimately intended to broaden and increase trade in services, including health services. It has no role in regulating health status or achieving greater equity of health provision. A key component of GATS relates to the harmonisation and mutual recognition of professional qualifications across borders, which, as in the EU, will increase migration opportunities, in a very gradual shift towards more global accreditation. GATS is restricted to temporary movements but in practice these are not easily distinguished (Bach 2003; Kingma 2006). Thus, 'with its inclusion in regional trade agreements and the GATS, mobility of the highly skilled has taken an important step out of the state-centered framework of national immigration policies, toward the market-led, multilateral framework of international trade' (Lavenex 2007: 41). In so doing, mobility moves further away from national regulation.

In different regions there has been some progress towards GATS objectives. In 2007 ASEAN set out a mutual recognition agreement that formulated goals for regional cooperation through the exchange of services. It will therefore probably lead to the migration of nurses from poorer to richer states, hitherto prevented by non-recognition of qualifications and linguistic and cultural constraints. Such intra-Asian movement may later extend into movement within the wider APEC community (Manning and Sidorenko 2007; Arunanondchai and Fink 2007). Similarly, the establishment of a Caribbean single market economy at the end of 2008 should lead to greater mobility within the Caribbean region, and more migration of nurses from poorer to richer states, for example, from Guyana, St Vincent and Grenada to Barbados and the Bahamas. Migration is not constrained by language in much of the Caribbean. Although arguments have been made that this will be beneficial for the region as a whole (Hosein and Thomas 2007: 328–9; Yan 2006; Salmon et al. 2007), those states that are presently poorly served, notably Jamaica, Trinidad and Guyana, are likely to be disadvantaged further, while 'the danger is that each country competes with the other with the risk of selling what they have at bargain basement prices' (Caribbean Commission on Health and Development 2006: 77). Although the 15-member Caribbean Community (CARICOM) will 'provide some degree of ease for frustrated nurses as they move from one territory within the intra-regional agreement to another territory in the region in search of greener pastures' (Hosein and Thomas 2007: 329), the wider benefits are not evident. As codes seek greater controls over migration and GATS seeks to facilitate movement, two significant institutional shifts are competing with and challenging each other.

MANAGED MIGRATION: A NEO-LIBERAL SOLUTION?

The more legalistic developments involved in codes and under GATS are a response to, or have gone on in parallel with, greater interest in migration on the part of source countries. In this century a more controversial response to health-worker migration has become more widespread, based on 'the Philippines model': a deliberate strategy of producing significantly more health workers than are required locally on the basis that many will migrate (and others resign), and that migration can be beneficial. The 'Philippines model' centres on the assumptions that many SHWs will migrate anyway, most training is in the private sector, enough SHWs are available locally, and remittances are greater than the cost of training, so there is a net national benefit from migration. Many countries have sponsored overseas migration, and provided training and orientation programmes, but primarily of unskilled and semi-skilled workers, whereas the Philippines has been the acknowledged global leader in the export of SHWs.

The 'Philippines model' has been remarkably pervasive. In Ghana the vice-chancellor of the University of Ghana has stated that Africa, and specifically Ghana, can make economic gains from the brain drain by training more doctors, nurses and other professionals for export. He argued that 'We must not look at international migration only from the negative point of view. India, the Philippines and other countries support their economies well through international migration.' He noted that Ghana received more than $2 billion per year through official remittances from Ghanaians working abroad, so that if more professionals were trained for export, the volume of remittances would increase tremendously. He also indicated that the university would require substantial extra funding for laboratories to enable it to take in an extra intake of medical students (www.ghanaweb. com, 26 January 2005). Similar positive perspectives on the economic outcomes of the migration of health workers are near the core of policies directed at managed migration.

In China and Indonesia, where the Philippines is seen as a 'successful pioneer model', migration of SHWs has been advocated as a valuable policy despite the recognition of significant human resource shortages in regional areas (Gordon 2005: 372; Suwandono et al. 2005; Fang 2007), although in both countries the rush to export was slowed by a lack of training staff, language and the need to modify curricula. While not specifically targeting SHWs, China has thus 'made significant business investments in the training of workers for export', and nurses have been part of this. China has followed the Philippines in negotiating international labour supply agreements, with such countries as Saudi Arabia and the UK. In 2002 a centre was established in Beijing for nurse accreditation in the USA. Overseas Chinese workers were idiosyncratically viewed as a 'brain bank' and 'brain power stored abroad' (Kingma 2006: 82, 83). In South Africa and parts of Asia, labour export has been a private sector activity; India has suggested that it might become an exporter of nurses, much like the Philippines, because of large-scale 'nursing unemployment' (quoted in Yeates 2009: 180). Some of the states that emerged from the former Soviet Union have similarly sought to follow the Philippines model (Aiken et al. 2004: 75). Global financial crisis has further encouraged external orientation.

Several Caribbean states have recognised the extreme difficulty of unilateral change, and the futility of Canute-like attempts to stem migration or significantly change the international context of recruitment, but have argued for forms of 'managed migration' that involve regional activities (including the standardisation of nurse certification across the region), domestic marketing strategies that aggressively sell nursing as a valuable profession, providing more effective salary structures, and also special incentive schemes to encourage skilled workers to return at least on a temporary basis (and share their skills and expertise). Managed migration would ideally be structured within a context of reciprocity and 'human capital replenishment', where recipient countries invest in the training programmes of source countries, as is beginning in parts of the Caribbean: 'a long-term and more sustainable solution would be to enlarge training facilities to meet the expanding demand in labour importing countries' (Nurse 2004: 4, Salmon et al. 2007). In 2002, a regional health strategy was endorsed that planned for the emigration of a certain proportion of the region's health professionals, and the rotating and short-term migration of others. A key component was the negotiation of new linkages with recruiting countries, specifically the USA, where nurses are trained within the region but the cost of that training is reimbursed by the USA. New nursing schools have been established, primarily to produce nurses for export, as in St Vincent, with the majority going to work for hospital partners in the USA, who would pay for the training costs (Connell 2007a), but with constraints on how long nurses might stay overseas before returning, effectively contract labour migration revised. However, there are doubts over the general willingness of recruiting countries to enter into expensive, long-term contracts, and the outcomes of the Caribbean experiment remain to be assessed.

A similar scheme was mooted whereby Pacific island states might collectively support a training programme for about 150–200 nurses, established in conjunction with a hospital in a major destination. The economic assumption was that the private benefits and costs would be split between the nurses and their families and the government, with the government receiving taxes and perhaps training fees (ADB 2005). Where local economic development opportunities are relatively few, it has even been argued that 'Pacific governments must invest in preparing their youth to earn skilled jobs in the global market place . . . Otherwise, much like our primary commodities, Pacific island workers will be exported cheap and unprocessed' (Chand 2008a: 41). Kiribati, one of the smallest and poorest countries in the world, has entered into an agreement for groups of students to undertake nursing degree courses in Australia, funded by Australia's aid agency, AusAID, whose 'development specialist' has stated that 'We expect quite a few of the students will take advantage of the global shortage in nursing skills. It's a highly transportable profession.' Hence 'some students after graduation will of course return to Kiribati but those who find employment in other countries will most likely send home remittances' (*Focus*, 23(1), 2008: 33). While this may differ from managed migration, in having no key agreement, it constitutes a thinly disguised form of Australian recruitment, albeit with Kiribati anxious to be involved.

Significantly, at the same time that a growing number of countries have begun to contemplate, and organise, formal labour exports, there is growing evidence that the Philippines, with a population of about 97 million, has almost literally 'sold out', since the migration of SHWs now affects the functioning of the health system, especially in regional areas (Chapter 7). For small countries particularly, where labour reservoirs are restricted, this 'second-generation' problem suggests an ominous precedent. None the less, the rise of MOUs and GATS, widespread interest in more managed migration, with its remittance outcome, and the quest for education at 'international' and thus marketable standards, indicate that growing numbers of countries are oriented to migration rather than seeking to stem the tide. Ghana's attempt to train more doctors, almost certain to migrate, after the loss of many more, prompted one comment: 'they have a leaky bucket now. In desperation they are building a bigger leaky bucket' (Mullan 2007: 441). As the contemporary tribulations of the Philippines indicate, individuals and households may be more significant beneficiaries than nations.

IN A POLICY VACUUM?

In an ideal world the need for SHWs would be reduced by steadily improving health, but that is unlikely. Indeed, the simultaneous transition towards HIV/AIDS, NCDs and longer life expectancies has increased the need for SHWs, demanded larger budgets, drawn attention to vacancies and stimulated migration. Global increases in the extent of migration, and interest in sponsored or managed migration, have occurred despite doubts over the willingness of recipient countries to develop more ethical recruitment systems that would support reciprocity and compensation. Recipient countries have found it easier, and much cheaper, to become 'free-riders' and recruit SHWs overseas, as they first did in the 1940s. Intensification in the competition for SHWs has meant more widespread recruiting, rather than addressing the 'more difficult' causes of attrition and shortage, which are linked to wages and working conditions. They have consequently taken few policy directions that would slow migration. The abstractions of the London Declaration are at some distance from reality.

In the source countries, seemingly paradoxically, there has been both widespread acceptance of the need to develop subtle and wide-ranging policy packages to encourage recruitment and retention, and simultaneous interest in more managed migration. As Marilyn Lorenzo has said, 'Even if we fix all the policies within the Philippines it will not amount to much. We cannot stop migration; we just want to manage it more effectively' (pers. comm. 2005). Policies that might redress and reduce migration are implausible for numerous states, where economic growth is slight, public policy formation has proved difficult, employment conditions are unlikely ever to be comparable with those in developed countries, and the relatively recent loss of SHWs is one part of wider migration streams that, for half a century, have provided real gains from remittances for the households of migrants. In various states, including some of those most affected by migration, state regulation is as much concerned with encouraging as preventing migration. Rather than a policy vacuum, there is a surfeit of sometimes conflicting policies.

Policy packages have been elaborated many times, developing themes first raised in the 1970s. Despite widespread and longstanding recognition of the potential utility of particular policy directions, limited implementation has resulted from a lack of finance, professional resistance (to nurse practitioners and others), the lack of political will and management to implement and monitor plans effectively, and alternative national priorities. Ineffective management has often been singled out as a 'binding constraint to scaling up health services and achieving the MDGs', especially in rural and remote areas (Egger and Ollier 2007: 1), where even senior staff may lack management training. Management is crucial where mentoring, support and recognition are as valuable as financial incentives. Yet health managers are almost as prone to migrate internationally as they are locally. In Malawi, middle management is particularly migration prone;

hence the capacity and discipline of the public service have markedly declined since the early 1990s (Palmer 2006). The task of managing health systems then becomes even more difficult. Substantial gulfs separate plans from reality. Policy formation does not constitute implementation, and effective plans are beyond short-term government lifetimes. Even the best policies take time to hone and implement (Pong 2008). In-country education with a local curriculum reduces attrition and migration more effectively than overseas education, but its practice challenges the cultures of migration. Nepotism and regionalism likewise challenge the virtues of meritocracy.

Nowhere is without opportunities for improved policy directions, no problems are wholly intractable and most of the key elements of policy are well known. Yet public health sector funding is rarely a national priority, as governments globally seek to reduce public expenditure and outsource key functions. Underpinning any hope of long-lasting success is the need for global monetary and financial policies different from those that have contributed to the structural dependence of developing countries. No technocratic solutions, whether incremental wage gains, improved roads or malaria nets, can overcome structural disadvantages.

The rise of migration has challenged any lingering notions of self-sufficiency and various components of globalisation, restructuring and neo-liberalism have been diametrically opposed to more idealistic notions centred on national self-reliance. Indeed, as was pointed out some time ago, the whole idea of the national production of doctors, in the USA at least, was and is very distinct from the lack of national self-sufficiency in almost anything, notably energy (Feldstein and Butter 1978). Although the UK has moved much closer to self-sufficiency, at least in nurses, in this century this has been relatively unusual. To demand, therefore, that the major recipients of SHWs restructure their training programmes challenges a philosophical evolution where the public sector is of gradually waning significance and internationalisation is at the core of policies in areas such as trade and even environmental management. In a world where public sector solutions are against the flow of contemporary history, the will to discourage migration is fading.

Where there have been extended success stories, the lessons may be contextual and only infrequently transferable. Geography usually matters. In remote Australia, retaining a rural health workforce has been achieved in part by 'inspirational leadership' (Humphreys et al. 2008: S78). Such leadership may just as often be absent. Moreover, in Australia rural health workers are well organised institutionally and politically: an outcome of a 'rural political voice [and a] rural medical identity' (McEwin and Cameron 2007: 45) that created valuable and necessary empowerment. Much the same has been recommended, less hopefully, for the very different Mali (van Dormael et al. 2008). Such local organisation may be much more valuable than global codes and declarations that set out distant, albeit important, but often abstract goals. It is perhaps uniquely true of health workers that a degree of idealism is expected of them and of no other component of the workforce. As Isaacs has written of the need for doctors to serve in rural areas: 'such a program serves as a gentle reminder to young doctors of their social responsibilities' (2007: 582). Yet while health workers are supposed to have attachments and responsibilities to particular places, primarily countries but also regions of origin, and to display this through caring about and for their fellow nationals, they are also implicitly part of international communities that share tacit knowledge about the nature of a health career, so that brain-drain mobility is achieved essentially because of the global circulation of knowledge (Raghuram 2009a, 2009b) and thus within dual cultures of migration. To expect that moral responsibility be tied to place, and the place is the nation-state of origin, demands much of migrants. Idealism becomes a challenging basis on which to establish a modern health care system, and a greater challenge to wider structures of the circulation of knowledge and capital. In the end the key solution is as simple and as challenging as ensuring that health receives a rather greater effective share of the national budget. But that is at least in part a critical function of global uneven development.

10. The enigma of globalisation

In a long-term reversal of fortune, for half a century there has been substantial international migration of skilled health workers to more developed countries, initially particularly from Asian countries, and subsequently from sub-Saharan Africa and small island states. Migration has been constantly in flux, depending on market demands, domestic pressures, recruitment, economic and political crises, and perceptions of amenable destinations. While still centred on global and local uneven development, it has become more complex, more global yet also more intra-regional, absorbing most countries, many as both sources and recipients, and increasingly dominated by women. Only South America stands partly aloof as neither source nor recipient. Intensified competition has exacerbated the concerns of those countries that lose workers from fragile health systems, yet economic challenges have resulted in more strategic external orientation.

Globalisation is inherently uneven, differing in economic, social and political terms and between places. Countries most affected by emigration are not the least developed countries, but relatively poorly performing economies, with inadequate resources to counteract the costs. Migrant numbers, however, have been greatest from larger Asian countries. International flows are also intra-regional, as something of a two-tier system has emerged: from poorer states to other nearby states, and onwards to the metropoles. Developing and developed countries, the South and the North, are increasingly linked through migration in what has gradually become a global health care chain, moving along 'steps' and 'escalators' through the Gulf and (mainly) European (OECD) states, often culminating in the USA, as it does for many other skilled workers. These 'steps' loosely correspond to those of the hierarchical core, semi-periphery and periphery of Wallerstein's world system (Ishi 1988; Xiang 2007). Formerly colonial and post-colonial, contemporary migration transcends linguistic, cultural, political and even institutional barriers.

The international migration of SHWs has increased because perceptions of inadequate local conditions and uneven development have grown, migrant 'host' populations are generally increasing in metropolitan states, demand has expanded and recruitment intensified. Health skills are valuable marketable commodities within international migration: 'passports to prosperity'. Yet, paradoxically, fewer people are being attracted to health careers, although high levels of unemployment and the lure of overseas opportunities provide some certainty of supply in developing countries. Otherwise jobs in health are more likely to be perceived as poorly paid, dirty, difficult or simply old-fashioned. They may even sometimes be dangerous, as HIV/AIDS retains its virulence, compared with a wider range of opportunities, especially for women, in the private sector. Attrition rates are high, and older workers rather than high-school graduates are increasingly the new recruits. Such conjunctures pose significant problems for retaining health workforces.

Shortages of SHWs exist in most countries but, significantly, in many developed countries, where wealth, education levels and salaries are relatively high, and have been remedied by migration, rather than improved retention and recruitment. The principal occupational flows are of nurses, partly because numerically they are the largest part of the health workforce and partly because migration is an attractive option for relatively poorly paid professionals. The evidence and impact of their losses are greatest, while there is less obvious evidence of serious outcomes from losses of doctors, or the relatively smaller stocks of allied health workers, although the loss of just a few of these can place health systems in jeopardy.

Attrition and migration rates have both increased in this century, accompanying the widespread downsizing (or stabilising) of public service numbers in both developed and developing countries: the widespread retreat of the welfare state or, more simply, the retreat of the state. Privatisation of health care, sometimes linked to externally imposed restructuring, has increased inequity and created parallels to international migration with internal migration into the urbanised private sector. Despite enhanced aid, the effects of migration and privatisation are compounded by withering budgets, especially where health care has no necessary priority, resources are poorly aligned to outcomes, accountability is lacking and few incentives support the effective delivery of services. Consequently, even when workers are there, their real contributions are much reduced and they may even be unemployed: a 'pseudo-crisis' that is not insignificant, and exists in source and recipient countries. As the public sector is neglected and shrinks, what was once solid slowly melts into air.

OUTCOMES AND IMPACTS

Migration is not usually an overflow, nor probably has it ever been, but a definite loss in terms of national needs, with certain negative social, economic and health outcomes. In a number of countries where ratios of health workers to people are not increasing, life expectancies too are no longer increasing, even though recent decades have generally witnessed rising life expectancies. Accelerated migration has come at a time of financial pressures, resulting from national economic development problems alongside population ageing, changing consumer expectations and increased chronic disease burdens, in a context of market-driven values, economic efficiency and competition. Migration is just one critical element in health care provision. The impact of loss (including attrition), although data are still substantially selective and anecdotal, is evident in more costly but less effective health care systems, especially in remote areas, lower productivity, overwork, frustration and depleted morale, only partly compensated by return migration, replacement or remittances. A brain drain remains in place.

Low densities of SHWs correlate closely with inadequate health outcomes, most evident in tropical states where densities are lowest, disease burdens greatest and health least adequate. SHWs should be most useful in poorer countries and remote regions, where needs are demonstrably greatest, yet too often health care systems in such places are underfunded and poorly managed. Those who work and live there are marginalised, and prefer not to stay for long, unless that has always been their home. Policy decisions rarely favour them and failures of 'housekeeping' limit the effective delivery of goods and services. Rising costs of transport, and of oil, suggest the potential for a deterioration of rural infrastructure and services (as is presently occurring in several developing countries). Simultaneously, as patients in rural areas make individual rational choices to migrate or move to urban areas for medical care, so the collective ability to demand more effective regional services is reduced.

Migration has tended to be problematic for various countries as the care chain becomes more global and hierarchical. Skilled migration itself has become more selective, so that pure numbers disguise the impact on the quality of care. The costs of global mobility are unevenly borne by the poorer source countries, with the primary benefits elsewhere. Migration emerges from inequality, contributes to it (especially as skilled migrants ply their skills elsewhere), stimulating an institutionalisation of social and economic inequality that may ultimately entrench social problems (Wilkinson and Pickett 2009). Training health workers is expensive; hence migration remains perverse, a subsidy from the poor to the rich, and a consolidation of the inverse care law at a new international scale.

The migration and recruitment of female care givers and nurses – and, to a much lesser extent, male doctors – redistributes care to countries that are less willing to provide it. Yet, despite being highly valued, such workers experience discrimination and disadvantage in the lower echelons of the workforce. Conventionally, the global care chain has been linked to the migration of women, as unskilled domestic workers and care givers have been employed in general child care and elder care, where migrants are poorly paid, often exploited and beyond the reach of ethical principles, labour legislation, unionisation and even kindness. Migrant male doctors fare better than female nurses. The 'emotional' and family context of nurse migration, and the extent of deskilling and devaluing rather than empowerment, emphasise that SHWs are predominantly women, unlike so many other skilled migrants. The global care chains in which SHWs are embedded may extend geographically beyond those of the unskilled, but parallel them in being tangential to the activities of those 'economic powerhouses' where male migrants are employed, and where the 'real work' of globalisation occurs (cf. Kofman and Raghuram 2006), in contrast to women 'merely' ensuring the health of destination countries.

A GLOBAL ISSUE

Initial international migration streams from developing countries were mainly of unskilled workers: a proletariat for the manufacturing and unskilled services sector. While many migrants are still destined for such positions, the migration of health workers has been part of an emerging duality – where skilled workers are relatively easily able to migrate, but unskilled workers much less so – as the global economy has taken on new dimensions.

Migration of health workers has usually occurred in a context where other forms of migration have been common, often culturally established and which effectively legitimise newer skilled migration. In many countries long characterised by migration, a dual culture of migration is centred on both indigenous cultures of reciprocity and care, and on a desire for superior skills and their contemporary economic consequences. Migration strategies may therefore be developed and enabled over many years, rather than being short-term responses to the catalysts of 'inadequate wages and poor working conditions' so widely presumed to be the causes of migration. Indeed, the migration of doctors from India must be seen in such a broad historical context of colonial and post-colonial practices that adequate comprehension requires 'a genealogical approach' (Raghuram 2009b: 111). Much as Choy has argued in the context of Filipino nurses, the desire to migrate 'cannot be reduced to an economic logic, but rather reflects individual *and collective* desire for a unique form of social, cultural and economic success obtainable only outside the national borders' (2003: 7; my italics). International migration may even have a quasi-autonomous existence, centred on evolving transnational kinship structures.

None the less, within the fluctuating international structures of uneven development, an economic 'logic' positions migration in a loosely neo-classical context of relatively low incomes (and the perception, and knowledge, of higher wages overseas), poor promotion prospects, inflexible and difficult hours, the lack of continuing educational opportunities, limited training facilities, weak management, supervision, appreciation and mentoring, shortages of supplies and equipment and poor working environments. Structures and institutions shape human agency, beyond the simple polarities of 'push' and 'pull' factors, contributing to the commodification of even skilled labour as an international 'reserve army'.

Outside the health sector, parallel problems of service provision exist in such areas as transport and education. Frustrations over incomes and working conditions are universal but most evident in developing countries – a situation that also says much about the need for 'good housekeeping' and management. Public spending cuts have sometimes reduced the capacity for management, and managers also migrate, making 'good governance' more challenging, and its reach over the private sector more difficult to achieve, even in the wake of global financial crisis.

A corresponding range of potential, yet partial, solutions to excessive international (and regional) migration has been suggested – better wages, incentives, working conditions, management and supervision – to the extent that the 'package' has become as familiar and positive as 'apple pie and motherhood', yet rarely effectively implemented. Measures have been all too often 'reactive, piecemeal and non-integrated' (Wibulpolprasert and Pachanee 2008: 14). Putting in place a system that is meaningful and morally attractive, with teamwork and new skill mixes, where economic incentives are lacking, is difficult. Scaling up has domestic opponents. Even though developing countries can provide more effective health care systems, no 'magic bullets' compensate for lack of consistent investment and the structural deficiencies that characterise many health systems (Mathauer and Imhoff 2006: 16). There is a striking disjuncture between understanding what needs to be done, and implementing policies and practices to achieve that outcome, where national and local autonomy are being eroded by globalisation, and public trust evaporates.

Many source countries have sought to implement national policies on wage rates, incentives and working conditions, but comparable wages are out of reach of developing countries, and marginal changes are inadequate or all too easily cancelled out by national economic development problems, intermittent social and political instability and intensified recruitment. Access to the Internet enables instantaneous communication and health workers can effectively recruit themselves, and cross new borders, being better informed and better able to choose than at any time in the past.

In the face of uneven integration into the global system, substantial demands are placed on source countries, especially where economies are stagnating. That has resulted in some seeking to turn seemingly inevitable migration into a more structured and managed outcome, despite the more evidently negative outcomes of the 'Philippines model', where any sense of 'overflow' is no longer evident. In a fluctuating global economy, where small developing countries especially cannot easily influence global outcomes, 'managed migration' is both euphemistic and optimistic. There is a Janus face to migration policy and practice.

Developing countries cannot act alone. Since migration cannot be ended, and source countries have only limited scope for substantial policy change that will improve the number, status and effectiveness of local health workers, the onus has shifted on to recipient countries. They can ensure that the global care chain becomes less inevitable and inequitable, and reparation for losses incurred in sending countries is more evident while they themselves move closer towards self-reliance. As populations age, demand for care mounts, local supplies of health workers dwindle and technology offers little, that will not be easy. Most recipient countries have been reluctant to even establish effective ethical codes of recruitment practice, or any form of compensation or technology transfer, beyond generalised aid delivery, and source countries have not always effectively benefited from such aid. (It is ironic that countries that receive the largest numbers of SHWs from HIV-affected areas are those that have been the most proactive in HIV/AIDS funding.) Despite occasional 'good intentions', minimal evidence exists of almost any presently recipient country (the UK, Netherlands and Norway stand almost alone) taking realistic steps to increase national market supply, or substantially modify a migration system that provides substantial national economic benefits. Even as codes were being proclaimed a success in the UK, it was still possible to conclude that 'nursing is likely to remain a safe career choice for foreigners hoping to emigrate to the UK' (Batata 2005: 9), and, by extension, even more so to other destinations. Ultimately, almost any solution requires multilateral consensus as much as national or bilateral approaches.

In the midst of both global financial uncertainties and the steady privatisation of public sectors, developing more self-reliant national workforces in either source or recipient countries is improbable (even though global financial crisis provides some support for national regulation), unless it is forced upon countries by recession, in a world where moves towards reduced global trade barriers, including those in services (hence GATS), still prevail. Without 'controls' over other skilled workers (whether teachers, airline pilots, footballers or IT specialists), any justification for 'health exceptionalism' is reduced. Yet, remarkably, even the strongest proponents of unfettered international migration have drawn the line at SHWs (e.g. Legrain 2007). Recruitment has been in place for over half a century, from the Empire Windrush voyage of 1948 (which brought the first migration stream from the Caribbean to the UK) and, coincidentally in the same year, the Exchange Visitor Program that enabled Filipino nurses to transform their caps into passports and move to the USA (Choy 2003). Hundreds of recruitment agencies tout the advantages of migration, and their alluring advertisements grace readily available professional magazines and web pages.

Only political and cultural issues (which, for example, slowed Japan's acceptance of immigration) have discouraged migration on a larger scale. Inertia, language and cultural differences, family connections, notions of duty and unacknowledged qualifications prevent health care systems in many source countries from worsening further. Although every survey undertaken, even at times of accelerated migration, has stressed that the vast majority of health workers would prefer to work in their home countries, as long as the conditions were right, such conditions have rarely been achieved.

THE OUTWARD URGE

Increasing pressures for migration in most parts of the world are evident in dramatic journeys of refugees to penetrate the outer barriers of 'Fortress Europe', the construction of barriers between Mexico and the USA, even the legal excision of Australian offshore islands to discourage 'boat people' and others, and the widespread naval patrolling of coastal waters. In the wake of 9/11 of 2001 – and in response to the 2008 global financial crisis – the politics of migration has become ever more contested, with landscapes of migration becoming increasingly territorialised, securitised and penalised (Raghuram 2009a) and thus increasingly dominated by skilled workers. Skilled workers are not immune to or apart from such pressures, although they are best placed to succeed, in circumstances where the EU contemplates a 'blue card', analogous to the 'green card' in the USA, to facilitate their migration within what has increasingly become a 'global war for talent' (Cerna 2008). The growing focus on migration in China, sometimes locally referred to as 'leave the country fever', following the examples of the Philippines and India, is also evident in a new 'outward urge' in most independent Pacific island states, which incorporates a range of 'departure strategies', so following similar trends in the Caribbean (Connell 2009). Cultures of migration have been enhanced.

With limited national and local opportunities, demanding working conditions and increased familiarity with other countries, migration has become an established option and a potential realisation of household dreams: the outcome of a dual culture of migration that begins at home, is accentuated in school and consolidated in the workforce. Experiences and perceptions of the wider world, its values and its material rewards underlie the migratory experience and, in an electronic era, where more numerous kin and colleagues are overseas, knowledge of distant places is no longer fragmentary. Migration is now more than ever an appropriate and legitimate means to economic and social well-being, rather than a rupture and discontinuity with past experiences.

Even when they have sought to do so, source countries have not been able to discourage migration, which is widely perceived as a human right. Several remittance-dependent countries, such as Cape Verde, Samoa and the Philippines, have not challenged migration because of its valuable economic role. Indeed, Cape Verde entered into a pilot partnership with the EU in 2009 based on a 'circular migration' model, with liberal repeat migration provisions, to assure a migration quota. Other states like Kiribati, Tuvalu and Vanuatu have sponsored international migration streams that spill over into the health sector. Unions (like the Fiji Nursing Association) have supported the rights of members to better their circumstances by migration while also pressing governments to act locally to improve working conditions. Migration is increasingly inherent in national political economies.

Migration primarily occurs for economic reasons, and demonstrates sensitivity to income disparities, but situated in a social context that emphasises duty, service and reciprocity, resulting in sustained contacts across the diaspora and significant remittance flows. Remittances have partly replaced the morality of return. For most SHWs, income is an influence on decisions to join the health profession, and a key influence on decisions to leave it and/or migrate. Migrants stress extended family contexts, as education is directed towards income-generating opportunities where the rewards flow back home: embedded in the 'roots' of social relationships and nurtured in the 'routes' taken to achieve overseas success. The notion of a 'transnational corporation of kin' is alluring in the sense of an extended family, exercising some degree of self-interest, nepotism and strategic decision-making within an international moral economy (Connell 2009). Social norms ensure that as long as there are kin at home, remittances will reach them. What for health care is perverse migration is a private gain for the families of migrants, despite social costs, just as migrants endure discrimination and deskilling, because there is a logic to migration and its economic benefits, steadily transforming and extending cultures so that migration becomes increasingly ubiquitous and normative, and households increasingly transnational. International migration now constitutes a rather less hesitant solution to development issues: a globalisation from below that will nevertheless always be both uneven and unsatisfying, as its resolution lies elsewhere. Simultaneously it poses particular problems for the public health sectors of many source countries.

Contraction of the world, through migration, electronics and their consequences, from remittances to new cosmopolitan and hybrid, hyphenated identities, has widened international ties yet ultimately ensured that symbolically and practically migrants rarely abandon home. As Marshall has phrased it, while 'people are no longer bound to places, they are still bound up in them' (2004: 145), so that migrant SHWs remain intricately enmeshed in social networks which ensure that, however long they have been away, they have essentially 'gone away without leaving' (Nietschmann 1979: 22). Migration is an arena of multiple uncertainties – linked to national and global financial crises, political shifts, household changes and evolving health systems – but also situated within the indefinable process of assimilation, which may be marked by issues of racism, citizenship and residence, family separations and contradictory structures of social mobility, quite different in destinations from those at home. In such contexts Indian nurses have been described, even after two decades in the USA, as having 'a foot here, a foot there, and a foot nowhere' (DiCicco-Bloom 2004: 28). Unsurprisingly, circular migration is preferred, but return can be an elusive dream and, particularly for doctors, may merely be empty rhetoric.

Greater competition for workers between states, and intensified efforts at recruitment by governments and specialised recruitment agencies, have followed migration in becoming more demand driven. Developed countries long ago outgrew their immediate resource bases and reached far beyond their national borders in a relentless search for new resource frontiers and continued growth; that process has now extended to human resources. The concomitant shift towards more skilled migration has created a new dimension of inequality. The poor are less easily able to move (although that was actually never easy) whereas the relatively rich (or at least those who have acquired training and marketable skills) are actively courted and recruited. The more skills the better. There is growing international competition not just for the 'creative class' (Florida 2005) but for a wide range of skilled workers. In boom times the IT industry was even characterised by 'body shopping', where recruitment agencies and consultancies sought out international labour, and 'benching', where so many workers were recruited that the excess were temporarily unemployed (Xiang 2007). Such international processes, analogous to the recruitment of SHWs, parallel the complexities and organisational structures involved in the global outsourcing of a significant part of the human resource needs of health systems.

It is now possible to recognise the rise of the 'competition state' whose task is to make economic (and other) activities within the state more competitive on global terms, but in a context of reduced government spending, and the deregulation and geographical expansion of labour markets, so adapting national economies to the global economy, in a neo-liberal formulation that withers away social democracy and the welfare state. Indeed, the state becomes less vertical and more horizontal, less bound by space, and less focused on the public sector, as its global reach extends. The competition state is itself therefore 'an authoritative agent of globalisation, embedding that process in its domestic practices as well as its international and transnational linkages' (Evans 2005: 76), through which it actively competes for both natural and human resources. While competition is most obviously seen in the drive for foreign investment, it is apparent in the quest for labour, above all by developed countries but, conversely, in the active promotion of migration in various developing countries. While the state's role is usually (and correctly) seen to be one of regulating migration by restriction, its growing converse is that of enabling and encouraging selective migration: a greater liberalisation of migration and a more flexible multilateralism (exemplified by the intended 'frictionless mobility' of GATS, but also by new MOUs and the whole loose concept of 'managed migration'). Skilled migration has thus 'become an important element in the external economic policy of the competition state' (Lavenex 2007: 34), within which social policy is used to 'create flexible enterprising workers suited to a globalising, knowledge based economy' (Jessop 2002: 168). Beyond the state, professions such as nurses are not merely organised at a national level but, in Europe at least, into a European Federation of Nurses' Associations. Underpinning this is job market flexibility, the gradual global harmonisation of qualifications (and thus the internationalisation of the professions, especially within regional blocs) so that they are internationally transferable, and its accompaniment in increasing local demands for 'international standards' of training.

GLOBAL CHAINS, CONVEYOR BELTS AND CAROUSELS

If economic growth were not substantially greater in the developed countries of 'the North' than in the developing countries of the globalised South, the context of uneven development in which much international migration occurs would no longer exist. There is, however, little prospect of significant changes in global economic and social imbalances; hence migration is likely to remain an attractive proposition, where two cultures are dominant, wages and working conditions remain highly unequal, recruitment intensifies and kin are overseas. This is enhanced through the gradual institutionalisation of migration, formally involving states, recruitment agencies, unions and professional organisations. As states extended their global reach, so migrants reached new destinations.

The rhetoric and even intermittent practice of self-reliance in developing countries, at national and household levels, have largely disappeared and, in most cases, have simply disguised a situation of growing dependence on external sources of funding, whether from aid, remittances or investment. While accelerated migration – or at least the demand for it – has been partly a response to economic vicissitudes and the political and social instability that this engenders, it has long been an effective strategy for diversification. More localised migration has given way to international and intra-regional migration (and movements into the private sector), as 'steps' have metaphorically speeded up to become 'escalators' and 'carousels' taking workers to distant shores. What were once quite localised and temporary movements – to mines, plantations or seasonal agricultural opportunities – have taken place over greater distances, across even more distinct cultural realms and with longer-term consequences.

Even as states increase their reach and control over migration, greater stress on the role of diasporas has placed a substantial burden on migrants, not least because their remittances support households, rather than the nations they moved away from. Indeed, the states that are best placed to benefit from remittances are those with 'higher quality political and economic policies and institutions' (Catrinescu et al. 2009: 81). The social and emotional costs of such a new form of 'international self-reliance' are thus uneven and inherently problematic. In what may be seen as either a 'virtuous or vicious cycle' (Yeates 2009: 183), the remittances of nurses consequently fuel the next wave of nurse migration.

Global mobility has become increasingly common – although remarkably few people actually leave their home countries – and in many countries it has become built into the socioeconomic system, or at least into wider household expectations. In a growing number of states, migration is unexceptional and may be encouraged as a more effective means of income generation than anything available at home. For more than 20 years some smaller Pacific, and more recently Caribbean, island states have been seen as MIRAB states, where MIgration, Remittances and Aid are important components of an increasingly Bureaucratic economy, compared with trade or tourism (Bertram and Watters 1985; Connell and Conway 2000).

At a time of aid fatigue, demographic structures have changed as states, individuals and international agencies (such as the World Bank) have attached new and increased significance to migration, remittances and the role of the diaspora. In such circumstances, where migration has brought substantial economic gains, the migration of SHWs is just one part of much wider migration streams. Competition between states for SHWs is consequently more evident than cooperation in the development of regulatory mechanisms for minimising the negative impacts of migration.

The new focus on migration in development discourse (perhaps alongside the shift towards managed migration) would seem to some a measure of the manner in which migration has gone from being regarded as a problem for development in source countries to an opportunity for, if not necessarily an alternative to, national development (Faist 2008; Piper 2009). In the context of the migration of SHWs, the much-vaunted potential 'win–win–win' outcome, where migrants, source and destination countries all benefit, is rarely evident. Asymmetry, with destinations the primary beneficiaries and individual migrants and their households lesser beneficiaries, and source countries gaining rather less, is the norm.

Local circumstances are subsumed in the growing interdependence of states, regions, social groups and institutions, and such interdependence poses problems for policy formation and planning. States are far from equal – 'failed states' are a recently recognised phenomenon – and powerful states are more easily able to control and benefit from globalisation, in almost any form, including migration. Such power structures tend to ensure that benefits are captured and localised, where asymmetrical globalisation emphasises that 'labour markets tend to reward those who already possess substantial "human capital" or the means to acquire it' (Labonté and Schrecker 2007a: 2). Precisely because asymmetry also results from other facets of globalisation, whether trade or financial markets, the resolution of crises and global inequalities in health care ultimately lies beyond the health sector, involving global reforms in international trade, more effective development assistance, extending debt relief and recognising health as a human right, an investment rather than a cost. Such policies might 'blunt the negative impact of the emerging global marketplace' (Labonté and Schrecker 2007b: 15), although formidable and overwhelming barriers stand in their way within an increasingly open, deregulated and competitive global economy.

While it is reasonable to presume that the migration of skilled health workers is an inescapable facet of the modern world, how that migration will evolve and with what outcomes is quite uncertain, within a contemporary global care chain now extending far beyond the old order of national, loosely self-reliant welfare states. Ultimately, migration is always fluid, indeterminate and ambivalent; hence planning for workforces is problematic, as the carousels move onwards. However, education and health care are the most cyclically stable employment sectors (both expanding slightly in the USA in 2008) and both are predominantly female. Following the 2008 global financial crisis, and despite its tribulations, the Philippines sought more actively to deploy overseas workers to 'ensure a supply of remittances, and increasingly emphasised the role of health workers for whom the market was expected to remain constant' (*Jakarta Post*, 10 February 2009). On the other side of the Pacific, the former financial trader 'Mr Brush is retraining as a nurse. That might not impress those of his friends who are still rating commercial mortgage-backed securities on New York's State Street Plaza. But in turning to a traditionally female job, Mr Brush is trying to escape a very male recession' (*Financial Times*, 19 April 2009). In Africa, Botswana was seeking to recruit doctors from a new global source: North Korea. Meanwhile Czech nurses were being discouraged from migration by the lure of plastic surgery. Migration will surely continue and, although it may be increasingly structured and managed, the geometry of power, combined with an 'outward urge' in many developing countries, will ensure that its outcomes will almost certainly be no less uneven and asymmetrical than they have ever been. None of global health care, equity or social justice are likely to be well served.

References

Abel-Smith, B. (1987), 'The price of unbalanced health manpower', in Z. Bankowski and A. Mejia (eds), *Health Manpower Out Of Balance*, Geneva: Council for International Organizations of Medical Sciences, pp. 110–23.

Aboderin, I. (2007), 'Contexts, motives and experiences of Nigerian overseas nurses: understanding links to globalization', *Journal of Clinical Nursing*, **16**, 2237–45.

Adams, R. (2009), 'The determinants of international remittances in developing countries', *World Development*, **37**, 93–103.

Adano, U. (2008), 'The health worker recruitment and deployment process in Kenya: an emergency hiring program', *Human Resources for Health*, **6** (19), 1–3.

Adkoli, B. (2006), 'Migration of health workers: perspectives from Bangladesh, India, Nepal, Pakistan and Sri Lanka', *Regional Health Forum*, **10**, 49–58.

Aglionby, J. (2006), 'Health of Burma tribes "worst in the world"', *The Guardian*, 7 September.

Agwu, K. and Llewelyn, M. (2009), 'Compensation for the brain drain from developing countries', *The Lancet*, **373**, 1665–6.

Aiken, L., Buchan, J., Sochalski, J. et al. (2004), 'Trends in international nurse migration', *Health Affairs*, **23**, 69–77.

Aiken, L., Clarke, S., Sloane, D. et al. (2001), 'Nurses' reports on hospital care in five countries', *Health Affairs*, **20**, 43–53.

Aiken, L., Crake, S., Sloane, D. et al. (2002), 'Hospital nurse staffing and patient mortality, nurse burnout and job dissatisfaction', *Journal of the American Medical Association*, **288**, 1987–93.

Aitken, J. and Kemp, J. (2003), 'HIV/AIDS, equity and health sector personnell in southern Africa', Harare: EQUINET Discussion Paper No. 12.

Akhtar, R. and Izhar, N. (1994), 'Spatial inequalities and historical evolution in health provision. Indian and Zambian examples', in D. Phillips and Y. Verhasselt (eds), *Health and Development*, London: Routledge, pp. 216–33.

Akl, E., Maroun, N., Major, S. et al. (2007), 'Why are you draining your brain? Factors underlying decisions of graduating Lebanese medical students to migrate', *Social Science and Medicine*, **64**, 1278–84.

Alexis, O. and Vydelingum, V. (2009), 'Experiences in the UK National Health Service: the overseas nurses' workforce', *Health Policy*, **90**, 320–28.

Alexis, O., Vydelingum,V. and Robbins, I. (2006), 'Overseas nurses' experiences of equal opportunities in the NHS in England', *Journal of Health, Organisation and Management*, **2**, 130–39.

Alexis, O., Vydelingum,V. and Robbins, I. (2007), 'Engaging with a new reality: experiences of overseas minority ethnic nurses in the National Health Service', *Journal of Clinical Nursing*, **16**, 2221–8.

Ali, Z. (2006), 'How many doctors do we need in Sudan?', *Sudanese Journal of Public Health*, **1**, 180–91.

Alimoglu, M. and Donmez, L. (2005), 'Daylight exposure and the other predictors of burnout among nurses in a university hospital', *International Journal of Nursing Studies*, **42**, 549–55.

Al-Jarallah, K., Moussa, M., Hakeem, S. and Al-Khanfar, F. (2009), 'The nursing workforce in Kuwait to the year 2020', *International Nursing Review*, **56**, 65–72.

Alkire, S. and Chen, L. (2004), '"Medical exceptionalism" in international migration: should doctors and nurses be treated differently?', Joint Learning Initiative Working Paper 7–3, Harvard University.

Allan, H. (2007), 'The rhetoric of caring and the recruitment of overseas nurses: the social production of a care gap', *Journal of Clinical Nursing*, **16**, 2204–12.

Alonso-Garbayo, A. and Maben, J. (2009), 'Internationally recruited nurses from India and the Philippines in the United Kingdom: the decision to emigrate', *Human Resources for Health*, **7** (37), 1–11.

Alubo, S. (1990), 'Debt crisis, health and health services in Africa', *Social Science and Medicine*, **31**, 639–48.

Aly, Z. and Taj, F. (2008), 'Why Pakistani medical graduates must remain free to migrate', *PLoSMedicine*, **5** (1), 6–8.

Aminuzaman, S. (2006), 'Migration of skilled nurses from Bangladesh: an exploratory study', Brighton: Development Research Centre on Migration, Globalisation and Poverty, University of Sussex.

Anand, S. and Barnighausen, T. (2004), 'Human resources and health outcomes: cross country econometric study', *The Lancet*, **364**, 1603–9.

Anand, S. and Barnighausen, T. (2007), 'Health workers and vaccination coverage in developing countries: an econometric analysis', *The Lancet*, **369**, 1277–85.

Anand, S., Fan, V., Zhang, J. et al. (2008), 'China's human resources for health: quantity, quality and distribution', *The Lancet*, **372**, 1774–81.

Anderson, B. and Isaacs, A. (2007), 'Simply not there: the impact of international migration of nurses and midwives – perspectives from Guyana', *Journal of Midwifery and Women's Health*, **52**, 392–7.

Anderson, T. (2008), 'Solidarity aid: the Cuba-Timor Leste health programme', *International Journal of Cuban Studies*, **1** (2), 1–13.

Anon (2005), 'Vacation, adventure and surgery?', *CBS News*, 4 September (www.cbsnews.com/stories).

Anon (2008), 'Only one doctor left at Phuket hospital', *Bangkok Post*, 1 October.

Anwar, I., Sami, M., Akhtar, N. et al. (2008), 'Inequity in maternal health care services: evidence from home-based skilled-birth-attendant programmes in Bangladesh', *Bulletin of the WHO*, **86**, 252–9.

Arah, O. (2007), 'The metrics and correlates of physician migration from Africa', *BMC Public Health*, **7** (83), 1–7.

Arah, O., Ogbu, U. and Okeke, C. (2008), 'Too poor to leave, too rich to stay: developmental and global health correlates of physician migration to the United States, Canada, Australia, and the United Kingdom', *American Journal of Public Health*, **98**, 148–54.

Arends-Kuenning, M. (2006), 'The balance of care: trends in the wages and employment of immigrant nurses in the US between 1990 and 2000', *Globalizations*, **3**, 333–48.

Arunanondchai, J. and Fink, C. (2007), *Trade in Health Services in the ASEAN Region*, Washington: World Bank Policy Research Working Paper 41417.

Asian Development Bank (1996), *Tonga. Economic Performance and Selected Development Issues*, Manila: ADB.

Asian Development Bank (2002), *Vanuatu. Economic Performance and Challenges Ahead*, Manila: ADB.

Asian Development Bank (2005), *Towards a New Pacific Regionalism*, Manila: ADB.

Astor, A., Akhtar, T., Matallana, M.A. et al. (2005), 'Physician migration: views from professionals in Colombia, Nigeria, India, Pakistan and the Philippines', *Social Science and Medicine*, **61**, 2492–500.

Auerbach, D., Buerhaus, P. and Staiger, D. (2007), 'Better late than never: work force supply implications of late entry into nursing', *Health Affairs*, **26**, 178–85.

Awases, M., Gbary, A., Nyoni, J. and Chatora, R. (2004), *Migration of Health Professionals in Six Countries*, Brazzaville: WHO.

Bach, S. (2003), *International Migration of Health Workers*, Geneva: ILO.

Bach, S. (2004), 'Migration patterns of physicians and nurses: still the same story?', *Bulletin of the WHO*, **82**, 624–5.

Bach, S. (2008), 'International mobility of health professionals: brain drain or brain exchange?', in A. Solimano (ed.), *The International Mobility of Talent*, Oxford: Oxford University Press, pp. 202–35.

Badr, E. (2005), 'Brain drain of health professionals in Sudan: magnitude, challenges and prospects for solution', unpub. MA thesis, University of Leeds.

Badr, E. (2007), *Human Resources for Health (HRH) Strategic Work Plan for Sudan (2008–2012)*, Khartoum: National Human Resources Observatory for Health.

Baer, L., Gesler, W. and Konrad, T. (2000), 'The wineglass model: tracking the locational histories of health professionals', *Social Science and Medicine*, **50**, 317–29.

Baird, V. (2005), 'Out of Africa', *New Internationalist*, **379**, June, 9–28.

Bakeea, M. (1991), 'Kiribati', in M. Bray (ed.), *Ministries of Education in Small States*, London: Commonwealth Secretariat, pp. 247–64.

Bala, P. (1991), *Imperialism and Medicine in Bengal*, New Delhi: Sage.

Baldassar, L. (2007), 'Transnational families and aged care: the mobility of care and the migrancy of ageing', *Journal of Ethnic and Migration Studies*, **33**, 275–97.

Ball, R. (1996), 'Nation building or dissolution: the globalization of nursing – the case of the Philippines', *Pilipinas*, **27**, 67–92.

Ballard, K., Robinson, S. and Laurence, P. (2004), 'Why do general practitioners from France choose to work in London practices? A qualitative study', *British Journal of General Practice*, **54**, 747–52.

Balon, A., Mufti, R., Williams, M. and Riba, M. (1997), 'Possible discrimination in recruitment of psychiatry residents', *American Journal of Psychiatry*, **154**, 781–8.

Barclay, L., Fenwick, J., Nielson, F. et al. (1998), *Samoan Nursing. The Story of Women Developing a Profession*, Sydney: Allen and Unwin.

Barnett, J. (1988), 'Foreign medical graduates in New Zealand 1973–79: a test of the exacerbation hypothesis', *Social Science and Medicine*, **26**, 1049–60.

Barnett, J. (1991), 'Geographical implications of restricting foreign medical immigration: a New Zealand case study, 1976–87', *Social Science and Medicine*, **33**, 459–70.

Barnighausen, T. and Bloom, D. (2009a), '"Conditional scholarships" for HIV/AIDS health workers: educating and retaining the workforce to provide antiretroviral treatment in sub-Saharan Africa', *Social Science and Medicine*, **68**, 544–51.

Barnighausen, T. and Bloom, D. (2009b), 'Financial incentives for return of service in underserved areas: a systematic review', *BMC Health Services Research*, **9** (86), 1–17.

Barron, D. and West, E. (2005), 'Leaving nursing: an event-history analysis of nurses' careers', *Journal of Health Services Research and Policy*, **10**, 150–57.

Bartsch, W. (1974), *The Skill Drain from Fiji. Situation and Possible Remedies*, Suva: Central Planning Office.

Baru, R. (2005), 'Commercialization and the public sector in India: implications for values and aspirations', in M. Mackintosh and M. Koivusalo (eds), *Commercialization of Health Care*, Basingstoke: Palgrave Macmillan, pp. 101–16.

Batata, A. (2005), 'International nurse recruitment and NHS vacancies: a cross-sectional analysis', *Globalization and Health*, **1** (7), 1–10.

Beaverstock, J. and Smith, J. (1996), 'Lending jobs to global cities: skilled international labour migration, investment banking and the City of London', *Urban Studies*, **33**, 1377–94.

Bell, H. (1999), *Frontiers of Medicine in the Anglo-Egyptian Sudan 1899–1940*, Oxford: Clarendon Press.

Bertram, I. and Watters, R. (1985), 'The MIRAB economy in South Pacific microstates', *Pacific Viewpoint*, **26**, 497–520.

Betancourt, J., Green, A., Carrillo, J. and Ananeh-Firempong, O. (2003), 'Defining cultural competence: a practical framework for addressing racial/ethnic disparities in health and health care', *Public Health Reports*, **118**, 293–302.

Bhagwati, J. (1976), *The Brain Drain and Taxation: Theory and Empirical Analysis*, Amsterdam: North-Holland.

Bhagwati, J. and Hamada, K. (1974), 'The brain drain, international integration of markets for professionals and unemployment. A theoretical analysis', *Journal of Development Economics*, **77**, 19–42.

Bhargava, A. and Docquier, F. (2008), 'HIV pandemic, medical brain drain, and economic development in Sub-Saharan Africa', *World Bank Economic Review*, **2**, 345–66.

Bhutta, Z., Nundy, S. and Abbasi, K. (2004), 'Is there hope for South Asia?', *British Medical Journal*, **328**, 777–8.

Bilefsky, D. (2009), 'If plastic surgery won't convince you, what will?', *New York Times*, 25 May.

Birch, M. (2009), 'Implementing equity: the Commission on Social Determinants of Health', *Bulletin of the WHO*, **87**, 3.

Birks, M., Chapman, Y. and Francis, K. (2009), 'Women and nursing in Malaysia', *Journal of Transcultural Nursing*, **20**, 116–23.

Bloch, A. (2005), 'Emigration from Zimbabwe: migrant perspectives', *Social Policy and Administration*, **40**, 67–87.

Blythe, J., Baumann, A., Rhéaume, A. and McIntosh, K. (2009), 'Nurse migration to Canada. Pathways and pitfalls of workplace integration', *Journal of Transcultural Nursing*, **20**, 202–10.

Bohning, W. (1982), *Towards a System of Recompense for International Labour Migration*, Geneva: ILO.

Bouras, G. (1986), *A Foreign Wife*, Melbourne: Penguin.

Bower, F. and McCullough, C. (2004), 'Nurse shortage or nursing shortage: have we missed the real problem?', *Nursing Economics*, **22**, 200–203.

Braine, T. (2008), 'Mexico's midwives enter the mainstream', *Bulletin of the WHO*, **86**, 244–5.

Brown, D. (1997), 'Workforce losses and return migration to the Caribbean. A case study of Jamaican nurses', in P. Pessar (ed.), *Caribbean Circuits. New Directions in the Study of Caribbean Migration*, Center for Migration Studies, New York, pp. 197–223.

Brown, L., Schultz, J., Forsberg, A. et al. (2002), 'Predictors of retention among HIV/hemophilia health care professionals', *General Hospital Psychiatry*, **24**, 48–54.

Brown, R. and Connell, J. (2004), 'The migration of doctors and nurses from South Pacific island nations', *Social Science and Medicine*, **58**, 2193–210.

Brown, R. and Connell, J. (2006), 'Occupation-specific analysis of migration and remittance behaviour: Pacific island nurses in Australia and New Zealand', *Asia-Pacific Viewpoint*, **47**, 133–48.

Brown, R., Foster, J. and Connell, J. (1995), 'Remittances, savings and policy formation in Pacific Island states', *Asian and Pacific Migration Journal*, **4**, 169–85.

Brunt, A. and Morris-Tafatu, C. (2002), *Review of NZODA Scholarships and Training in Niue*, Niue.

Brush, B. (2008), 'Global nurse migration today', *Journal of Nursing Scholarship*, **40**, 20–25.

Brush, B. and Sochalski, J. (2007), 'International nurse migration: lessons from the Philippines', *Policy, Politics and Nursing Practice*, **8**, 37–46.

Brush, B. and Vasupuram, R. (2006), 'Nurses, nannies and caring work: importation, visibility and marketability', *Nursing Inquiry*, **13**, 181–5.

Buchan, J. (2002), *Here to Stay? International Nurses in the UK*, London: Royal College of Nursing.

Buchan, J. (2008), 'New opportunities. United Kingdom recruitment of Filipino nurses', in J. Connell (ed.), *The International Migration of Health Workers*, New York and London: Routledge, pp. 47–61.

Buchan, J. and dal Poz, M. (2002), 'Skills mix in the health care workforce: reviewing the evidence', *Bulletin of the WHO*, **80**, 575–80.

Buchan, J. and Dovlo, D. (2004), *International Recruitment of Health Workers to the United Kingdom*, London: Department for International Development.

Buchan, J., McPake, B., Mensah, K. and Rae, G. (2009), 'Does a code make a difference – assessing the English code of practice on international recruitment', *Human Resources for Health*, **7** (33), 1–8.

Buchan, J., Parkin, T. and Sochalski, J. (2004), *International Nurse Mobility: Trends and Policy Implications*, Geneva: WHO, ICN and RCN.

Buchan, J. and Perfilieva, G. (2006), *Health Worker Migration in the European Region*, Copenhagen: WHO.

Buchan, J. and Seccombe, I. (2005), *Past Trends, Future Imperfect? A Review of the UK Nursing Labour Market in 2004 to 2005*, London: Royal College of Nursing.

Bump, M. (2006), *Ghana. Searching for Opportunities at Home and Abroad*, Washington, DC: Migration Research Institute.

Bunnag, S. (2008), 'Universities hit by "brain drain"', *Bangkok Post*, 11 December, 1.

Bunting, M. (2008), 'Pregnancy should not be a death sentence', *Guardian Weekly*, 4 July, 19.

Burnham, G., Lafta, R. and Doocy, S. (2009), 'Doctors leaving 12 tertiary hospitals in Iraq, 2004–2007', *Social Science and Medicine*, **69**, 172–7.

Butterworth, K., Hayes, B. and Neupane, B. (2008), 'Retention of general practitioners in rural Nepal: a qualitative study', *Australian Journal of Rural Health*, **16**, 201–6.

Buve, A., Foaster, S., Mbwili, C. et al. (1994), 'Mortality among female nurses in the face of the AIDS epidemic: a pilot study in Zambia', *AIDS*, **8**, 396.

Cameron, A., Ewen, M., Ross-Degnan, D. et al. (2009), 'Medicine prices, availability and affordability in 36 developing and middle-income countries: a secondary analysis', *The Lancet*, **373**, 240–49.

Carey, M. (2009), '"It's a bit like being a robot or working in a factory": does Braverman help explain the experiences of state social workers in Britain since 1971?', *Organization*, **16**, 505–27.

Caribbean Commission on Health and Development (2006), *Report of the Caribbean Commission on Health and Development*, Kingston: PAHO and Caribbean Community Secretariat.

Catrinescu, N., Leon-Ledesma, M., Piracha, M. and Quillin, B. (2009), 'Remittances, institutions and economic growth', *World Development*, **37**, 81–92.

Cavagnero, E., Lane, C., Evans, D. and Carrin, G. (2008), 'Development assistance for health: should policy makers worry about its macroeconomic impact?', *Bulletin of the WHO*, **86**, 864–70.

Cavender, A. and Alban, M. (1998), 'Compulsory medical service in Ecuador: the physician's perspective', *Social Science and Medicine*, **47**, 1937–46.

Celik, S., Celik, Y., Agirbas, I. and Ugurluoglu, O. (2007), 'Verbal and physical abuse against nurses in Turkey', *International Nursing Review*, **54**, 359–66.

Cembrowicz, S., Ritter, S. and Wright, S. (2002), 'Attacks on doctors and nurses', in J. Shepherd (ed.), *Violence in Health Care*, Oxford: Oxford University Press, pp. 118–54.

Cerna, L. (2008), 'Towards an EU Blue Card? The delegation of national high skilled immigration policies to the EU level', Oxford: ESRC Centre for Migration, Policy and Society Working Paper No. 65.

Chaguturu, S. and Vallabhaneni, S. (2005), 'Aiding and abetting – nursing crises at home and abroad', *New England Journal of Medicine*, **353**, 1761–3.

Chaloff, J. (2008), 'Mismatches in the formal sector, expansion in the informal sector: immigration of health professionals to Italy', Paris: OECD Health Working Paper No. 34.

Chan, M., Luk, A., Leong, S. et al. (2008), 'Factors influencing Macao nurses' intentions to leave current employment', *Journal of Clinical Nursing*, **18**, 893–901.

Chand, S. (2008a), 'Biceps or the brain: investing in our most valuable resource!', *Islands Business*, **34** (6), 40–41.

Chand, S. (2008b), 'Train and trap to trap and trash', *The Lancet*, **371**, 1576.

Chand, S. and Clemens, M. (2008), 'Skilled emigration and skill creation: a quasi-experiment', Washington, DC: Center for Global Development Working Paper No. 152.

Chaudhury, N. and Hammer, J. (2003), 'Ghost doctors: absenteeism in Bangladeshi health facilities', Washington: World Bank Policy Research Working Paper No. 3065.

Chen, L. and Boufford, J. (2005), 'Fatal flows – doctors on the move', *New England Journal of Medicine*, **353**, 1850–52.

Cheng, M. (2009), 'The Philippines' health worker exodus', *The Lancet*, **373**, 111–12.

Chikanda, A. (2004), 'Skilled health professionals' migration and its impact on health care delivery in Zimbabwe', Oxford: Centre on Migration, Policy and Society Working Paper No. 4.

Chikanda, A. (2008), 'The migration of health professionals from Zimbabwe', in J. Connell (ed.), *The International Migration of Health Workers*, New York and London: Routledge, pp. 110–28.

Choate, M. (2008), *Emigrant Nation. The Making of Italy Abroad*, Cambridge, MA: Harvard University Press.

Chomitz, K. Setiadi, G. and Azwar, A. (1998), 'What do doctors want? Developing strategies for doctors to serve in Indonesia's rural and remote areas', Washington, DC: World Bank Policy Research Working Paper No. 1888.

Choo, V. (2003), 'Philippines losing its nurses, and now maybe its doctors', *The Lancet*, **361**, 1356.

Chory-Assad, R. and Tamborini, R. (2001), 'Television doctors: an analysis of physicians in fictional and non-fictional television programs', *Journal of Broadcasting and Electronic Media*, **45**, 499–521.

Choy, C. (2003), *Empire of Care. Nursing and Migration in Filipino American History*, Durham, NC: Duke University Press.

Christensen, P.M. (1995), *Infant Nutrition and Child Health on Tarawa, Kiribati*, Sydney: University of New South Wales Pacific Studies Monograph No. 15.

Chung, G. (2007), 'The feminisation of migration and transnational nurses: the fifty Korean nurses that left for Brisbane', unpub. paper to American Sociological Association, New York.

Clark, P. Stewart, J. and Clark, D. (2006), 'The globalization of the labour market for health-care professionals', *International Labour Review*, **145**, 37–64.

Clemens, M. (2007), 'Do visas kill? Health effects of African health professional emigration', Washington, DC: Center for Global Development Working Paper No. 114.

Clemens, M. and Pettersson, G. (2008), 'New data on African health professionals abroad', *Human Resources for Health*, **6** (1), 1–11.

Cohen, J. (2004), *The Culture of Migration in Southern Mexico*, Austin, TX: University of Texas Press.

Commonwealth Secretariat (2004), *Migration of Health Workers from Commonwealth Countries*, London: Commonwealth Secretariat.

Connell, J. (1997), 'Health in Papua New Guinea: a decline in development', *Australian Geographical Studies*, **35**, 271–93.

Connell, J. (2006), 'Medical tourism: sea, sun, sand . . . and surgery', *Tourism Management*, **27**, 1093–100.

Connell, J. (2007a), 'Local skills and global markets? The migration of health workers from Caribbean and Pacific island states', *Social and Economic Studies*, **56**, 67–95.

Connell, J. (2007b), 'At the end of the world. Holding on to health workers in Niue', *Asian and Pacific Migration Journal*, **16**, 179–97.

Connell, J. (2008a), 'Tummy tucks and the Taj Mahal? Medical tourism and the globalisation of health care', in D. Martin and A. Woodside (eds), *Advancing Tourism Management*, Wallingford: CABI, pp. 232–44.

Connell, J. (2008b), 'Niue: embracing a culture of migration', *Journal of Ethnic and Migration Studies*, **34**, 1021–40.

Connell, J. (2009), *The Global Health Care Chain: From the Pacific to the World*, New York: Routledge.

Connell, J. and Brown, R. (2004), 'The remittances of migrant Tongan and Samoan nurses in Australia', *Human Resources for Health*, **2** (2), 1–21.

Connell, J. and Conway, D. (2000), 'Migration and remittances in island microstates: a comparative perspective on the South Pacific and the Caribbean', *International Journal of Urban and Regional Research*, **24**, 52–78.

Connell, J. and Stilwell, B. (2006), 'Merchants of medical care: recruiting agencies in the global health care chain', in C. Kuptsch (ed.), *Merchants of Labour*, Geneva: ILO, pp. 239–53.

Connell, J. and Voigt-Graf, C. (2006), 'Towards autonomy? Gendered migration in Pacific Island states', in K. Ferro and M. Wallner (eds), *Migration Happens. Reasons, Effects and Opportunities of Migration in the South Pacific*, Vienna: Lit Verlag, pp. 43–62.

Connell, J., Zurn, P., Stilwell, B. et al. (2007), 'Sub-Saharan Africa: beyond the health worker migration crisis?', *Social Science and Medicine*, **64**, 1876–91.

Conradson, D. and Latham, A. (2005), 'Friendship, networks and trans-nationality in a world city: Antipodean transmigrants in London', *Journal of Ethnic and Migration Studies*, **31**, 287–305.

Cooke, H. (2006), 'Seagull management and the control of nursing work', *Work, Employment and Society*, **20**, 223–43.

Coomber, B. and Barriball, K. (2007), 'Impact of job satisfaction on intent to leave and turnover for hospital-based nurses: a review of the research literature', *International Journal of Nursing Studies*, **44**, 297–314.

Cooper, R. (2008), 'The U.S. physician workforce: where do we stand?', Paris: OECD Health Working Paper No. 37.

Cooper, R. and Aiken, L. (2006), 'Health services delivery: reframing poli-cies for global migration of nurses and physicians – a U.S. perspective', *Policy, Politics and Nursing Practice*, **7**, 66S–70S.

Coory, M. (2004), 'Aging and healthcare costs in Australia: a case of policy based evidence?', *Medical Journal of Australia*, **180**, 581–3.

Cuban, S. (2008), 'Home/work: the roles of education, literacy and learn-ing in the networks and mobility of professional women migrant carers in Cumbria', *Ethnography and Education*, **3**, 81–96.

Culley, L., Dyson, S., Ham-ying, S. and Young, W. (1999), 'Caribbean nurses: racisms, resistances and healing narratives', in S. Roseneil and J. Seymour (eds), *Practising Identities. Power and Resistance*, Basingstoke: Macmillan, pp. 155–79.

Cumbi, A., Pereira, C., Malalane, R. et al. (2007), 'Major surgery delega-tion to mid-level health practitioners in Mozambique: health profes-sionals' perceptions', *Human Resources for Health*, **5** (27), 1–9.

Cutchin, M. (1997), 'Physician retention in rural communities: the perspective of experiential place integration', *Health and Place*, **3**, 25–41.

Czupryniak, L. and Loba, J. (2005), 'Route of corruption in Poland's health-care system', *The Lancet*, **365**, 1620.

Dalmia, S. (2006), 'Migration and Indian doctors', *Indian Journal of Surgery*, **68**, 280–82.

Daniel, P., Chamberlain, A. and Gordon, F. (2001), 'Expectations and experiences of newly recruited Filipino nurses', *British Journal of Nursing*, **10**, 254–65.

Daniels, N. (2008), *Just Health. Meeting Health Needs Fairly*, New York: Cambridge University Press.

Danishevski, K. (2005), 'Human resources for health in Russia', in C. Dubois, E. Nolte and M. McKee (eds), *Human Resources for Health in Europe*, London: Open University Press, pp. 117–32.

Daviaud, E. and Chopra, M. (2008), 'How much is not enough? Human resource requirements for primary health care: a case study from South Africa', *Bulletin of the WHO*, **86**, 46–51.

Day, G., Minichiello, V. and Madison, J. (2006), 'Nursing morale: what does the literature reveal?', *Australian Health Review*, **30**, 516–24.

Denham, L. and Shaddock, A. (2004), 'Recruitment and retention of rural allied health professionals in developmental disability services in New South Wales', *Australian Journal of Rural Health*, **12** (1), 28–9.

Denoon, D. (1989), *Public Health in Papua New Guinea: Medical Possibility and Social Constraint, 1884–1984*, Cambridge: Cambridge University Press.

DiCicco-Bloom, B. (2004), 'The racial and gendered experiences of immigrant nurses from Kerala, India', *Journal of Transcultural Nursing*, **15**, 26–33.

Dieleman, M., Cuong, P., Anh, L. and Martineau, T. (2003), 'Identifying factors for job motivation of rural health workers in North Viet Nam', *Human Resources for Health*, **1** (10), 1–10.

Dodani, S. and LaPorte, R. (2005), 'Brain drain from developing countries: how can brain drain be converted to wisdom gain?', *Journal of the Royal Society of Medicine*, **98**, 487–91.

Dore, R. (1976), *The Diploma Disease*, London: Allen and Unwin.

van Dormael, M., Dugas, S., Kone, Y. et al. (2008), 'Appropriate training and retention of community doctors in rural areas: a case study from Mali', *Human Resources for Health*, **6** (25), 1–8.

Dovlo, D. (2003), 'The brain drain and retention of professionals in Africa', unpub. paper to Conference on Improving Tertiary Education in Sub-Saharan Africa, Accra.

Dovlo, D. (2004), 'Using mid-level cadres as substitutes for internationally mobile health professionals in Africa', *Human Resources for Health*, **2** (7), 1–12.

Dovlo, D. (2005), 'Wastage in the health workforce: some perspectives from African countries', *Human Resources for Health*, **3** (6), 1–9.

Dovlo, D. (2006), 'Ghanaian health workers on the causes and consequences of migration', in K. Tamas and J. Palme (eds), *Globalizing Migration Regimes: New Challenges in Transnational Cooperation*, Aldershot: Ashgate, pp. 118–27.

Dovlo, D. and Nyonator, F. (1999), 'Migration by graduates of the University of Ghana Medical School: a preliminary rapid appraisal', *Human Resources for Health*, **3**, 40–51.

Doyal, L. (1979), *The Political Economy of Health*, London: Pluto Press.

Drager, S., Gedik, G. and dal Poz, M. (2006), 'Health workforce issues and the global fund to fight AIDS, tuberculosis and malaria', *Human Resources for Health*, **4** (23), 1–12.

Dugger, C. (2004), 'An exodus of African nurses puts infants and the ill in peril', *New York Times*, 12 July.

Dumont, J. and Meyer, J. (2004), 'The international mobility of health professionals: an evaluation and analysis based on the case of South Africa', in OECD, *Trends in International Migration*, Paris: OECD, pp. 150–205.

Dumont, J. and Zurn, P. (2007), 'Immigrant health workers in OECD countries in the broader context of highly skilled migration', in OECD, *International Migration Outlook*, Paris, OECD, pp. 162–228.

Durey, A. (2005), 'Settling in: overseas trained GPs and their spouses in rural Western Australia', *Rural Sociology*, **15**, 38–54.

Dussault, G. and Franceschini, M. (2006), 'Not enough there, too many here: understanding geographical imbalances in the distribution of the health workforce', *Human Resources for Health*, **4** (12), 1–16.

Duverne, A., Carnet, D., d'Athis, P. and Quantin, C. (2008), 'Caractéristiques et motivations des médecins français ayant choisi d'émigrer en Grande Bretagne', *Revue d'Epidémiologie et de Santé Publique*, **56**, 360–73.

Dyer, S., McDowell, L. and Batnitzky, A. (2008), 'Emotional labour/ body work: the caring labours of migrants in the UK's National Health Service', *Geoforum*, **39**, 2030–38.

Egger, D. and Ollier, E. (2007), 'Managing the Health Millennium Development Goals – the challenges of management strengthening', Geneva: WHO/HSS Working Paper No. 8.

El-Jardali, F., Dimassi, H., Dumit, N. et al. (2009), 'A national cross-sectional study on nurses' intentions to leave and job satisfaction in Lebanon: implications for policy and practice', *BMC Nursing*, **8** (3), 1–13.

El-Jardali, F., Dumit, N., Jamal, D. and Mouro, G. (2008a), 'Migration of Lebanese nurses: a questionnaire survey and secondary data analysis', *International Journal of Nursing Studies*, **45**, 1490–500.

El-Jardali, F., Jamal, D., Jaafar, M. and Rahla, Z. (2008b), 'Analysis of health professionals' migration: a two country case study for the United Arab Emirates and Lebanon', Beirut: American University of Beirut (mimeo).

Engels, B. and Connell, J. (1983), 'Indian doctors in Australia: costs and benefits of the brain drain', *Australian Geographer*, **15**, 308–18.

Espiritu, Y. (2005), 'Gender, migration and work: Filipina health care professionals to the United States', *Revue Européenne des Migrations Internationales*, **21**, 55–75.

Evans, M. (2005), 'Neoliberalism and policy transfer in the British competition state: the case of welfare reform', in S. Soederberg, G. Menz and P. Cerny (eds), *Internalizing Globalization*, Basingstoke: Palgrave, pp. 69–89.

van Eyck, K. (2004), *Women and International Migration in the Health Sector*, Ferney-Voltaire: Public Services International.

van Eyck, K. (2005), *Who Cares? Women Health Workers in the Global Labour Market*, Ferney-Voltaire: Public Services International.

Faini, R. (2007), 'Remittances and the brain drain: do more skilled migrants remit more?', *World Bank Economic Review*, **21**, 177–91.

Faist, T. (2008), 'Migrants as transnational development agents: an inquiry into the newest round of the migration–development nexus', *Population, Space and Place*, **14**, 21–42.

Fang, Z. (2007), 'Potential of China in global nurse migration', *Health Services Research*, **42**, 1419–28.

Favell, A., Feldblum, M. and Smith, M. (2006), 'The human face of global mobility: a research agenda', in M. Smith and A. Favell (eds), *The Human Face of Global Mobility*, New Brunswick, NJ: Transaction Publishers, pp. 1–25.

Feldstein, P. and Butter, I. (1978), 'The foreign medical graduate and public policy: a discussion of the issues and options', *International Journal of Health Services*, **8**, 541–58.

Fendall, N. (1972), *Auxiliaries in Health Care*, New York: Johns Hopkins Press.

Finau, S., Wainoqolo, I. and Cuboni, G. (2004), 'Health transition and globalization in the Pacific: vestiges of colonialism?', *Perspectives on Global Development and Technology*, **3**, 109–29.

Findlay, A. and Stewart, E. (2002), *Skilled Labour Migration from Developing Countries*, ILO International Migration Papers No. 55, Geneva: ILO.

Flahault, D. (1978), 'Primary health care by non-physicians', in T. Hall and A. Mejia (eds), *Health Manpower Planning*, Geneva: WHO, pp. 177–99.

Florida, R. (2005), *The Flight of the Creative Class. The New Global Competition for Talent*, New York: Harper.

Folbre, N. (2006), 'Nursebots to the rescue? Immigration, automation and care', *Globalizations*, **3**, 349–60.

Folbre, N. and Nelson, J. (2000), 'For love or money – or both?', *Journal of Economic Perspectives*, **14**, 123–40.

Foner, N. (2001), *Islands in the City. West Indian Migration to New York*, Berkeley, CA: University of California Press.

Fong, M. (2003), 'A review of options for achieving an adequate and cost-effective supply of appropriately qualified nurses for the Fijian health system', unpub. paper to WHO Meeting on Migration of Skilled Health Personnel in Pacific Island Countries, Nadi.

Fongwa, M. (2002), 'International health care perspectives: the Cameroon example', *Journal of Transcultural Nursing*, **13**, 325–30.

Forcier, M., Simoens, S. and Giuffrida, A. (2004), 'Impact, regulation and health policy implications of physician migration in OECD countries', *Human Resources for Health*, **2** (12), 1–11.

Forsyth, C. (2008), 'The crisis in healthcare in rural Bolivia', *LatinAm/ Caribbean Affairs* (http://latinamcaribbeanaffairs.suite101.com/article, accessed 17 October 2008).

Forti, E., Martin, K., Jones, R. and Herman, J. (1995), 'Factors influencing retention of rural Pennsylvania family physicians', *Journal of American Board of Family Practice*, **8**, 469–74.

Franco, L., Bennett, S., Kanfer, R. and Stubbledine, P. (2004), 'Determinants and consequences of health worker motivation in hospitals in Jordan and Georgia', *Social Science and Medicine*, **58**, 343–55.

Freedman, D. (2008), 'Tales from the South Pacific', *Australian Volunteer*, Summer, 22–3.

Freund, P. (1987), 'Environment, disease and health service utilization: a comparative study with Zambia', in R. Akhtar (ed.), *Health and Disease in Tropical Africa. Geographical and Medical Viewpoints*, Chur: Harwood, pp. 469–86.

Fullilove, M. (2008), *World Wide Webs. Diasporas and the International System*, Sydney: Lowy Institute.

Furler, J., Harris, E., Chondros, P. et al. (2002), 'The inverse care law revisited: impact of disadvantaged location on accessing longer GP consultation times', *Medical Journal of Australia*, **177**, 80–83.

Fusitu'a, P. (2000), 'My island homes: Tonga, migration and identity', unpub B.A. (Honours) thesis, University of Sydney.

Gaidzanwa, R. (1999), *Voting With Their Feet: Migrant Zimbabwean Nurses and Doctors in the Era of Structural Adjustment*, Uppsala: Nordiska Africainstitutet Research Report No. 111.

Galak, M. (2009), 'Doctors of the second freshness. Why does Australia not have enough doctors?', *Quadrant*, **53** (6), 30–36.

Gamlen, A. (2008), 'The emigration state and the modern geographical imagination', *Political Geography*, **27**, 840–56.

Gardiner, M., Sexton, R., Kearns, H. and Marshall, K. (2006), 'Impact of support initiatives on retaining rural general practitioners', *Australian Journal of Rural Health*, **14**, 196–201.

Garrett, L. (2007), 'The challenge of global health', *Foreign Affairs*, **86** (1), 14–38.

George, S. (2005), *When Women Come First. Gender and Class in Transnational Migration*, Berkeley, CA: University of California Press.

George, T., Rozario, K., Jeffrin, A. et al. (2007), 'Non-European Union doctors in the National Health Service: why, when and how do they come to the United Kingdom of Great Britain and Northern Ireland?', *Human Resources for Health*, **5** (6), 1–6.

Gerein, N., Green, A. and Pearson, S. (2006), 'The implications of shortages of health professionals for maternal health in Sub-Saharan Africa', *Reproductive Health Matters*, **14** (27), 40–50.

Gesler, W. and Gage, G. (1987), 'Health care delivery for under five children in rural Sierra Leone', in R. Akhtar (ed.), *Health and Disease in Tropical Africa. Geographical and Medical Viewpoints*, Chur: Harwood, pp. 427–68.

Gilles, M., Wakerman, J. and Durey, A. (2008), '"If it wasn't for OTDs, there would be no AMS": overseas-trained doctors working in rural and remote Aboriginal health settings', *Australian Health Review*, **32**, 655–63.

Gish, O. (1969a), 'Emigration and the supply and demand for medical manpower: the Irish case', *Minerva*, **7**, 668–79.

Gish, O. (1969b), 'Foreign born midwives in the United Kingdom: a case of the skill drain', *Social and Economic Administration*, **3**, 39–51.

Gish, O. (1971), *Doctor Migration and World Health*, London: Bell.

Gish, O. and Godfrey, M. (1979), 'A reappraisal of the "brain drain" with special reference to the medical profession', *Social Science and Medicine*, **13C**, 1–11.

Global Health Workforce Alliance (2008), *Scaling Up, Saving Lives*, Geneva: WHO.

Golbasi, Z., Kelleci, M. and Dogan, S. (2008), 'Relationships between coping strategies, individual characteristics and job satisfaction in a sample of hospital nurses: cross-sectional questionnaire survey', *International Journal of Nursing Studies*, **45**, 1800–806.

Goldfarb, R., Havrylyshyn, O. and Mangum, S. (1984), 'Can remittances compensate for manpower outflows? The case of Philippine physicians', *Journal of Development Economics*, **15**, 1–17.

Goodman, B. (2005), 'Overseas recruitment and migration', *Nursing Management*, **12** (8), 32–7.

Gordon, S. (2005), *Nursing Against the Odds*, Ithaca, NY: ILR Press.

Gorman, S. and Hohmuth-Lemonick, E. (2009), 'At work with Malawi's nurses', *American Journal of Nursing*, **109** (6), 26–30.

Gourlay, J. (2003), *Florence Nightingale and the Health of the Raj*, Aldershot: Ashgate.

Grant, H. (2006), 'From the Transvaal to the Prairies: the migration of South African Physicians to Canada', *Journal of Ethnic and Migration Studies*, **32**, 681–95.

Grigulis, A., Prost, A. and Osrin, D. (2009), 'The lives of Malawian nurses: the stories behind the statistics', *Transactions of the Royal Society of Tropical Medicine and Hygiene*, **103**, 1195–6.

Groutsis, D. (2009), 'Recruiting migrant nurses to fill the gaps: the contribution of migrant women in the nursing care sector in Greece', *Journal of International Migration and Integration*, **10**, 49–65.

Hadley, M., Blum, L., Mujaddid, S. et al. (2007), 'Why Bangladeshi nurses avoid "nursing": social and structural factors on hospital wards in Bangladesh', *Social Science and Medicine*, **64**, 1166–77.

Hagey, R., Choudhry, U., Guruge, S. et al. (2001), 'Immigrant nurses' experience of racism', *Journal of Nursing Scholarship*, **33**, 389–94.

Hagopian, A., Thompson, M., Fordyce, M. et al. (2004), 'The migration of physicians from sub-Saharan Africa to the United States of America: measures of the African brain drain', *Human Resources for Health*, **2** (17), 1–10.

Hagopian, A., Ofosu, A., Fatusi, A. et al. (2005), 'The flight of physicians from West Africa: views of African physicians and implications for policy', *Social Science and Medicine*, **61**, 1750–60.

Hamilton, K. and Yau, J. (2004), *The Global Tug-of-War for Health Workers*, Washington: Migration Policy Institute.

Hamnett, M. and Connell, J. (1981), 'Diagnosis and cure: the resort to traditional and modern medical practitioners in the North Solomons', *Social Science and Medicine*, **15B**, 489–98.

Han, G. and Humphreys, J. (2005), 'Overseas-trained doctors in Australia: community integration and their intention to stay in a rural community', *Australian Journal of Rural Health*, **13**, 236–41.

Hancock, P. (2008), 'Nurse migration: the effects on nursing education', *International Nursing Review*, **55**, 258–64.

Hansdotter, F. (2007), *Why do Nurses leave Zambia and How Can They be Retained?*, Stockholm: Karolinska Institute.

Hardill, I. and Macdonald, S. (2000), 'Skilled international migration: the experience of nurses in the UK', *Regional Studies*, **34**, 681–92.

Harper, S., Aboderin, I. and Ruchieva, I. (2008), 'The impact of the out-migration of female care workers on informal family care in Nigeria and Bulgaria', in J. Connell (ed.), *The International Migration of Health Workers*, New York and London: Routledge, pp. 163–71.

Harrison, M. (1998), 'Female physicians in Mexico: migration and mobility in the lifecourse', *Social Science and Medicine*, **47**, 455–68.

Hawkes, M., Kolenko, M., Shockness, M. and Diwaker, K. (2009), 'Nursing brain drain from India', *Human Resources for Health*, **7** (5), 1–2.

Hawthorne, L. (2001), 'The globalisation of the nursing workforce: barriers confronting overseas qualified nurses in Australia', *Nursing Inquiry*, **8**, 213–29.

Hayes, L., O'Brien-Pallas, L., Duffield, C. et al. (2006), 'Nurse turnover: a literature review', *International Journal of Nursing Studies*, **43**, 237–63.

Hays, R., Veitch, P., Cheers, B. and Crossland, L. (1997), 'Why rural doctors leave their practices', *Australian Journal of Rural Health*, **5**, 198–203.

Healy, G. and Oikelome, F. (2007), 'A global link between national diversity policies? The case of the migration of Nigerian physicians into the UK and USA', *International Journal of Human Resources Management*, **18**, 1917–33.

Hedson, J. (2000), 'Teleconsultations in Pohnpei State, Federated States of Micronesia', *Pacific Health Dialog*, **7** (2), 46–50.

Hegney, D., Plank, A. and Parker, V. (2003), 'Workplace violence in nursing in Queensland', *International Journal of Nursing Practice*, **9**, 261–8.

Henry, L. (2007), 'Institutionalised disadvantage: older Ghanaian nurses' and midwives' reflections on career progression and stagnation in the NHS', *Journal of Clinical Nursing*, **16**, 2196–203.

Hintermann, C. and Reeger, U. (2005), 'On nurses and newsvendors. Asian immigrants in the Vienna labour market', in E. Spaan, F. Hillmann and T. van Naerssen (eds), *Asian Migrants and European Labour Markets*, London: Routledge, pp. 56–79.

Ho, C. (2008), 'Chinese nurses in Australia. Migration, work and identity', in J. Connell (ed.), *The International Migration of Health Workers*, New York and London: Routledge, pp. 147–62.

Hoadley, S. (1980), 'Aid, politics and hospitals in Western Samoa', *World Development*, **8**, 443–55.

Hochschild, A. (1983), *The Managed Heart. Commercialization of Human Feeling*, Berkeley, CA: University of California Press.

Hooker, K. and Varcoe, J. (1999), 'Migration and the Cook Islands', in J.

Overton and R. Scheyvens (eds), *Strategies for Sustainable Development. Experiences from the Pacific*, Sydney: UNSW Press, pp. 91–9.

Horn, J. (1977), 'The medical brain drain and health priorities in Latin America', *International Journal of Health Services*, **7**, 425–42.

Hosein, R. and Thomas, C. (2007), 'Caribbean single market economy (CSME) and the intra-regional migration of nurses', *Global Social Policy*, **7**, 316–38.

Hugo, G. (2009), 'Care worker migration, Australia and development', *Population, Space and Place*, **15**, 189–203.

Huish, R. (2009), 'How Cuba's Latin American School of Medicine challenges the ethics of physician migration', *Social Science and Medicine*, **69**, 301–4.

Humphreys, J. (1985), 'A political economy approach to the allocation of health care resources: the case of remote areas in Queensland', *Australian Geographical Studies*, **23**, 222–42.

Humphreys, J. (1988), 'Social provision and service delivery: problems of equity, health and health care in rural Australia', *Geoforum*, **19**, 323–38.

Humphreys, J., Wakerman, J., Wells, R. et al. (2008), '"Beyond workforce": a systemic solution for health service provision in small rural and remote communities', *Medical Journal of Australia*, **188** (8), S77–S80.

Humphries, N., Brugha, R. and McGee, H. (2008), 'Overseas nurse recruitment: Ireland as an illustration of the dynamic nature of nurse migration', *Health Policy*, **87**, 264–72.

Humphries, N., Brugha, R. and McGee, H. (2009a), 'Sending money home. A mixed methods study of remittances sent by migrant nurses in Ireland', *Human Resources for Health*, **7** (66).

Humphries, N., Brugha, R. and McGee, H. (2009b), '"I won't be staying here for long": a qualitative study on the retention of migrant nurses in Ireland', *Human Resources for Health*, **7** (68), 1–12.

Hunsberger, M., Baumann, A., Blythe, J. and Crea, M. (2008), 'Sustaining the rural workforce: nursing perspectives on worklife challenges', *Journal of Rural Health*, **25**, 17–25.

Hussey, P. (2007), 'International migration patterns of physicians to the United States: a cross-national panel analysis', *Health Policy*, **84**, 298–307.

Iganski, P. and Mason, D. (2002), *Ethnicity, Equality of Opportunity and the British National Health Service*, Aldershot: Ashgate.

Ihekweazu, C., Anya, I. and Anosike, E. (2005), 'Nigerian medical graduates: where are they now?', *The Lancet*, **365**, 1847–8.

Iredale, R. (2000), 'Skilled migration policies in the Asia-Pacific region', *International Migration Review*, **34**, 882–906.

Iredale, R. (2001), 'The migration of professionals: theories and typologies', *International Migration*, **39**, 7–26.

Isaacs, A. (2007), 'Insufficient rural doctors: Maslow's theory and the need for social accountability', *Australian and New Zealand Journal of Public Health*, **31**, 582.

Ishi, T. (1987), 'Class conflict, the state and linkage: the international migration of nurses from the Philippines', *Berkeley Journal of Sociology*, **32**, 281–95.

Ishi, T. (1988), 'International linkage and national class conflict: the migration of Korean nurses to the United States', *Amerasia Journal*, **14**, 23–50.

Iyun, B. (1989), 'An assessment of a rural health programme on child and maternity care: the Ogbomoso community health care programme, Oyo State, Nigeria', *Social Science and Medicine*, **29**, 933–8.

Iyun, B. (1994), 'Health care in the Third World: Africa', in D. Phillips and Y. Verhasselt (eds), *Health and Development*, London: Routledge, pp. 249–58.

Jackson, D. (2008), 'The aging nursing workforce: how can we avoid a retirement brain drain?', *Journal of Clinical Nursing*, **17**, 2949–50.

Jackson, R. (2009), 'A cold wind in Iceland', *Financial Times*, 10 October, 17.

James, K. (2003), 'Is there a Tongan middle class? Hierarchy and protest in contemporary Tonga', *The Contemporary Pacific*, **15**, 309–36.

Janus, K., Amelung, V., Gaitanides, M. and Schwartz, F. (2007), 'German physicians on strike – shedding light on the roots of physician dissatisfaction', *Health Policy*, **82**, 357–65.

Jeffrey, R. (1979), 'Recognising India's doctors: the institutionalization of medical dependency (1918–39)', *Modern Asian Studies*, **13**, 301–26.

Jerety, J. (2008), 'Primary health care: Fiji's broken dream', *Bulletin of the WHO*, **86**, 166–7.

Jessop, B. (2002), *The Future of the Capitalist State*, Cambridge: Polity Press.

Jinks, C., Ong, B. and Paton, C. (2000), 'Mobile medics? The mobility of doctors in the European Economic Area', *Health Policy*, **54**, 45–64.

Joint Learning Initiative (2004), *Human Resources for Health. Overcoming the Crisis*, Cambridge: Harvard University Press.

Jones, A., Sharpe, J. and Sogren, M. (2004), 'Children's experiences of separation from parents as a consequence of migration', *Caribbean Journal of Social Work*, **3**, 89–109.

Jones, M. (2004), 'Heroines of lonely outposts or tools of the empire? British nurses in Britain's model colony: Ceylon, 1878–1948', *Nursing Inquiry*, **11**, 148–60.

Jones, P. (2008), 'Doctor and physician assistant distribution in rural and remote Texas counties', *Australian Journal of Rural Health*, **16**, 389.

Joorabchi, B. (1973), 'Physician migration: brain drain or overflow? With special reference to the situation in Iran', *British Journal of Medical Education*, **7**, 44–7.

Jorgensen, S. (2008), 'Some perspectives on the geographies of poverty and health: a Ghanaian context', *Norsk Geografisk Tidsskrift*, **62**, 241–50.

Joseph, A. and Martin-Matthews, A. (1994), 'Caring for elderly people', in D. Phillips and Y. Verhasselt (eds), *Health and Development*, London: Routledge, pp. 168–81.

Joyce, R. and Hunt, C. (1982), 'Philippine nurses and the brain drain', *Social Science and Medicine*, **16**, 1223–33.

Jumpa, M., Jan, S. and Mills, A. (2007), 'The role of regulation in influencing income-generating activities among public sector doctors in Peru', *Human Resources for Health*, **5** (5), 1–8.

Kandel, W. and Massey, D. (2002), 'The culture of Mexican migration: a theoretical and empirical analysis', *Social Forces*, **80**, 981–1004.

Kangasniemi, M., Winters, L. and Commander, S. (2007), 'Is the medical brain drain beneficial? Evidence from overseas doctors in the UK', *Social Science and Medicine*, **65**, 915–23.

Kaushik, M., Jaiswal, A., Shah, N. and Mahal, A. (2008), 'High-end physician migration from India', *Bulletin of the WHO*, **86**, 40–45.

Ken, C. (2008), 'Training islanders a top priority', *Islands Business*, **34** (3), 42–3.

Khadria, B. (2007), 'International nurse recruitment in India', *Health Services Research*, **42**, 1429–36.

Khalik, A., Broyles, R. and Mwachofi, A. (2008), 'Global nurse migration: its impact on developing countries and prospects for the future', *World Health and Population*, **10** (3), 5–23.

Kida, T. and Mackintosh, M. (2005), 'Public expenditure allocation and incidence under health care market liberalization: a Tanzanian case study', in M. Mackintosh and M. Koivusalo (eds), *Commercialization of Health Care*, Basingstoke: Palgrave Macmillan, pp. 267–83.

Kienene, T. (1993), 'Health care', in H. van Trease (ed.), *Atoll Politics. The Republic of Kiribati*, Suva: Institute of Pacific Studies, pp. 250–57.

Kimani, D. (2005), 'Brain drain robs Africa's health sector of $552 bn', *The East African*, **7** February, p. 42.

Kinfu, Y., dal Poz, M., Mercer, H. and Evans, D. (2009), 'The health worker shortage in Africa: are enough physicians and nurses being trained?', *Bulletin of the WHO*, **87**, 225–30.

King, M. (1967), *Medical Care in Developing Countries*, Nairobi: Oxford University Press.

King, R. (2000), 'Generalizations from the history of return migration', in

B. Ghosh (ed.), *Return Migration. Journey of Hope or Despair*, Geneva: International Organization for Migration, pp. 7–56.

Kingham, T., Kamara, T., Cherian, M. et al. (2009), 'Quantifying surgical capacity in Sierra Leone', *Archives of Surgery*, **144**, 122–7.

Kingma, M. (2006), *Nurses on the Move. Migration and the Global Health Care Economy*, Ithaca, NY: Cornell University Press.

Kirigia, J., Gbary, A., Muthuri, L. et al. (2006), 'The cost of health professionals' brain drain in Kenya', *BMC Health Services Research*, **6** (89), 1–10.

Kissah-Korsah, K. (2008), 'Spatial accessibility to orthodox health care facilities in the Ajumako-Enyan-Essiam and Upper Denkyira districts in the central region of Ghana', *Norsk Geografisk Tidsskrift*, **62**, 203–9.

Kittay, E., Jennings, B. and Wasunna, A. (2005), 'Dependency, difference and the global ethic of longterm care', *Journal of Political Philosophy*, **13**, 443–69.

Kline, D. (2003), 'Push and pull factors in international nurse migration', *Journal of Nursing Scholarship*, **35**, 107–11.

Kober, K. and van Damme, W. (2006), 'Public sector nurses in Swaziland: can the downturn be reversed?', *Human Resources for Health*, **4** (13), 1–11.

Kofman, E. and Raghuram, P. (2006), 'Gender and global labour migrations: incorporating skilled workers', *Antipode*, **38**, 282–303.

Kolawole, B. (2009), 'Ontario's internationally educated nurses and waste in human capital', *International Nursing Review*, **56**, 184–90.

Koloto, A. (2003), *National Survey of Pacific Nurses and Nursing Students*, Auckland: Koloto and Associates.

Kopetsch, T. (2009), 'The migration of doctors to and from Germany', *Journal of Public Health*, **17**, 33–9.

Krajewski-Siuda, K., Romaniuk, P., Madaj, B. et al. (2008), 'Brain drain threat – Polish students are not satisfied with labor market options for health professionals in Poland', *Journal of Public Health*, **16**, 347–51.

Kristiansen, I. and Forde, O. (1992), 'Medical specialists' choice of location: the role of geographical attachment in Norway', *Social Science and Medicine*, **34**, 57–62.

Kronfol, N., Sibai, A. and Rafeh, N. (1992), 'The impact of civil disturbances on the migration of physicians: the case of Lebanon', *Medical Care*, **30**, 208–15.

Kruk, M., Prescott, M., de Pinho, H. and Galea, S. (2009), 'Are doctors and nurses associated with coverage of essential health services in developing countries? A cross-sectional study', *Human Resources for Health*, **7** (27), 1–9.

Kuan, P. (1970), 'Medical education in Taiwan', *British Journal of Medical Education*, **4**, 164–7.

Kwok, R., Law, Y., Li, K. et al. (2006), 'Prevalence of workplace violence against nurses in Hong Kong', *Hong Kong Medical Journal*, **12**, 6–9.

Labonté, R., Packer, C. and Klassen, N. (2006), 'Managing health professionals' migration from sub-Saharan Africa to Canada: a stakeholder inquiry into policy options', *Human Resources for Health*, **4** (22), 1–15.

Labonté, R. and Schrecker, T. (2007a), 'Globalization and social determinants of health: the role of the global market place', *Globalization and Health*, **3** (6), 1–17.

Labonté, R. and Schrecker, T. (2007b), 'Globalization and social determinants of health: promoting health equity in global governance', *Globalization and Health*, **3** (7), 1–15.

Laleman, G., Kegels, G., Marchal, B. et al. (2007), 'The contribution of international health volunteers to the health workforce in sub-Saharan Africa', *Human Resources for Health*, **5** (19), 1–9.

Lanfranchi, P. and Taylor, M. (2001), *Moving with the Ball. The Migration of Professional Footballers*, Oxford: Berg.

Larsen, J., Allan, H., Bryan, K. and Smith, P. (2005), 'Overseas nurses' motivations for working in the UK: globalization and life politics', *Work, Employment and Society*, **19**, 349–68.

Larsson, E., Atkins, S., Chopra, M. and Ekstrom, A. (2009), 'What about health system tightening and the internal brain drain?', *Transactions of the Royal Society of Tropical Medicine and Hygiene*, **103**, 533–4.

Laurant, M., Reeves, D., Hermens, R. et al. (2009), 'Substitution of doctors by nurses in primary care', *The Cochrane Library*, **3**, 1–42.

Lavenex, S. (2007), 'The competition state and highly skilled migration', *Society*, **44** (2), 32–41.

Lazaridis, G. (2000), 'Filipino and Albanian women migrant workers in Greece: multiple layers of oppression', in F. Anthias and G. Lazaridis (eds), *Gender and Migration in Southern Europe*, Oxford: Berg, pp. 49–80.

Leckie, J. (2000), 'Gender and work in Fiji: constraints to re-negotiation', in A. Jones, P. Herda and T. Suaalii (eds), *Bitter Sweet. Indigenous Women in the Pacific*, Dunedin: University of Otago Press, pp. 73–92.

Legrain, P. (2007), *Immigrants. Your Country Needs Them*, London: Abacus.

Lehmann, U., Dieleman, M. and Martineau, T. (2008), 'Staffing remote rural areas in middle- and low-income countries: a literature review of attraction and retention', *BMC Health Services Research*, **8** (19), 1–10.

Léonard, C., Stordeur, S. and Roberfroid, D. (2009), 'Association between physician density and health care consumption: a systematic review of the evidence', *Health Policy*, **91**, 121–34.

LeSergent, C. and Haney, C. (2005), 'Rural hospital nurses' stressors and coping strategies: a survey', *International Journal of Nursing Studies*, **42**, 315–24.

Likupe, G. (2006), 'Experiences of African nurses in the UK National Health Service: a literature review', *Journal of Clinical Nursing*, **15**, 1213–20.

Lillis, S., St George, I. and Upsdell, R. (2006), 'Perceptions of migrant doctors joining the New Zealand medical workforce', *New Zealand Medical Journal*, **119** (1229), 1–9.

Lipley, N. and Stokes, B. (1998), 'A real solution to nursing shortages?', *Nursing Standard*, **12** (34), 12–13.

Lipton, M. (1977), *Why Poor People Stay Poor. Urban Bias in World Development*, London: Temple Smith.

Little, L. (2005), 'Nurse migration: a Canadian study', *Health Services Research*, **42**, 1336–53.

Loewenson, R. (2004), 'Epidemiology in the era of globalization: skills transfer or new skills?', *International Journal of Epidemiology*, **33**, 1144–50.

Long, L. and Mensah, K. (2007), 'MIDA Ghana Health Project evaluation', mimeo.

Lorenzo, M. (2006), 'Migration of health workers: country case study Philippines', Geneva: ILO Working Paper No. 236.

Lorenzo, M., Galvez-Tan, J., Icamina, K. and Javier, L. (2007), 'Nurse migration from a source country: Philippine country case study', *Health Services Research*, **42**, 1406–18.

Lu, H., While, A. and Barriball, L. (2005), 'Job satisfaction among nurses: a literature review', *International Journal of Nursing Studies*, **42**, 211–27.

Luck, M., Fernandes, M. and Ferrinho, P. (2000), 'At the other end of the brain-drain: African nurses living in Lisbon', *Studies in Health Service Organisation and Policy*, **16**, 157–69.

Luna, L. (1998), 'Culturally competent health care: a challenge for nurses in Saudi Arabia', *Journal of Transcultural Nursing*, **9** (2), 8–14.

Lusale, D. (2007), 'Why do Zambian healthworkers migrate abroad?', *Bulletin of the Medicus Mundi Switzerland*, **104**, 97–103.

Lutua, K. (2002), 'Salaries and conditions of employment for nurses, nurse practitioners and midwives – a Fijian perspective', unpub. paper to 11th South Pacific Nurses Forum, Vila.

Lyttleton, C. (2005), 'Market bound. Relocation and disjunction in Northwest Laos', in S. Jatrana, M. Toyota and B. Yeoh (eds), *Migration and Health in Asia*, London: Routledge, pp. 41–60.

McCourt, W. and Awases, M. (2007), 'Addressing the human resources crisis: a case study of the Namibian health service', *Human Resources for Health*, **5** (1), 1–13.

McCoy, D., Bennett, S., Witter, S. et al. (2008), 'Salaries and incomes of health workers in sub-Saharan Africa', *The Lancet*, **371**, 675–81.

McEwin, K. and Cameron, I. (2007), *The 1987 NSW Rural Doctors' Dispute. The Dispute that Changed the Face of Rural Medicine*, Newcastle, NSW: Rural Doctors Network.

McGregor, J. (2007), 'Joining the BBC (British bottom cleaners): Zimbabwean migrants and the UK care industry', *Journal of Ethnic and Migration Studies*, **33**, 801–24.

McKendry, R., Wells, G., Dale, P. et al. (1996), 'Factors influencing the emigration of physicians from Canada to the United States', *Canadian Medical Association Journal*, **154**, 171–81.

McKenna, H., Thompson, D. and Watson, R. (2007), 'Health care assistants – an oxymoron?', *International Journal of Nursing Studies*, **44**, 1283–4.

Mackintosh, M., Mensah, K., Henry, L., and Rowson, M. (2006), 'Aid, restitution and international fiscal redistribution in health care: implications of health professionals' migration', *Journal of International Development*, **18**, 757–70.

MacLachlan, M. (2006), *Culture and Health. A Critical Perspective Towards Global Health*, Chichester: Wiley & Sons.

McLean, G., Sutton, M. and Guthrie, B. (2006), 'Deprivation and quality of primary care services: evidence for persistence of the inverse care law from the United Kingdom', *Journal of Epidemiology and Community Health*, **60**, 917–22.

Macpherson, C. (1994), 'Changing patterns of commitment to island homelands: a case study of Western Samoa', *Pacific Studies*, **17**, 83–116.

Macpherson, C. (2004), 'Transnationalism and transformation in Samoan society', in V. Lockwood (ed.), *Globalization and Culture Change in the Pacific Islands*, Upper Saddle River, NJ: Pearson Prentice Hall, pp. 165–81.

Mahler, S. (1998), 'Theoretical and empirical contributions to a research agenda for transnationalism', in M. Smith and L. Guarnizo (eds), *Transnationalism from Below*, New Brunswick, NJ: Transaction Publishers, pp. 65–100.

Malvarez, S. and Castrillon Agudelo, C. (2005), 'Overview of the nursing workforce of Latin America', Geneva: Issue Paper No. 6, International Council of Nurses.

Manning, C. and Sidorenko, A. (2007), 'The regulation of professional migration: insights from the health and IT sectors in ASEAN', *The World Economy*, **30**, 1084–113.

Marcus, G. (1981), 'Power on the extreme periphery: the perspective of Tongan elites in the modern world system', *Pacific Viewpoint*, **22**, 48–64.

Mareckova, M. (2004), 'Exodus of Czech doctors leaves gap in health care', *The Lancet*, **363**, 1443–6.

Maron, N. and Connell, J. (2008), 'Return to Nukunuku. Employment, identity and return migration in Tonga', *Asia-Pacific Viewpoint*, **49**, 168–84.

Marshall, M. (2004), *Namoluk Beyond the Reef. The Transformation of a Micronesian Community*, Boulder, CO: Westview.

Martineau, T., Decker, K. and Bundred, P. (2002), 'Briefing note on international migration of health professionals: levelling the playing field for developing country health systems', Liverpool: Liverpool School of Tropical Medicine.

Masango, S., Gathu, K. and Sibandze, S. (2008), 'Retention strategies for Swaziland's health sector workforce: assessing the role of non-financial incentives', Harare: EQUINET Discussion Paper No. 68.

von Massow, F. (2001), *Access to Health and Education Services in Ethiopia*, Oxford: Oxfam.

Mathauer, I. and Imhoff, I. (2006), 'Health worker motivation in Africa: the role of non-financial incentives and human resource management tools', *Human Resources for Health*, **4** (24), 1–17.

Mathauer, I., Imhoff, I. and Korte, R. (2004), 'Staff motivation: the impact of non-financial incentives and quality management tools', Berlin: Deutsche Gesellschaft für Technische Zusammenarbeit (GTZ).

Mathews, M., Rourke, J. and Park, A. (2006), 'National and provincial retention of medical graduates of Memorial University of Newfoundland', *Canadian Medical Association Journal*, **175**, 357–60.

Matsumotu, M., Okayama, M., Inoue, K. and Kajii, E. (2005), 'Factors associated with rural doctors' intention to continue a rural career: a survey of 3072 doctors in Japan', *Australian Journal of Rural Health*, **13**, 219–25.

Matsumotu, M., Okayama, M. and Kajii, E. (2004), 'Rural doctors' satisfaction in Japan: a nationwide survey', *Australian Journal of Rural Health*, **12** (2), 40–48.

Mayta-Tristan, P., Dulanto-Pizzorni, A. and Miranda, J. (2008), 'Low wages and brain drain: an alert from Peru', *The Lancet*, **371**, 1577.

Meek, J. (2009), 'Sleeping with one eye open', *Guardian Weekly*, 12 June, 25–7.

Mejia, A. (1978), 'International migration of professional health manpower', in T. Hall and A. Mejia (eds), *Health Manpower Planning*, Geneva: WHO, pp. 255–76.

Mejia, A. (1987), 'Nature of the challenge of health manpower imbalance', in Z. Bankowski and A. Mejia (eds), *Health Manpower Out Of Balance*, Geneva: Council for International Organizations of Medical Sciences, pp. 34–87.

Mejia, A., Pizurski, H. and Royston, E. (1979), *Physician and Nurse Migration: Analysis and Policy Implications*, Geneva: WHO.

Meng, Q., Yuan, J., Jing, L. and Zhang, J. (2009), 'Mobility of primary health care workers in China', *Human Resources for Health*, **7** (24), 1–5.

Mensah, K. (2005), 'International migration of health care staff: extent and policy responses, with illustrations from Ghana', in M. Mackintosh and M. Koivusalo (eds), *Commercialization of Health Care*, Basingstoke: Palgrave Macmillan, pp. 201–15.

Mensah, K., Mackintosh, M. and Henry, L. (2005), *The 'Skills Drain' of Health Professionals from the Developing World: A Framework for Policy Formation*, London: Medact.

Mick, S., Lee, S. and Wodchis,W. (2000), 'Variations in geographical distribution of foreign and domestically trained physicians in the United States: "safety nets" or "surplus exacerbation"', *Social Science and Medicine*, **50**, 185–202.

Miho, D. (2007), 'Palau. Nursing a system back to health', *Pacific*, **32** (5), 45.

Millar, J. and Salt, J. (2007), 'In whose interests? IT migration in an interconnected world economy', *Population, Space and Place*, **13**, 41–58.

Millen, J. (2008), 'Health worker shortages and HIV/AIDS: responses and linkages', *Practicing Anthropology*, **30** (4), 8–12.

Miller, E., Laugesen, M., Lee, S. and Mick, S. (1998), 'Emigration of New Zealand and Australian physicians to the United States and the international flow of medical personnel', *Health Policy*, **43**, 253–70.

Mills, A. and Shillcutt, S. (2004), 'Communicable diseases', in B. Lomborg (ed.), *Global Crises, Global Solutions*, Cambridge: Cambridge University Press, pp. 62–114.

Mills, E., Schabas, W., Volmink, J. et al. (2008), 'Should active recruitment of health workers from sub-Saharan Africa be viewed as a crime?', *The Lancet*, **371**, 685–8.

Mimura, C., Griffiths, P. and Norman, I. (2009), 'What motivates people to enter professional nursing?', *International Journal of Nursing Studies*, **46**, 603–5.

Mitchell, A., Bossert, T., Yip, W. and Mollahaliloglu, S. (2008), 'Health worker densities and immunization coverage in Turkey: a panel data analysis', *Human Resources for Health*, **6** (29), 1–23.

Moran, A., Nancarrow, S. and Butler, A. (2005), '"There's no place like home". A pilot study of perspectives of international health and social care professionals working in the UK', *Australia and New Zealand Health Policy*, **2** (25), 1–9.

Morgan, R. (2005), *Addressing Health Worker Shortages: Recruiting Retired Nurses to Reduce Mother-to-Child Transmission in Guyana*, Arlington, VA: Family Health International.

Mountford, A. (1997), 'Can a brain drain be good for growth in the source economy?', *Journal of Development Economics*, **53**, 287–303.

Mullan, F. (2004), *A Legacy of Pushes and Pulls: An Examination of Indian Physicians'* Emigration, Bethesda, MD: George Washington University.

Mullan, F. (2005), 'The metrics of the physician brain drain', *New England Journal of Medicine*, **353**, 1810–18.

Mullan, F. (2006), 'Doctors for the world: Indian physician emigration', *Health Affairs*, **25**, 380–93.

Mullan, F. (2007), 'Doctors and soccer players – African professionals on the move', *New England Journal of Medicine*, **356**, 440–43.

Mullan, F. and Frehywot, S. (2007), 'Non-physician clinicians in 47 sub-Saharan African countries', *The Lancet*, **370**, 2158–63.

Mullan, F., Frehywot, S. and Jolley, L. (2008), 'Aging, primary care, and self-sufficiency: health care workforce challenges ahead', *Journal of Law, Medicine and Ethics*, **36**, 703–8.

Mullan, F., Politzer, R. and Davis, C. (1995), 'Medical migration and the physician workforce: international medical graduates and American medicine', *Journal of the American Medical Association*, **273**, 1521–7.

Munga, M. and Maestad, O. (2009), 'Measuring inequalities in the distribution of health workers: the case of Tanzania', *Human Resources for Health*, **7** (4), 1–12.

Mutizwa-Mangiza, D. (1998), 'The impact of health sector reform on public sector health worker motivation in Zimbabwe', Partnerships for Health Reform Working Paper No. 4, Bethesda: Abt Associates.

Muula, A. and Broadhead, R. (2001), 'The Australian contribution towards medical training in Malawi', *Medical Journal of Australia*, **175**, 42–7.

Muula, A. and Maseko, F. (2006), 'How are health professionals earning their living in Malawi?', *BMC Health Services Research*, **6** (97), 1–12.

Muula, A., Mfutso-Bengo, J., Makoza, J. and Chatipwa, E. (2003), 'The ethics of developed nations recruiting nurses from developing countries: the case of Malawi', *Nursing Ethics*, **10**, 433–8.

Muula, A., Panulo, B. and Maseko, F. (2006), 'The financial losses from the migration of nurses from Malawi', *BMC Nursing*, **5** (9), 1–6.

Mwaniki, D. and Dulo, C. (2008), 'Migration of health workers in Kenya:

the impact on health service delivery', Harare: EQUINET Discussion Paper No. 55.

Nair, S. (2007), 'Globalization and livelihoods: the perspective of women nurses in Delhi', *Asian Journal of Women's Studies*, **13** (4), 34–56.

Ndetei, D. (2008), 'Retention or migration of mental health workers: psychiatrists in Kenya', *Global Social Policy*, **8**, 311–14.

Neelankantan, S. (2003), 'India's global ambitions', *Far Eastern Economic Review*, **6**, November, 52–4.

Nguyen, L., Ropers, S., Nderitu, E., et al. (2008), 'Intent to migrate among nursing students in Uganda: measures of the brain drain in the next generation of health professionals', *Human Resources for Health*, **6** (5), 1–11.

Nguyen, V. and Peschard, K. (2003), 'Anthropology, inequality, and disease: a review', *Annual Review of Anthropology*, **32**, 447–74.

Nietschmann, B. (1979), 'Ecological change, inflation and migration in the far western Caribbean', *Geographical Review*, **69**, 1–24.

Nieves, J. and Stack, K. (2008), 'Puerto Rico's physician migration', *Revista Panamericana de Salud Publica*, **24** (2), 147–8.

Noree, T., Chokchaichan, H. and Mongkolporn, V. (2005), *Abundant for the Few, Shortage for the Majority: The Inequitable Distribution of Doctors in Thailand*, Bangkok: International Health Policy Program.

North, N. (2007), 'International nurse migration: impacts on New Zealand', *Policy, Politics and Nursing Practice*, **8**, 220–28.

Norwegian Directorate of Health (2009), *Migration and Health. Challenges and Trends*, Oslo: Directorate of Health.

Novak, J. (2009), 'Gendered perceptions of migration among skilled female Ghanian nurses', *Gender and Development*, **17**, 269–80.

Nurse, K. (2004), 'Migration and development in the Caribbean', *Focal Point*, March, 3–5.

Oberoi, S. and Lin, V. (2006), 'Brain drain of doctors from southern Africa: brain gain for Australia', *Australian Health Review*, **30**, 25–33.

O'Brien, P. and Gostin, L. (2009), 'Health worker shortages and inequalities: the reform of United States policy', *Global Health Governance*, **2** (2), 1–26.

O'Brien, T. (2007), 'Overseas nurses in the National Health Service: a process of deskilling', *Journal of Clinical Nursing*, **16**, 2229–36.

O'Brien-Pallas, L. and Wang, S. (2006), 'Innovations in health care delivery: responses to global nurse migration – a research example', *Policy, Politics and Nursing Practice*, **7** (3), 49S–57S.

O'Connor, T. and Hooker, R. (2007), 'Extending rural and remote medicine with a new type of health worker: physician assistants', *Australian Journal of Rural Health*, **15**, 346–51.

OECD (2005), *Trends in International Migration*, Paris: OECD.

OECD (2008), *The Looming Crisis in the Health Workforce. How Can OECD Countries Respond?*, Paris: OECD.

Ogilvie, L., Mills, J., Astle, B. et al. (2007), 'The exodus of health professionals from sub-Saharan Africa: balancing human rights and societal needs in the twenty-first century', *Nursing Inquiry*, **14**, 114–24.

Ojo, K. (1990), 'International migration of health manpower in sub-Saharan Africa', *Social Science and Medicine*, **31**, 631–7.

Okafor, S. (1987), 'Inequalities in the distribution of health care facilities in Nigeria', in R. Akhtar (ed.), *Health and Disease in Tropical Africa. Geographical and Medical Viewpoints*, Chur: Harwood, pp. 383–401.

Olshansky, S. and Ault, A. (1986), 'The fourth stage of the epidemiologic transition: the age of delayed degenerative diseases', *Milbank Memorial Fund Quarterly*, **49**, 509–38.

Olumwallah, O. (2002), *Disease in the Colonial State: Medicine, Society and Change among the AbaNyole of Western Kenya*, Westport, CT: Greenwood.

Oman, K., Moulds, R. and Usher, K. (2009), 'Specialist training in Fiji: why do graduates migrate, and why do they remain? A qualitative study', *Human Resources for Health*, **7** (9), 1–10.

Omeri, A. and Atkins, K. (2002), 'Lived experiences of immigrant nurses in New South Wales, Australia: searching for meaning', *International Journal of Nursing Studies*, **39**, 495–505.

Ong, P. and Azores, T. (1994), 'The migration and incorporation of Filipino nurses', in P. Ong, E. Bocacich and L. Cheng (eds), *The New Asian Immigration in Los Angeles and Global Restructuring*, Philadelphia, PA: Temple University Press, pp. 164–95.

Oommen, T. (1989), 'India: "brain drain" or migration of talent?', *International Migration*, **27**, 411–22.

Opiniano, J. (2003), 'Migration part of being a nurse – study', *CyberDyaryo*, 2 April (www.cyberdyaryo.com).

Ospina, H. (2006), 'Cuba exports health', *Le Monde Diplomatique*, **52**, 10.

Osunkoya, B. (1974), 'Postgraduate medical education in developing countries', *British Journal of Medical Education*, **8**, 69–73.

Oulton, J. (1998), 'International trade and the nursing profession', in S. Zarilli and C. Kinnon (eds), *International Trade in Health Services*, Geneva: WHO and United Nations, pp. 125–32.

Owusu-Daaku, F., Smith, F. and Shah, R. (2008), 'Addressing the workforce crisis: the professional aspirations of pharmacy students in Ghana', *Pharmacy World and Science*, **30**, 577–83.

Pablico, M. (1972), 'A survey on attitude of Filipino nurses towards nursing profession in the Philippines', *Philippine Journal of Nursing*, **41** (3), 107–14.

Padareth, A., Chamberlain, C., McCoy, D. et al. (2003), 'Health personnell in southern Africa: confronting maldistribution and brain drain', Harare: EQUINET Discussion Paper No. 3.

Pak, S. and Tukuitonga, C. (2006), 'Towards brain circulation: building the health workforce capacity in the Pacific Region', Wellington: NZAID.

Palese, A., Barba, M. and Mesaglio, M. (2008), 'The career path of a group of Romanian nurses in Italy: a 3-year follow-up study', *International Nursing Review*, **55**, 234–9.

Palmer, D. (2006), 'Tackling Malawi's human resources crisis', *Reproductive Health Matters*, **14** (27), 27–39.

Pandya, S. (1969), 'Brain drain in medicine', *The Times of India*, 9 November.

Pantenburg, H. (2009), 'Responding to violence and lack of basic healthcare', *InterAction*, **5**, May, 10–11.

Parker, S. (2004), 'African nursing shortage puts health care system on verge of collapse', *VOA News.com* (www.voanews.com/Focus/article.cfm?objectID=C9090F8D-C858-4Fbb-AB9).

Parkhouse, J. (1979), *Medical Manpower in Britain*, Edinburgh: Longman.

Parrenas, R. (2001), *Servants of Globalization: Women, Migration and Domestic Work*, Stanford, CA: Stanford University Press.

Parrenas, R. (2002), 'The care crisis in the Philippines: children and transnational families in the new global economy', in B. Ehrenreich and A. Hochschild (eds), *Global Woman. Nannies, Maids and Sex Workers in the New Economy*, New York: Metropolitan Books, pp. 39–54.

Pastor, W., Huset, R. and Lee, M. (1989), 'Job and life satisfaction amongst rural physicians', *Minnesota Medicine*, **72**, 215–23.

Patel, V. (2003), 'Recruiting doctors from poor countries: the great brain robbery?', *British Medical Journal*, **327**, 926–8.

Pathman, D., Williams, E. and Konrad, T. (1996), 'Rural physician satisfaction: its sources and relationship to retention', *Journal of Rural Health*, **12**, 366–77.

Pearce, J., Dorling, D., Wheeler, B. et al. (2006), 'Geographical inequalities in health in New Zealand, 1980–2001: the gap widens', *Australian and New Zealand Journal of Public Health*, **30**, 461–6.

Pell, J., Pell, A., Norrie, J. et al. (1997), 'Effects of socioeconomic deprivation on waiting times for cardiac surgery: retrospective cohort study', *British Medical Journal*, **314**, 669–72.

Percot, M. (2005), 'Les infirmières indiennes émigrées dans les pays du

Golfe: de l'opportunité à la stratégie', *Revue Européenne des Migrations Internationales*, **21**, 29–54.

Percot, M. (2006), 'Indian nurses in the Gulf: from job opportunity to life strategy', in A. Agrawal (ed.), *Migrant Women and Work*, New Delhi: Sage, pp. 155–76.

Percot, M. and Rajan, S. (2007), 'Female emigration from India. Case study of nurses', *Economic and Political Weekly*, **42**, 318–25.

Perrin, M., Hagopian, A., Sales, A., and Huang, B. (2007), 'Nurse migration and its implications for Philippine hospitals', *International Nursing Review*, **54**, 219–26.

Philippines Overseas Employment Administration (n.d.), *Filipino Medical Personnel*, POEA: Manila.

Phillips, D. (1996), 'The internationalisation of labour. The migration of nurses from Trinidad and Tobago', *International Sociology*, **11**, 109–27.

Phillips, R., Petterson, S., Fryer, G. and Rosser, W. (2007), 'The Canadian contribution to the US physician workforce', *Canadian Medical Association Journal*, **176**, 1083–7.

Pillay, R. (2009), 'Work satisfaction of professional nurses in South Africa: a comparative analysis of the public and private sectors', *Human Resources for Health*, **7** (15), 1–15.

Piper, N. (2009), 'The complex interconnections of the migration–development nexus: a social perspective', *Population, Space and Place*, **15**, 93–101.

Pittman, P., Folsom, A., Bass, E. and Leonhardy, K. (2007), *U.S.-Based International Nurse Recruitment*, Washington, DC: Academy Health.

Playford, D., Larson, A. and Wheatland, B. (2006), 'Going country: rural student placement factors associated with future rural employment in nursing and allied health', *Australian Journal of Rural Health*, **14**, 14–19.

Pond, B. and McPake, B. (2006), 'The health migration crisis: the role of four Organisation for Economic Cooperation and Development countries', *Lancet*, **367**, 1448–55.

Pong, R. (2008), 'Strategies to overcome physician shortages in northern Ontario: a study of policy implementation over 35 years', *Human Resources for Health*, **6** (24), 1–9.

Portes, A. (1978), 'Migration and underdevelopment', *Politics and Society*, **8**, 1–48.

Pratt, G. (1999), 'From registered nurse to registered nanny: discursive geographies of Filipina domestic workers in Vancouver, B.C.', *Economic Geography*, **75**, 215–36.

Price, S. (2008), 'Becoming a nurse: a meta-study of early professional socialization and career choice in nursing', *Journal of Advanced Nursing*, **65**, 11–19.

Raghuram, P. (2009a), 'Caring about "brain drain" migration in a postcolonial world', *Geoforum*, **40**, 25–33.

Raghuram, P. (2009b), 'Which migration? What development? Unsettling the edifice of migration and development', *Population, Space and Place*, **15**, 103–17.

Rahman, M. and Khan, R. (2007), 'Out-migration of health professionals from Bangladesh. Prospects of diaspora formation for homeland development', *Asian Population Studies*, **3**, 135–51.

Rai, S. (2003), 'Indians sought to staff US hospitals', *New York Times*, 10 February.

Ramo, W. (1991), 'Solomon Islands', in M. Bray (ed.), *Ministries of Education in Small States*, London: Commonwealth Secretariat, pp. 265–83.

Rasiah, R., Noh, A. and Tumin, M. (2009), 'Privatising healthcare in Malaysia: power, policy and profits', *Journal of Contemporary Asia*, **39**, 50–62.

Ravishankar, N., Gubbins, P., Cooley, R. et al. (2009), 'Global health funding soars, boosted by unprecedented private giving', *The Lancet*, **373**, 2113–24.

Rechel, B., Buchan, J. and McKee, M. (2009), 'The impact of health facilities on health care workers' well-being and performance', *International Journal of Nursing Studies*, **46**, 1025–34.

Record, R. and Mohiddin, A. (2006), 'An economic perspective on Malawi's medical "brain drain"', *Globalization and Health*, **2** (12), 1–8.

Reeves, R., West, E. and Barron, D. (2005), 'The impact of barriers to providing high-quality care on nurses' intentions to leave London hospitals', *Journal of Health Services Research and Policy*, **10**, 5–9.

Reid, U. (1999), *Human Resources Development for Health Project: Commonwealth Caribbean*, London: Commonwealth Secretariat.

Reynolds, R. (2002), 'An African brain drain: Igbo decisions to immigrate to the US', *Review of African Political Economy*, **92**, 273–84.

Ribas-Mateos, N. (2000), 'Female birds of passage: leaving and settling in Spain', in F. Anthias and G. Lazaridis (eds), *Gender and Migration in Southern Europe*, Oxford: Berg, pp. 173–98.

Richards, J. (2002), 'Rapid response: suction rather than drainage', *British Medical Journal*, **326**, 112–13.

Roach, S., Atkinson, D., Waters, A. and Jefferies, F. (2007), 'Primary health care in the Kimberley: is the doctor shortage much bigger than we think?', *Australian Journal of Rural Health*, **15**, 373–9.

Robinson, R. (2007), 'The costs and benefits of health worker migration from East and Southern Africa (ESA): A literature review', Harare: EQUINET Discussion Paper No. 49.

Robinson, S., Murrells, T. and Griffiths, P. (2008), 'Investigating the dynamics of nurse migration in early career: a longitudinal question-naire survey of variation in regional retention of diploma qualifiers in England', *International Journal of Nursing Studies*, **45**, 1064–80.

Robinson, V. and Carey, M. (2000), 'Peopling skilled international migra-tion: Indian doctors in the UK', *International Migration*, **38**, 89–108.

Rogerson, C. and Crush, J. (2008), 'The recruiting of South African health care professionals', in J. Connell (ed.), *The International Migration of Health Workers*, New York and London: Routledge, pp. 199–224.

Rokoduru, A. (2008), 'Transient greener pastures in managed temporary labour migration: Fiji nurses in the Marshall Islands', in J. Connell (ed.), *The International Migration of Health Workers*, New York and London: Routledge, pp. 171–80.

Rolfe, B., Leshabari, S., Rutta, F. and Murray, S. (2008), 'The crisis in human resources for health care and the potential of a "retired" work-force: case study of the independent midwifery sector in Tanzania', *Health Policy and Planning*, **23**, 137–49.

Ronaghy, H., Zeighami, B., Agah, T. et al. (1975), 'Migration of Iranian nurses to the United States: a study of one school of nursing in Iran', *International Nursing Review*, **22**, 87–8.

Ross, A. (2007), 'Success of a scholarship scheme for rural students', *South African Medical Journal*, **97**, 1087–90.

Ross, S., Polsky, D. and Sochalski, J. (2005), 'Nursing shortages and inter-national nurse migration', *International Nursing Review*, **52**, 253–62.

Rutten, M. (2009a), 'The economic impact of medical migration: a receiving country's perspective', *Review of International Economics*, **17**, 156–71.

Rutten, M. (2009b), 'The economic impact of medical migration: an over-view of the literature', *The World Economy*, **32**, 291–325.

Ryan, L. (2007), 'Who do you think you are? Irish nurses encountering ethnicity and constructing identity in Britain', *Ethnic and Racial Studies*, **30**, 416–38.

Ryan, L. (2008), '"I had a sister in England": family-led migration, social networks and Irish nurses', *Journal of Ethnic and Migration Studies*, **34**, 453–70.

Salmon, M., Yan., J, Hewitt, H. and Guisinger, V. (2007), 'Managed migration: the Caribbean approach to addressing nursing services capacity', *Health Services Research*, **42**, 1354–72.

Sarnsamak, P. (2009), 'Government should consider all sides of policy', *The Nation*, 14 January.

Schatz, J. (2008), 'Zambia's health-worker crisis', *The Lancet*, **371**, 638–9.

Scheffler, R., Liu, J., Kinfu, J. and dal Poz, M. (2008), 'Forecasting the global shortage of physicians: an economic and needs-based approach', *Bulletin of the WHO*, **86**, 516–25.

Schmid, K. (2003), *Emigration of Nurses from the Caribbean*, Santiago: Economic Commission for Latin America and the Caribbean.

Schrecker, T. and Labonté, R. (2004), 'Taming the brain drain: a challenge for public health systems in Southern Africa', *International Journal of Occupational and Environmental Health*, **10**, 409–15.

Scott, G. (2003), 'Situating Fijian transmigrants: towards racialised transnational social spaces of the undocumented', *International Journal of Population Geography*, **9**, 181–98.

Seboni, N. (2009), 'Proliferation of new health cadres: a response to acute shortage of nurses and midwives by sub-Saharan governments', *International Journal of Nursing Studies*, **46**, 1035–6.

Serneels, P., Lindelow, M., Gracia-Montalvo, J. and Barr, A. (2005), *For Public Service or Money. Understanding Geographical Imbalances in the Health Workforce*, Washington, DC: World Bank Policy Research Working Paper 3686.

Shapiro, K. (1987), 'Doctors or medical aides – the debate over the training of black medical personnel for the rural black population in South Africa in the 1920s and 1930s', *Journal of Southern African Studies*, **13**, 234–55.

Sharpston, M. (1972), 'Uneven geographical distribution of medical care: a Ghanaian case study', *Journal of Development Studies*, **8**, 205–22.

Shields, M. and Ward, M. (2001), 'Improving nurse retention in the National Health Service in England: the impact of job satisfaction on intentions to quit', *Journal of Health Economics*, **20**, 677–701.

Shisana, O., Hall, E., Maluleke, R. et al. (2004), 'HIV/AIDS prevalence among South African health workers', *South African Medical Journal*, **94**, 846–50.

Shuval, J. (1998), 'Credentialling immigrant physicians in Israel', *Health and Place*, **4**, 375–81.

Siebens, K., de Casterlé, B., Abraham, I. et al. (2006), 'The professional image of nurses in Belgian hospitals: a cross-sectional questionnaire survey', *International Journal of Nursing Studies*, **4**, 71–82.

Sinclair-Jones, J. (2000), 'E-medicine and e-work: the new international division of medical labour?', *Health Sociology Review*, **10** (1), 19–30.

Sitthi-amorn, C. and Somrongthong, R. (2000), 'Strengthening health research capacity in developing countries: a critical element for achieving health equity', *British Medical Journal*, **321**, 813–15.

Smigelskas, K., Starkeine, L. and Padaiga, Z. (2007), 'Do Lithuanian pharmacists intend to migrate?', *Journal of Ethnic and Migration Studies*, **33**, 501–9.

Smith, A. and Gray, L. (2009), 'Telemedicine across the ages', *Medical Journal of Australia*, **190** (1), 15–19.

Smith, J., Margolis, S., Ayton, J. et al. (2008), 'Defining remote medical practice', *Medical Journal of Australia*, **188**, 159–61.

Smith, P. and Mackintosh, M. (2007), 'Profession, market and class: nurse migration and the remaking of division and disadvantage', *Journal of Clinical Nursing*, **16**, 2213–20.

Smith, R. (2004), 'Access to healthcare via telehealth: experiences from the Pacific', *Perspectives on Global Development and Technology*, **3**, 197–211.

Sochalski, J. (2002), 'Nursing shortage redux: turning the corner on an enduring problem', *Health Affairs*, **21**, 157–64.

Solano, D. and Rafferty, A. (2007), 'Can lessons be learned from history? The origins of the British imperial nurse labour market: a discussion paper', *International Journal of Nursing Studies*, **44**, 1055–63.

Stagnitti, K., Schoo, A., Reid, C. and Dunbar, J. (2005), 'Retention of allied health professionals in the south-west of Victoria', *Australian Journal of Rural Health*, **13**, 364–5.

Stark, O. (2004), 'Rethinking the brain drain', *World Development*, **32**, 15–22.

Stevenson, D. (1987), 'Inequalities in the distribution of health care facilities in Sierra Leone', in R. Akhtar (ed.), *Health and Disease in Tropical Africa. Geographical and Medical Viewpoints*, Chur: Harwood, pp. 403–14.

Stilwell, B., Diallo, K., Zurn, P. et al. (2003), 'Developing evidence-based ethical policies on the migration of health workers: conceptual and practical challenges', *Human Resources for Health*, **1** (1), 1–13.

Stilwell, B., Diallo, K., Zurn, P. et al. (2004), 'Migration of health care workers from developing countries: strategic approaches to its management', *Bulletin of the WHO*, **82**, 595–600.

Stirling, A., Wilson, P. and McConachie, A. (2001), 'Deprivation, psychological distress and consultation length in general practice', *British Journal of General Practice*, **51**, 456–60.

Stock, R. (1987), 'Understanding health care behavior: a model, together with evidence from Nigeria', in R. Akhtar (ed.), *Health and Disease in Tropical Africa. Geographical and Medical Viewpoints*, Chur: Harwood, pp. 279–92.

Streefland, P. (2005), 'Public health care under pressure in sub-Saharan Africa', *Health Policy*, **71**, 375–82.

Stringhini, S., Thomas, S., Bidwell, P. et al. (2009), 'Understanding informal payments in health care: motivation of health workers in Tanzania', *Human Resources for Health*, **7** (53), 1–9.

Sudhir, A. and Barnighausen, T. (2004), 'Human resources and health outcomes: cross country economic study', *The Lancet*, **364**, 1603–9.

Suwandono, A., Muharso, Achadi, A. and Aryastami, K. (2005), 'Human resources on health (HRH), for foreign countries: a case of "nurse surplus" in Indonesia', Asian-Pacific Alliance on Human Resources for Health.

Syed, N., Khimani, F., Andrades, M. et al. (2008), 'Reasons for migration among medical students from Karachi', *Medical Education*, **42**, 61–8.

Talati, J. and Pappas, G. (2006), 'Migration, medical education and health care: a view from Pakistan', *Academic Medicine*, **81** (12), S55–S62.

Taylor, R. (1990), 'Problems of health administration in small states: observations from the Pacific', in Y. Ghai (ed.), *Public Administration and Management in Small States. Pacific Experiences*, Suva: Commonwealth Secretariat and USP, pp. 60–114.

Thomas, P. (2007), 'The international migration of Indian nurses', *International Nursing Review*, **53**, 277–83.

Thomas, P. (2008), 'Indian nurses – seeking new shores', in J. Connell (ed.), *The International Migration of Health Workers*, New York and London: Routledge, pp. 99–109.

Thomas-Hope, E. (1985), 'Return migration and its implications for Caribbean development', in R. Pastor (ed.), *Migration and Development in the Caribbean*, Boulder, CO: Westview, 157–77.

Thommasen, H. (2000), 'Physician retention and recruitment outside urban British Columbia', *British Columbia Medical Journal*, **42**, 304–8.

Thompson, M., Hagopian, A., Fordyce, M. and Hart, G. (2009), 'Do international medical graduates (IMGs) "fill the gap" in rural primary care in the United States? A national study', *Journal of Rural Health*, **25**, 124–34.

Thornley, K. (2003), 'What future for health care assistants: high road or low road?', in C. Davies (ed.), *The Future Health Workforce*, Basingstoke: Palgrave Macmillan, pp. 143–60.

Tountas, Y., Karnaki, P., Pavi, E. and Souliotis, K. (2005), 'The "unexpected" growth of the private health sector in Greece', *Health Policy*, **74**, 167–80.

Troy, P., Wyness, L. and McAuliffe, E. (2007), 'Nurses' experience of recruitment and migration from developing countries: a phenomenological approach', *Human Resources for Health*, **5** (15), 1–7.

Tudor Hart, J.T. (1971), 'The inverse care law', *The Lancet*, **297**, 405–12.

Turrittin, J., Hagey, R., Guruge, S. et al. (2002), 'The experiences of professional nurses who have migrated to Canada: cosmopolitan citizenship or democratic racism?', *International Journal of Nursing Studies*, **39**, 655–67.

Uba, L. (1992), 'Cultural barriers to health care for southeast Asian refugees', *Public Health Reports*, **107**, 544–8.

Upadhyay, A. (2003), 'Nursing exodus weakens developing world', *IPS News* (www.Ipsnews.net/migration/stories/exodus).

Usher, K. and Lindsay, D. (2003), 'The nurse practitioner role in Fiji: results of an impact study', *Contemporary Nurse*, **16** (1/2), 83–91.

Van de Poel, E., Hosseinpour, A., Speybroeck, N. et al. (2008), 'Socioeconomic inequality in malnutrition in developing countries', *Bulletin of the WHO*, **86**, 282–91.

de Veer, A., den Ouden, D. and Francke, A. (2004), 'Experiences of foreign European nurses in the Netherlands', *Health Policy*, **68**, 55–61.

Venning, P., Durie, A., Roland, M. et al. (2000), 'Randomised controlled trial comparing cost effectiveness of general practitioners and nurse practitioners in primary care', *British Medical Journal*, **320**, 1048–53.

Voigt-Graf, C. (2003), 'Fijian teachers on the move: causes, implications and policies', *Asia-Pacific Viewpoint*, **44**, 163–75.

Volqvartz, J. (2005), 'The brain drain', *The Guardian*, 11 March.

de Vos, P., de Ceukelaire, W., Bonet, M. and van der Stuyft, P. (2007), 'Cuba's international cooperation in health: an overview', *International Journal of Health Services*, **37**, 761–76.

Vujicic, M. and Zurn, P. (2006), 'The dynamics of the health labour market', *International Journal of Health Planning and Management*, **21**, 101–15.

Vujicic, M., Zurn P., Diallo, K. et al. (2004), 'The role of wages in the migration of health care professionals from developing countries', *Human Resources for Health*, **2** (3), 1–14.

Vullnetari, J. and King, R. (2008), '"Does your granny eat grass?" On mass migration, care drain and the fate of older people in rural Albania', *Global Networks*, **8**, 139–71.

Wasswa, H. (2008), 'Rich countries are accused of "snatching" doctors from poor ones', *British Medical Journal*, **336**, 579.

West, K. (1968), 'Physician brain-drain', *Medical Opinion and Review*, **4** (9), 36–45.

Whitehead, E., Mason, T. and Ellis, J. (2007), 'The future of nursing: career choices in potential student nurses', *British Journal of Nursing*, **16**, 491–6.

Wibulpolprasert, S. and Pachanee, C. (2008), 'Addressing the internal brain drain of medical doctors in Thailand: the story and lesson learned', *Global Social Policy*, **8**, 12–15.

Wibulpolprasert, S., Pachanee, C., Pitayarangsarit, S. and Hempisut, P. (2004), 'International service trade and its implications for human resources for health: a case study of Thailand', *Human Resources for Health*, **2** (10), 1–12.

Wibulpolprasert, S. and Pengpaibon, P. (2003), 'Integrated strategies to tackle the inequitable distribution of doctors in Thailand: four decades of experience', *Human Resources for Health*, **1** (12), 1–17.

Wickramasekara, P. (2003), *Policy Responses to Skilled Migration: Retention, Return and Circulation*, Geneva: ILO Perspectives on Labour Migration No. 5E.

Wilkinson, R. and Pickett, K. (2009), *The Spirit Level: Why More Equal Societies Almost Always Do Better*, London: Allen & Lane.

Williams, A. and Balaz, V. (2008), 'International return mobility, learning and knowledge transfer: a case study of Slovak doctors', *Social Science and Medicine*, **67**, 1924–33.

Wilson, N., Couper, I., de Vries, E. et al. (2009), 'A critical review of interventions to redress the inequitable distribution of health care professionals to rural and remote areas', *Rural and Remote Health*, **9**, 1–21.

Windeyer, C. (2002), 'Telehealth and the retention of health personnel in Western New South Wales', unpub B.A. (Honours) thesis, University of Sydney.

Winkelmann-Gleed, A. (2006), *Migrant Nurses. Motivation, Integration and Contribution*, Oxford: Radcliffe.

Wiskow, C. (2006), *Health Worker Migration Flows in Europe: Overview and Case Studies in Selected CEE Countries – Romania, Czech Republic, Serbia and Croatia*, Geneva: ILO.

World Bank (1994), *Health Priorities in the World Bank's Pacific Member Countries,* Washington, DC: World Bank.

World Bank (2007a), *Opportunities to Improve Social Services. Human Development in the Pacific Islands*, Washington, DC: World Bank.

World Bank (2007b), 'The Mongolian health system at a crossroads: an incomplete transition to a post-Semashkom model', Washington, DC: World Bank Paper No. 2007–1.

World Health Organization (2006a), *Working Together for Health*, Geneva: WHO.

World Health Organization (2006b), *Health Worker Shortages and the Response to AIDS*, Geneva: WHO.

World Health Organization (2007), *Atlas: Nurses in Mental Health 2007*, Geneva: WHO.

World Health Organization (2008a), *The Global Burden of Disease: 2004 Update*, Geneva: WHO.

World Health Organization (2008b), *Closing the Gap in a Generation*, Geneva: WHO.

Wuliji, T., Carter, S. and Bates, I. (2009), 'Migration as a form of workplace attrition: a nine-country study of pharmacists', *Human Resources of Health*, **7** (32), 1–10.

Xiang, B. (2007), *Global 'Body Shopping'. An Indian Labor System in the Information Technology Industry*, Princeton, NJ: Princeton University Press.

Xu, Y. (2003), 'Are Chinese nurses a viable source to relieve the US nursing shortage?', *Nursing Economics*, **21**, 269–74.

Xu, Y. (2007), 'Strangers in strange lands. A metasynthesis of lived experiences of immigrant Asian nurses working in Western countries', *Advances in Nursing Science*, **30**, 246–65.

Xu, Y., Gutierrez, A. and Kim, S. (2008), 'Adaptation and transformation through (un)learning: lived experiences of immigrant Chinese nurses in US healthcare environment', *Advances in Nursing Science*, **31**, E33–E47.

Xu, Y. and Kwak, C. (2006), 'Trended profile of internationally educated nurses in the United States: implications for the shortage and beyond', *Journal of Nursing Administration*, **30**, 522–5.

Yan, J. (2006), 'Health services delivery: reframing policies for global nursing migration in North America – a Caribbean perspective', *Policy, Politics and Nursing Practice*, **7** (3), 71S–75S.

Yeates, N. (2008), 'Here to stay? Migrant health workers in Ireland', in J. Connell (ed.), *The International Migration of Health Workers*, New York and London: Routledge, pp. 62–76.

Yeates, N. (2009), 'Production for export: the role of the states in the development and operation of global care chains', *Population, Space and Place*, **15**, 175–87.

Yi, M. and Jezewski, M. (2000), 'Korean nurses' adjustment to hospitals in the United States of America', *Journal of Advanced Nursing*, **32**, 721–9.

Yumkella, F. (2006), 'Retention of health workers in low-resource settings: challenges and responses', Chapel Hill, NC: The Capacity Project.

Zeytinoglu, I., Denton, M., Davies, S. et al. (2006), 'Retaining nurses in their employing hospitals and in the profession: effects of job preference, unpaid overtime, importance of earnings and stress', *Health Policy*, **79**, 57–72.

Zurn, P., dal Poz, M., Stilwell, B. and Adams, O. (2004), 'Imbalance in the health workforce', *Human Resources for Health*, **2** (13), 1–12.

Zurn, P., Dolea, C. and Stilwell, B. (2005), 'Nurse retention and recruitment: developing a motivated workforce', Geneva: ICN.

Zurn, P. and Dumont, J.-C. (2008), 'Health workforce and international migration: can New Zealand compete?', Paris: OECD Health Working Paper No. 33.

Zurn P., Vujicic, M., Diallo, K. et al. (2004), 'Planning for human resources for health: human resources for health and the production of health outcomes/outputs', *Cahiers de Sociologie et de Démographie Médicales*, **45**, 107–33.

Index